Methods in
Bronchial Mucology

Methods in Bronchial Mucology

Editors

Pier Carlo Braga, M.D.

Department of Pharmacology
University of Milan
School of Medicine
Milan, Italy

Luigi Allegra, M.D.

Institute of Respiratory Diseases
University of Milan
School of Medicine
Milan, Italy

Raven Press 📖 New York

Raven Press
1185 Avenue of the Americas
New York, New York 10036

Library of Congress Cataloging-in-Publication Data

Methods in bronchial mucology.

  Includes bibliographies and index.
  1. Mucus—Research—methodology. 2. Bronchi—
Secretions. I. Braga, Pier Carlo. II. Allegra, Luigi.
[DNLM: 1. Bronchi—secretion. 2. Mucus—analysis.
WF 500 M592]
QP215.M45 1988   616.2′3   86–42945
ISBN 0–88167–415–X

9 8 7 6 5 4 3 2 1

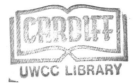

"ai nostri genitori"

Preface

In recent years, the number of investigations of bronchial mucus appears from the international literature to have increased logarithmically. There is interest in mucus in general and in bronchial mucus in particular not only on the part of pneumologists but also pharmacologists, surgeons, physicians, physicists, and medical engineers. This indicates the wide audience for this topic, and because of the characteristics of this unique biological material, we chose a multidisciplinary approach.

The interest of so many different specialists in bronchial mucology (we use the neologism "mucology" because now we can consider it to be a new discipline) means that varying approaches and techniques are used in its investigation. A specialist in his own discipline needs, for a better understanding of data and results, to know the specific techniques of investigation. From this requirement came our goal of providing in a unique source the main different experimental and clinical methods of investigation of mucus from the physical, chemical, biological, and clinical points of view, to reach a sort of state-of-the-art of the multidisciplinary approach to bronchial mucology.

Pier Carlo Braga
Luigi Allegra

Acknowledgments

This book would not have been possible without the help of all contributors. To each of these "mucologists," we wish to express our sincere thanks.

We are also deeply grateful to Camillo Corvi S.p.A., Italy, for its support and constant help and to Raven Press and Dr. Madeleine Hofmann for their assistance in publishing this volume.

Pier Carlo Braga
Luigi Allegra

Contents

2.5. Adhesivity Assessment

3. Chemical Methods of Analysis
3.1. Macromolecule and Ion Identification

3.5. Histochemical and Optical Methods

4. Biological Methods of Analysis

4.1. Ciliary Motion

4.2. Mucus Movements

4.3. In Vitro Methods

4.4. Electrophysiological Methods

5. Clinical Methods of Analysis

5.1. Mucus Transport and Clearance Measurement

Contributors

S. C. Afford
Clinical Teaching Block
General Hospital
Steelhouse Lane
Birmingham B4 6NH, UK

L. Allegra
Istituto di Tisiologia e Malattie
dell'Apparato Respiratorio
Ospedale Maggiore di Milano
Via F. Sforza 35
20100 Milano
Italy

G. Barbolini
Istituto di Anatomia e Istologia
  Patologica
Policlinico
Via del Pozzo
41100 Modena
Italy

A. Bisetti
Cattedra di Tisiologia e Malattie
Apparato Respiratorio
Università di Roma "La Supienza"
Istituto C. Forlanini
Piazza Forlanini 1
00151 Rome
Italy

D. B. Borson
Cardiovascular Research Institute
University of California–San
  Francisco
Box 0130
San Francisco, California 94143

R. Bossi
Istituto di Tisiologia e Malattie
dell'Apparato Respiratorio
Ospedale Maggiore di Milano
Via F. Sforza 35
20100 Milano
Italy

P. C. Braga
Dipartimento di Farmacologia,
  Chemioterapia, Tossicologia
Universita Degli Studi di Milano
Facoltà di Medicina
Via Vanvitelli 32
20129 Milano
Italy

S. W. Clarke
Department of Thoracic Medicine
The Royal Free Hospital
Pond Street
Hampstead
London NW3 2QC
UK

S. S. Davis
The University of Nottingham
University Park
Nottingham NG7 2RD
UK

C. F. Donner
Centro Medico di Riabilitazione
Divisione di Fisiopatologia Respira-
  toria
28010 Veruno (NO)
Italy

A. A. Gashi
Cardiovascular Research Institute
University of California–San
  Francisco
Box 0130
  San Francisco, California 94143

C. S. Kim
Mount Sinai Medical Center
Aerosol Research Laboratory
4300 Alton Road
Miami Beach, Florida 33140

M. King
Pulmonary Defense Group
317 Newton Research Bldg.
University of Alberta
Edmonton, AB T6G 2C2
Canada

M. T. Lopez-Vidriero
Boehringer Ingelheim Zentrale
  GMBH
Zentral Abteilung Medizinische
  Dienste
D-6507 Ingelheim am Rhein
Federal Republic of Germany

M. Lusuardi
Centro Medico di Riabilitazione
Divisione di Fisiopatologia Respira-
  toria
28010 Veruno (NO)
Italy

H. Matthys
Robert Koch Klinik
Medizinische Universitasklinik
Hugstetter Strasse 55
D-7800 Freiburg
Federal Republic of Germany

M. Moretti
Istituto di Tisiologia e Malattie
dell'Apparato Respiratorio
Policlinico
Via del Pozzo 71
41100 Modena
Italy

P. A. Mori
Istituto di Clinica e Malattie
dell'Apparato Respiratorio
Ospedale "G. Rasori"
Via Rasori 10
43100 Parma
Italy

J. A. Nadel
Cardiovascular Research Institute
University of California–San
  Francisco
Box 0130
San Francisco, California 94143

E. E. Odeblad
Department of Medical Biophysics
University of Umeå
S-90187 Umeå
Sweden

D. Olivieri
Istituto de Clinica e Malattie
dell'Apparato Respiratorio
Ospedale "G. Rasori"
Via Rasori 10
43100 Parma
Italy

D. Pavia
Department of Thoracic Medicine
The Royal Free Hospital
Pond Street
Hampstead
London NW3 2QG, UK

E. Puchelle
INSERM U 314
Faculte de Medecine
51, Rue Cognacq-Jay
51095 Reims Cedex
France

A. Silberberg
Department of Polymer Research
Weizmann Institute of Science
Rehovot 76100
Israel

R. A. Stockley
Lung Immunobiochemical Research
  Laboratory
The General Hospital
Steelhouse Lane
Birmingham B4 6NH, UK

J. M. Sturgess
Parke-Davis
2200 Eglinton Avenue East
Scarborough, Ontario M1L 2N3
Canada

A. Wanner
University of Miami
Division of Pulmonary Disease
4300 Alton Road
Miami, Florida 33101

J. G. Widdicombe
Department of Physiology
St. George's Hospital Medical School
Cranmer Terrace, Tooting
London SW17 ORE, UK

J. H. Widdicombe
Cardiovascular Research Institute
University of California–San
 Francisco
3rd & Parnassus Aves.
San Francisco, California 94143

D. B. Yeates
Section of Environmental and Occu-
 pational Medicine
Department of Medicine
University of Illinois at Chicago
1940 W. Taylor St.
Chicago, Illinois 60612

J. M. Zahm
INSERM U 314
Faculte de Medecine
51, Rue Cognacq-Jay
51095 Reims Cedex
France

1. Collecting and Measuring Methods

Methods in Bronchial Mucology,
edited by P. C. Braga and L. Allegra.
Raven Press, Ltd. © 1988.

1.1. Methods for Collecting and Measuring Airway Mucus in Animals

P. C. Braga

Department of Pharmacology, University of Milan, Milan, Italy

---

Methods
  Acute collection techniques
  Chronic collection techniques
  Discussion

Many diseases of the respiratory tract cause both qualitative and quantitative changes in the mucus that covers and protects the airway epithelium. Characteristics of mucus have been studied by pneumologists, pathologists, physiologists, biochemists, histologists, and pharmacologists, producing a copious literature.

The need for experimental studies in which different kinds of parameters are changed to understand both the physiology and pathology of bronchial mucus secretions and the need to test mucomodifying drugs have led to the development of several physicochemical methods.

To carry out this kind of experimental study, the first step is, of course, to collect bronchial mucus from laboratory animals, a procedure that, unlike collection from humans, often requires surgery. A chronological history of the development of methods for collecting respiratory tract fluid is presented in Table 1.

The techniques for collecting bronchial mucus differ in relation to the kind and size of the laboratory animal used. These techniques all have in common an operation

3

TABLE 1. *A chronology of methods for studying respiratory tract fluid[a]*

Year	Method	Author
1546	Output of sputum	Servetus (37)
1882	Mucus blotting	Rossbach (35)
1884	Laryngoscopic observation	James (20)
1910	CaCl$_2$ tubes	Henderson and Taylor (18)
1927	Intrapulmonary iodized oil	Ballon and Ballon (3)
1932	Pulmonary tissue water	Volmer (38)
1939	Sputum volume	Alstead (2)
1940	Cough screening	Connell et al. (12)
1941	Collection of respiratory tract fluid	Perry and Boyd (28)

[a] Modified by Boyd (5).

on the trachea, which is the final collector of mucus. A major subdivision can be made between acute and chronic collecting techniques.

METHODS

Acute Collection Techniques

Acute bronchial mucus collection often requires anesthetizing of the laboratory animal and subsequent surgery to expose the trachea for incision and intubation.

Mice

Measurement of phenol red concentration in respiratory tract washings of mice has been proposed to evaluate the changes in volume of respiratory tract mucus secretion (11). Phenol red (Fluka) was prepared as a 5% (w/v) solution in saline and was injected into mice intraperitoneally (i.p.) (500 mg/kg). Thirty minutes later, the animals were killed with carbon dioxide (CO$_2$). The whole trachea was dissected free of surrounding tissue and excised (always the same length). Each trachea was washed for 30 min in 1 ml of saline (15), then 0.1 ml 1 M/liter sodium hydroxide (NaOH) was added to the washing to stabilize the pH of the lavage fluid. The concentration of phenol red was measured photometrically at 546 nm (15). Within 30 min the basal secretion of phenol red into the trachea was about 0.60 µg (15). This method has been used to test drugs that affect mucus composition and secretion. Phenol red can act as a marker for both mucin and water secretion, but the reason for the observed correlation between increased phenol red and mucus secretion is still not known (15).

Other dyes, such as Evans blue and sodium florescein, also are reported to be eliminated in the respiratory tract fluids of mice (17). Sodium fluorescein, prepared as a 1% (w/v) solution, was injected subcutaneously (s.c.) (0.1 ml/10 g body weight).

After 30 min the animals were killed by vertebral dislocation. The trachea was cannulated by a needle, and 0.5 ml of Soerensen phosphate buffer, pH 7.4, was injected for pulmonary lavage. The lavage was repeated three times (17). Fluorescence was measured fluorimetrically (254 nm excitation, 415 nm emission). (For other details, see reference 17.)

Rats

Dye methods previously reported for mice also can be used for rats. Alcian blue was used to stain the normal bronchial tree. After chronic pretreatment with sulfur dioxide (SO_2), there were changes in bronchial coloration. Administration of drugs protected against the effects of SO_2 (31).

Rabbits

In 1941, Perry (27) described a method for collecting bronchial mucus from the rabbit. This method became a classic and has been used extensively (28). Many modifications of the original method have been published.

A rabbit, fasted for 24 hr, is anesthetized with urethane (1.1–1.4 g/kg, i.p.). The trachea is exposed by blunt dissection and half opened along the cartilage, 2 cm below the cricoid cartilage. One arm of a T cannula with a large enough diameter to slightly distend the trachea is inserted into the trachea from the lungs. The perpendicular arm is connected to an air outlet of a humidifier (temperature 35–38°C, relative humidity 80%), which is connected to a collection tube (Fig. 1). The rabbit is restrained in the supine position on a 60-degree inclined board with his head downward.

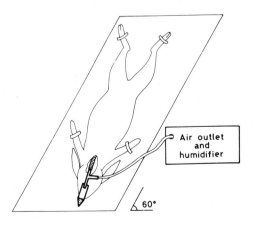

Air outlet and humidifier

60°

FIG. 1. Experimental setup of restrained supine rabbit. (From ref. 27.)

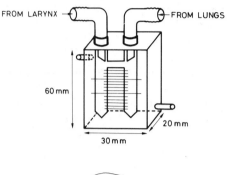

FROM LARYNX —   —FROM LUNGS

60 mm

20 mm

30 mm

FIG. 2. Mucus collecting box to be used in prone anesthetized rabbit.

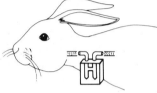

Modifications of the method of Perry mainly are concerned with the prevention of rebreathing and improvements in the production of conditioned air (7,8,13,14, 19,23,25,29). There were seasonal variations in the collected volume (the volume was lowest in September–October). The output of respiratory tract fluid declined with a decline in rectal temperature, and since urethane anesthesia induces a fall in body temperature in rabbits, the animals must be warmed to a constant temperature to avoid this kind of interference. A modification is the use of a collecting box, such as that shown in Fig. 2, in which no artificial humidification is used, but humidification is from the nose, in the natural way. In this case, the animal is not supine but prone (9,10).

The Perry and Boyd method has been used extensively to study the effects of sympathetic or parasympathetic agents and of different kinds of mucoactive drugs. The mucus production of rabbits with subacute bronchitis induced by long-term exposure to SO_2 also has been determined with this method (21,22).

Cats

The Perry and Boyd method can be used without modification for cats.

A method for collecting mucus from cats, using a segment of cervical trachea about 5 cm long isolated *in situ,* with nerve and blood supplies intact and a glass cannula inserted into each end, has been described (16). The animal breathed through a third cannula inserted into the cut caudal end of the cervical trachea. Mucus was collected from the segment by flushing 20 ml of Krebs-Henseleit solution with or without test substances through the rostral two cannulae, usually every 15 min (26). The tracheal segment remained full of physiological saline between washes.

Dogs

A method to collect mucus from the upper trachea and the nasopharynx in dogs in acute experiments has been proposed (30). The basic idea is the placement of materials in which mucus will accumulate in the upper trachea and the nasopharynx, without interference with the airways. The collecting trap is a plastic-coated glass fiber mesh that accumulates in its interstices mucus transported upward from the tracheobronchial tree. Since a portion of the mucus slips past such a device, it is necessary to place absorbent cotton attached to an airway just beneath the vocal cord (30).

Technical details also are reported in other articles (1), in which protein and mucoprotein composition (33) and the effects of cholinomimetic stimulation (34) were determined for tracheobronchial secretions collected by this method from intact dogs.

Chronic Collection Techniques

Rabbit

The possibility of inserting a chronic T-shaped cannula has been investigated (36). The cannula was inserted into the trachea under anesthesia and secured by silk surgical suture knots. The wound was sutured, the third arm was connected to a collecting tube, and after 3 days of antibiotic administration, the animals were ready for the experiment. On the fourth day after surgery, the mucus was collected at different times to control basal production, and on the fifth day drugs were administered and the amounts collected were compared with basal data.

Dog

In dogs, a segment of the cervical trachea can be separated for surgical construction of a subcutaneous tracheal pouch or a tracheal fistula. The surgical technique is about the same for both systems, the only difference being that the tracheal pouch is a closed system and the tracheal fistula is an open system.

Briefly, in the anesthetized dog (beagle, 9–11 kg), the cervical trachea was exposed by a midline skin incision and blunt dissection of the muscles. Hemostasis was usually unnecessary. A segment approximately 10 rings in length, with an intact blood and nerve supply, was transected (39). The cephalic and caudal parts

Fig 21.0

7×4

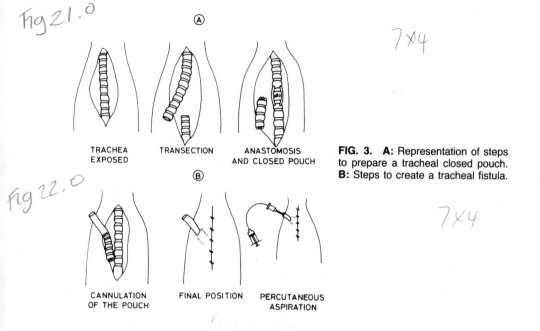

FIG. 3. A: Representation of steps to prepare a tracheal closed pouch. **B:** Steps to create a tracheal fistula.

Fig 22.0

7×4

of the trachea were anastomosed end-to-end with interrupted gut sutures to reestablish a patent airway (39). The isolated segment was closed at its caudal end with interrupted gut sutures (Fig. 3A). In the techniques described by Wardell (39,40), the mucosal surface of the cervical end of the isolated tracheal segment was sutured with interrupted silk sutures to the overlying subcutaneous tissue through a small incision in the cervical skin. Muscles and skin were sutured normally. In two or three weeks the skin healed over the small stoma, and a subcutaneous pouch of functioning tracheal tissue resulted.

Mucus samples (0.5 to 3 ml), usually free of microrganisms, can be collected once weekly for months through hypodermic needles. No pathological changes in histology of either pouch or reconstructed trachea mucosa were found.

By a surgical technique like that described, with the modification of anchoring a Silastic cannula to the outer surface of the proximal end of the tracheal segment with surgical mesh sutured in place, a tracheal fistula was constructed (41). With a funnel-shaped cannula placed exteriorly, which remained viable and functioning after 3 to 6 months, mucus could be collected by drainage. With this method 1.5 to 2.0 ml of tracheal fluid could be collected in 6 hr (41).

Ferret

A method that is a combination of the two previous techniques has been applied to the ferret, in which the tracheal pouch was prolonged with a Silastic cannula with a terminal plug to exteriorize the Silastic extension and facilitate entry into the pouch for collection (4) (Fig. 3B).

This technique also has been used successfully in the chicken (4).

Minipigs

Even in conscious minipigs (25 kg), tracheal pouches (six rings length) permanently cannulated at either end to provide a patent airway and exteriorized through the skin were established, and mucus samples were collected daily (24,32). Data on the action of drugs that affect tracheal mucus have been collected with this method (24,32).

DISCUSSION

Figure 4 summarizes the factors involved in collection of mucus for experimental studies. The parameters to be investigated are the chemical composition and the physical properties of bronchial mucus, their basal values, and their changes under pathological conditions and after drug administration. Many techniques have been proposed for the experimental animals generally used in the laboratory, and the only limit is the creativity of the researcher.

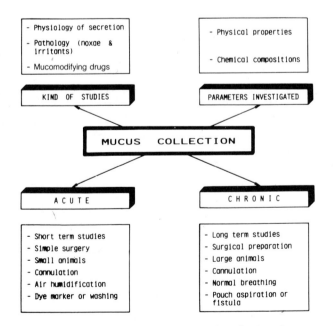

FIG. 4. Summary of the factors involved in collection of mucus.

Basically, and depending on the kind of experiment, mucus can be collected acutely or chronically. Acute experiments are short-term studies lasting some hours because the trachea is exposed and cannulated under anesthesia, with simple surgery and without asepsis. These kinds of experiments are frequently performed in small animals (low cost), and at the end of the experiment the animal is killed. The problems are the limitation of the collected quantities, obviously correlated with the size of the animal, and the fact that the chemical and physical properties of mucus are different from those of man and even from different species with different histomorphological characteristics. The variability is generally high, and large numbers of animals must be studied. Chronic studies have other problems. Surgical preparation of the animals, usually dogs, must be done in a proper room, and the animals must be allowed to recover. This means that the costs of experiments are high, and, for example, screening protocols for some drugs can cost a great deal. The advantages are that variability is low, each animal can be followed over a long period and can serve as its own control, and crossover studies can be performed. Moreover, the quantity of mucus is sufficient for both chemical and rheological studies.

REFERENCES

1. Adams, G. K., Ahronson, E. F., Reasor, M. J., and Proctor, D. F. (1976): Collection of normal canine tracheobronchial secretions. *J. Appl. Physiol.*, 40:247–249.
2. Alstead, S. (1939): Potassium iodide and ipecacuanha as expectorants. *Lancet*, 237:932–934.
3. Ballon, D. H., and Ballon, H. C. (1927): The effect of injection of Lipiodol and the rate of its disappearance in normal and diseased lungs. *Can. Med. Assoc. J.*, 17:410–416.
4. Barber, W. H., and Small P. A. Jr. (1977): Construction of an improved tracheal pouch in the ferret. *Am. Rev. Respir. Dis.*, 115:165–169.
5. Boyd, E. M. (1972): *Respiratory Tract Fluid.* Charles C Thomas, Springfield, IL.
6. Boyd, E. M. (1972): Studies on respiratory tract fluid. *Arzneimittelforsch.*, 22:612–616.
7. Boyd, E. M., and Boyd, C. E. (1964): Techniques for evaluating agents which affect respiratory tract fluid. In: *Animal and Clinical Pharmacologic Techniques in Drug Evaluation*, edited by P. E. Siegler and J. H. Moyer, p. 629. Year Book, Chicago.
8. Boyd, E. M., Hicks, R. N., and Trainor, A. V. (1956): Racemorphan, dextromethorphan and respiratory tract fluid. *Arch. Int. Pharmacodyn. Ther.*, 104:424–434.
9. Braga, P. C., Ferri, S., Magnoni, V., Lodi, F., and Marozzi, E. (1973): Farmacologia sperimentale dello iodopropilidenglicerolo. *International Round Table on Bronchial Hypersecretion*, pp. 1–7, Milan, Italy.
10. Braga, P. C., Marchioni, C. F., and Lodi, S. A. (1977): Rilievi clinici e sperimentali sull'azione dei mucolitici bronchiali. *III Europ. Congress of Chest Diseases*, pp. 211–212. Rome, Italy.
11. Chronic Bronchitis Research Group. (1977): The expectorant action of Farrerol. *Chin. Med. J.*, 3:259–265.
12. Connell, W. F., Johnston, G. N., and Boyd, E. M. (1940): On the expectorant action of resyl and other guaiacols. *Can. Med. Assoc. J.*, 42:220–223.
13. Cullumbine, N., and Dirnhuber, P. (1955): Oral and bronchial fluids in poisoning with anticholinesterases. *J. Pharm. Pharmacol.*, 7:580–585.
14. Eichler, O., Hobel, M., and Kammerer, P. (1964): Eine neue Versuchsanordnung zur Gewinnung von Bronchialsekret. *Arch. Int. Pharmacodyn. Ther.*, 148:172–180.
15. Engler, H., and Szelenyi, I. (1984): Thracheal phenol red secretion, a new method for screening muscosecretolytic compounds. *J. Pharmacol. Methods*, 11:151–157.
16. Gallagher, J. T., Kent, P. W., Passatore, M., Phipps, R. J., and Richardson, P. S. (1975): The

composition of tracheol mucus and nervous control of its secretion in the cat. *Proc. R. Soc. London [Biol.]*, 192:49–76.

17. Graziani, G., and Cazzulani, P. (1980): Su un metodo particolarmente indicato per lo studio dell'attività espettorante nei piccoli animali. *Farmaco [Prat.]*, 36:167–172.
18. Henderson, V. E., and Taylor, A. H. (1910): Expectorants. *J. Pharm. Exp. Ther.*, 2:153–164.
19. Hengelhorm, R., and Puschmann, S. (1971): Eine Methode zur Befenchtung der Aternluft in Tierexperiment. *Arzneimittelforsch.*, 21:1045–1046.
20. James, P. (1884): *The Therapeutics of the Respiratory Passages.* William Woods, New York.
21. Kasè, Y., Seo, H., Oyama, Y., et al. (1982): A new method for evaluating mucolytic expectorant activity and its application. I. Methodology. *Arzneimittelforsch.*, 32:368–373.
22. Kasè, Y., Seo, H., Oyama, Y., et al. (1982): A new method for evaluating mucolytic expectorant activity and its application. II. Application to two proteolytic enzymes, serratiopeptidose and seaprose. *Anzneimittelforsch.*, 32:374–378.
23. Mac Lachlan, M. L. (1943): On the expectorant action of paregoric. [Thesis for M.A. in Pharmacology]. Queen's University Library. Queen's University, Kingston, Ontario, Canada.
24. Marriott, C., Readman, A. S., and Turner, N. (1982): The effect of *S*-carboxymethylcysteine on the biochemistry of tracheal mucus. In: *Mucoregulation in Respiratory Tract Disorders,* Forum series 5, pp. 4–7. The Royal Society of Medicine, London.
25. Mendenhall, R. M., and Matzen, R. N. (1958): Apparatus for separation and expression of secretions in respiratory tract of experimental animals. *J. Appl. Physiol.*, 13:139–141.
26. Peatfield, A. C., and Richardson, P. S. (1982): The control of mucin secretion into the lumen of the cat trachea by α and β-adrenoceptors and their relative involvement during sympathetic nerve stimulation. *Eur. J. Pharmacol.*, 81:617–626.
27. Perry, W. F. (1941): Respiratory tract fluids. [Thesis for M.A. in Pharmacology]. Queen's University Library. Queen's University, Kingston, Ontario, Canada.
28. Perry, W. F., and Boyd, E. M. (1941): A method for studying expectorant action in animals by direct measurement of output of respiratory tract fluids. *J. Pharmacol. Exp. Ther.*, 73:65–77.
29. Plisnier, H. (1957): Etude comparative de l'action des derivés de l'opium et de diverses substances synthetiques à effet non morphinique sur les mécanismes de la toux, sur le bronchospasme, et sur la secretion bronchique. [Thesis]. Laboratoire de pharmacodynamie et de therapeutique. Université Libre de Bruxelles.
30. Proctor, D. F., Aharonson, E. F., Reasor, M. J., and Bucklen, K. R. (1973): A method for collecting normal respiratory mucus. *Bull. Physiopathol. Respir.*, 9:351–357.
31. Quevauviller, A., and Vu-Ngoc-Huyen (1966): Hypersecretion expérimentale du mucus bronchique chez le rat. I. Methode de appreciation anatomopathologique. *C.R. Soc. Biol.*, 160:1845–1849.
32. Readman, A. S., Marriott, C., and Barrett-Bee, K. (1982): The development of an *in vivo* model for the evaluation of drugs affecting tracheal mucus. *Adv. Exp. Med. Biol.*, 144:419–421.
33. Reasor, M. J., Adams, K., Proctor, D. F., and Rubin, R. J. (1978): Tracheobronchial secretions collected from intact dogs. I. Protein and mucous glycoprotein composition. *J. Appl. Physiol.*, 45:182–189.
34. Reasor, M. J., Cohen, D., Proctor, D. F., and Rubin, R. J. (1978): Tracheobronchial secretions collected from intact dogs. II. Effects of cholinomimetic stimulation. *J. Appl. Physiol.*, 45:190–194.
35. Rossbach, M. J. (1882): Uber die Behandlung des Hustens und Schleimauswurfs: eine Kritisch-experimentelle Studie. *Berl. Klin. Wochnschr.*, 19:281–284.
36. Scuri, R., Frova, C., Fantini, P. L., et al. (1980): Un nuovo metodo per lo studio della mucoproduzione nel coniglio. *Boll. Chim. Farm.*, 119:181–187.
37. Villanovanus (Servetus of Villanuwa), M. (1546): *Syroporum Universa Ratio ad Galeni Censuram Diligenter Expolita.* Guglielumus Ravilius, Lyons.
38. Vollmer, H. (1932): Untersuchungen uber Expektorantien und den Mechanismus ihrer Wirkung. *Klin. Wochnschr.*, 1:590–594.
39. Wardell, J. R. Jr., and Chakrin, L. W. (1970): The canine tracheal pouch model. *Arch. Intern. Med.*, 126:488–490.
40. Wardell, J. R. Jr., Chakrin, L. W., and Payne, B. J. (1970): The canine tracheal pouch: A model for use in respiratory mucus research. *Am. Rev. Respir. Dis.*, 10:741–754.
41. Yankell, S. L., Marshall, R., Kavanagh, B., De Palma, P. D., and Resnick, B. (1970): Tracheal fistula in dogs. *J. Appl. Physiol.*, 28:853–854.

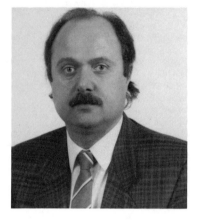

Pier Carlo Braga was born in Carpi (MO), Italy, in 1943. He received the degree of Doctor in Biological Sciences in 1968 and the M.D. degree in 1977 from the Università degli Studi of Milan, Italy. He is currently Associate Professor in the Department of Pharmacology, Chemotherapy and Toxicology of the University of Milan, School of Medicine, Milan, Italy. Fields of interest are pharmacology of mucoactive drugs, pharmacokinetics of antibiotics, and electrophysiological evaluation of antinociceptive drugs.

Methods in Bronchial Mucology,
edited by P. C. Braga and L. Allegra.
Raven Press, Ltd. © 1988.

1.2. Methods for Collecting and Measuring Airway Mucus in Humans

R. Bossi

Istituto di Tisiologia e Malattie dell'Apparato Respiratorio, Ospedale Maggiore di Milano, Milano, Italy

---

Methods
  Noninvasive methods
  Invasive methods
  Discussion

During recent years, collection of bronchial secretions has become increasingly important for complete diagnosis and more rational therapy of respiratory diseases. Since the clinical situation of each patient is correlated with bacteriological data (2,14) and physical and chemical properties (viscoelasticity, adhesiveness, glycoprotein composition, electrolyte concentration, enzymes, surfactant) (3,4,9), the importance of bronchial mucus evaluation and of the methods for collecting it is clear.

In many disease conditions characterized by mucus hypersecretion, such as chronic bronchitis, cystic fibrosis, and bronchiectasis, the rheological, biochemical, and microbiological evaluation (3,9,10,12) of well-collected mucus samples can supply a great deal of important information about the pathogenesis of the disease and help indicate the best therapy to modify the initial hypersecretion (3,8). In addition, some characteristics of bronchial secretion are negatively correlated with mucociliary clearance (11,16,17), since they worsen and reduce the mechanical defenses of the respiratory apparatus. This explains why clinicians and researchers

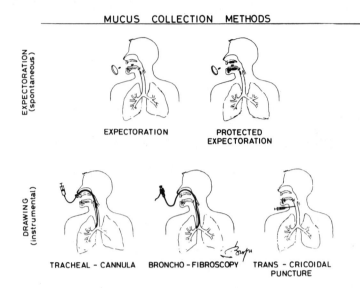

FIG. 1.   Schematic representation of noninvasive and invasive methods of mucus collection.

are interested in and have focused on mucus collection methods and on the possibility of studying chemical, biological, and rheological characteristics of mucus (3,6, 8–10).

Mucus collection methods can be divided into two general types, noninvasive methods and invasive methods (Fig. 1).

METHODS

Noninvasive Methods

Spontaneous Expectoration

This is the most natural and the simplest method, in which the patient expectorates after coughing. Under these conditions, however, bronchial mucus is contaminated by secretions of the nasal cavity and the posterior pharynx and by salivary secretions that mix with tracheal and bronchial mucus, thereby significantly altering the bacteriological, biochemical, and rheological study. Gargling with water or physiologic solutions (at least 200 ml) has been introduced recently to reduce salivary contamination. A modification of this collection method consists of stimulating coughing with the help of physiotherapeutic maneuvers based on postural drainage (Fig. 2).

This simple, noninvasive technique, although well tolerated by patients, is not otherwise satisfactory because of the possibility of quantitative and qualitative misinformation as a result of contamination of the bronchial mucus.

Protected Expectoration with Physiotherapy Using Postural Drainage

In this method (2,15), physiotherapeutic maneuvers based on thorax percussion, thorax vibration, and breathing exercise are used.

After rinsing of the oral cavity with saline, dental cotton rolls (diameter 18 mm, length 45 mm) are placed between the cheek and the gum at the lower and upper maxillary levels and under the tongue at the outlets of the parotid, submaxillary, and sublingual salivary glands; a total of five rolls is used. The patient is told to cough, and sputum is collected (Fig. 3).

As many investigators have reported (2,15,16), mucus collected by this technique is ideally free of salivary contamination, and the technique is relatively simple and easy and is well tolerated by the patient. The major inconvenience is dryness of the mouth after placing the rolls. Occasionally, the rolls cause nausea.

This noninvasive technique, routinely applicable, has given highly reproducible rheological measurements (viscoelasticity) and mucociliary transport of secretions.

FiG 23 .0

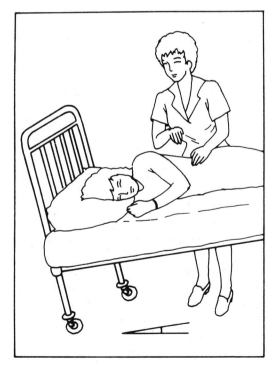

FIG. 2. Clapping maneuver during postural drainage.

9x7

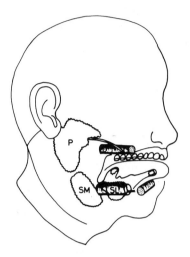

FIG. 3. Dental cotton rolls positioned over the orifices of salivary glands. (P) parotid; (SL) sublingual; (SM) submaxillary.

With this technique, we can obtain bacteriological analyses of sputum similar to those obtained with the invasive method of transtracheal aspiration.

Invasive Methods

Aspiration by Endotracheal Intubation

Tracheal intubation can be performed with a flexible tube through the patient's nose or mouth (5). The material is aspirated by suction and is collected into a test tube connected in series to the suction apparatus. This technique is fairly invasive and it is not well tolerated by patients. Coughing attacks or increasing respiratory distress may occur. The evident disadvantage is mucus contamination during endotracheal intubation by secretions produced in the nasal or the oral cavity.

This technique is helpful for unconscious or comatose patients but otherwise is not very reproducible, and it is certainly not simple to do routinely.

Transtracheal Aspiration

In this method (1), the patient lies down, with the head hyperextended. After local anesthesia of the cricoid, a 14-gauge needle is introduced. Coughing and swallowing usually follow cricoid membrane puncture. When the needle is fixed in the lower part, a thin plastic catheter is inserted into the trachea. Aspiration is performed with a syringe connected to the outside end of the needle (Fig. 4). A small quantity of physiological solution can be used if it is not possible to aspirate any material. This maneuver may cause the patient to cough. In addition, dilution of the secretion by physiological solution modifies the viscoelasticity of the secretion and interferes with rheological study. Several studies (1,2,5) have demonstrated

Fig 24

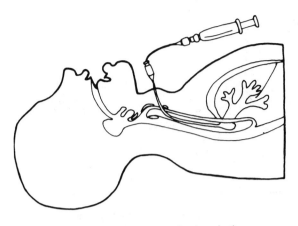

8 X 6

FIG. 4. Setup for transtracheal aspiration.

that saline inhibits some bacteria, especially pneumococci, and for this reason, the bacteriological study of the bronchial secretion sample when saline is used will not give a true picture of the bacteria present.

With this technique, it is possible to induce lethal reactions in very hypoxic patients or cause subcutaneous bleeding in patients who have coagulation disorders. Temporary expectoration of blood, occasional subcutaneous emphysema, and bacterial contamination of the respiratory tract by the needle may occur. The disadvantages of transtracheal aspiration are evident. It is very invasive, and there can be bacterial contamination by the needle, attacks of coughing, difficulty in taking a sufficient mucus sample for some analyses (e.g., rheological evaluation needs at least 0.8–1.0 ml and bacteriological study at least 300–400 µl), and possible modification of the rheological properties of mucus when using saline.

A technique similar to this can be used for tracheostomized patients. However, since tracheostomy prevents warming and humidification of the inspired air, mucus hypersecretion and bacterial contamination are frequent.

Aspiration by Bronchofibroscopy

Bronchofibroscopy, proposed by Ikeda in 1967 (8), is widely used and has mostly replaced traditional bronchoscopy because it is easier, it is better tolerated by the patients, and it increases the likelihood of accurate diagnosis. For the technical description of bronchofibroscopy, the reader is referred to specialized literature. The endoscopic tube is usually inserted through the nasal cavity or the oral cavity (Fig. 5), so examination can begin from the rhinopharyngeal cavity and proceed to segmental and subsegmental branches of the tracheobronchial tree, including those of the lower lobes. Large-sized bronchofibroscopes have a 6 mm diameter with a 2 to 2.6 mm inner channel through which one can take secretion samples, introduce special brushes for tracheobronchial epithelium brushing or a biopsy forceps, or infuse drugs.

Fig 25

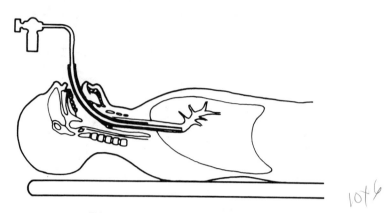

10f6

FIG. 5. Bronchofibroscopy setup.

The patient must be pretreated with 10 mg morphine and 0.5 mg atropine. Morphine strengthens the effect of the local anesthetic, and atropine decreases salivary and bronchial gland hypersecretion. Local preanesthesia is used, the most widely used agents being 2% lidocaine solution (mean dose 8 ml), 1% oxybucaine solution (mean dose 8 ml), or 1% tetracaine solution (mean dose 6 ml).

The principal aim of bronchofibroscopy is diagnosis. Mucus is obtained to look for pathogenic organisms or neoplastic cells, for biochemical and immunological tests, and for rheological examinations (viscoelasticity, adhesiveness, spinability).

The disadvantages of this method are invasiveness and the necessity of using local anesthetics that may have toxic effects, such as trembling, dizziness, anxiety, myoclonic spasms, cerebral hypoxia, in some cases followed by respiratory or circulatory failure. Bronchofibroscopy should be performed in the hospital, and the instrument is expensive. The most obvious disadvantage is that when it is necessary to collect repeated mucus samples during the same day, sampling by broncofibroscopy cannot be repeated more than once.

The advantages of the method are reproducibility, fairly good patient compliance, obtaining biopsy specimens without general anesthesia and bronchial or alveolobronchiolar washings, which often help to characterize the type of cells, even neoplastic ones, and the possibility of epithelial brushing (5,13,18). Bronchial mucus can be collected with very little likelihood of salivary contamination, thus providing reliable rheological data.

DISCUSSION

The methods for collecting bronchial mucus in humans are of two kinds, invasive and noninvasive (Fig. 6). The invasive methods—endotracheal intubation, aspiration by transcricoidal puncture, and aspiration by bronchofibroscopy—are preferable when chemical, cytological, and bacteriological diagnoses are not certain. The considerable disadvantages are the expense of the instruments, the need for a specialized staff, the poor patient compliance, the possibility of unexpected collateral effects, and the impossibility of test repetitions during the same day.

The noninvasive methods—spontaneous expectoration, spontaneous expectoration after physiotherapy, and protected expectoration after physiotherapy—are not expensive, are easier to use, and are repeatable, with good toleration by the patient even when mucus has to be collected more than once during the same day. Protected expectoration (15) allows repeated mucus sample collection largely free of salivary contamination (2,15), so that it can be used for bacteriological, cytological, and rheological studies (15,16).

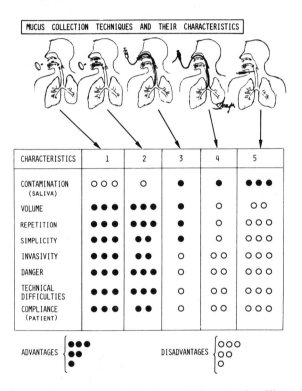

FIG. 6. Comparison of mucus collection techniques. (1) Expectoration; (2) protected expectoration; (3) tracheal cannula; (4) bronchofibroscopy; (5) transcricoidal puncture.

REFERENCES

1. Bartlett, J. G. (1977): Diagnostic accuracy of transtracheal aspiration. Bacteriologic studies. *Am. Rev. Respir. Dis.,* 115:777–782.
2. Beck, G., Puchelle, E., Laroche, D., Mongel, D., and Sadoul, P. (1982): Bacteriologie quantitative des expectorations recueillies par une technique simple limitant la contamination salivaire. *Bull. Eur. Physiopathol. Respir.,* 18:885–892.
3. Davis, S. S. (1973): Rheological examination of sputum and saliva and the effect of drugs. In:

Rheology of Biological Systems, edited by H. L. Gabelnick and M. Litt, p. 158. Charles C Thomas, Springfield, IL.

4. Giordano, A. M., Holsclaw, D., and Litt, M. (1978): Mucus rheology and mucociliary clearance: Normal physiologic state. *Am. Rev. Respir. Dis.,* 118:245–249.
5. Haas, H., Morris, J. F., Samson, S., Kolbourn, J. P., and Kim, P. J. (1977): Bacterial flora of the respiratory tract in chronic bronchitis: Comparison of transtracheal fiberbronchoscopic and oropharyngeal sampling methods. *Am. Rev. Respir. Dis.,* 116:41–47.
6. Iravani, J., and Norris-Melville, G. (1976): A simple method for the determination of the thread-forming property of tracheobronchial secretions. *Respiration,* 33:289–293.
7. King, M. (1979): Interrelation between mechanical properties of mucus and mucociliary transport: Effect of pharmacologic interventions. *Biorheology,* 16:57–68.
8. Ikeda, S. (1967): *Atlas of Flexible Bronchofibroscopy.* University Park Press, Baltimore, MD.
9. Lopez-Vidriero, M. T., and Reid, L. (1980): Respiratory tract fluid: Chemical and physical properties of airway mucus. *Eur. J. Respir. Dis.,* 61:21–27.
10. Marriot, C., and Irons, L. (1974): A study of the rheology and biochemistry of saliva and tracheobronchial gels. *Biroheology,* 11:119–124.
11. Meyer, F. A. (1976): Mucus structure: Relation to biological transport function. *Biorheology,* 13:49–58.
12. Meyer, F. A., Eliezer, N., Silberberger, A., Vered, J., Sharon, N., and Sade, J. (1973): An approach to the biochemical basis for the transport function of epithelial mucus. *Bull. Eur. Physiopathol. Respir.,* 9:250–272.
13. Pecora, D. V. (1963): A comparison of transtracheal aspiration with other methods of determining the bacterial flora of the lower respiratory tract. *N. Engl. J. Med.,* 269:664–667.
14. Puchelle, E., Beck, G., and Thevenin, F. (1977): Bactériologie quantitative des expectoration chez les bronchiteux chroniques. *Respiration,* 34:220–231.
15. Puchelle, E., Tournier, J. M., Zahm, J. M., and Sadoul, P. (1984): Rheology of sputum collected by a simple technique limiting salivary contamination. *J. Lab. Clin. Med.,* 103:347–353.
16. Puchelle, E., Zahm, J. M., and Duvivier, C. (1983): Spinability of bronchial mucus. Relationship with viscoelasticity and mucus transport properties. *Biorheology,* 20:239–243.
17. Puchelle, E., Zahm, J. M., Girard, F., et al. (1980): Mucociliary transport *in vivo* and *in vitro.* Relations to sputum properties in chronic bronchitis. *Eur. J. Respir. Dis.,* 61:254–261.
18. Wimberley, N., Faling, L. J., and Bartlett, J. G. (1979): A fiberoptic bronchoscopy technique to obtain uncontaminated lower airway secretions for bacterial culture. *Am. Rev. Respir. Dis.,* 119:337–343.

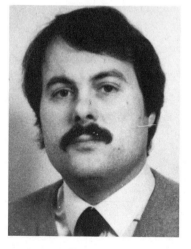

Roberto Bossi was born in 1947 in Milan, Italy. He received the M.D. degree in 1973 from the University of Milan, Italy. He is currently Hospital Assistant in the Pulmonary Division of Garbagnate Hospital, Italy. His interests are in mucociliary clearance, physiopathology of cough, and pharmacokinetics.

Methods in Bronchial Mucology,
edited by P. C. Braga and L. Allegra.
Raven Press, Ltd. © 1988.

1.3. Methods for Collecting and Measuring Mucus from Specific Sources

J. G. Widdicombe

*Department of Physiology, St. George's Hospital Medical School,
London, United Kingdom*

Methods
    Micropipetting of submucosal glands
    Tantalum dust hillock method
    Whole trachea *in vitro* method
Results
Discussion

Many methods for assessing mucus secretion suffer from one or both of two limitations. Some do not measure volume flow of output, which is presumably one of the important characteristics of airway mucus, at least in relation to airway obstruction. Thus methods depending on biochemical analysis or radiolabeling of glycoproteins at best give indirect evidence of the volume of mucus containing the constituents. Other methods can assess volume flow accurately but cannot relate this precisely to the source of the fluid; this limitation applies to such methods as the collection of respiratory tract fluid or sputum, in which the airway mucus may be contaminated by transudate and saliva, respectively.

This chapter describes three methods that do not suffer from these limitations, since volume of mucus can be measured accurately from defined sources. However, as will be discussed, they have their own limitations: the techniques are rather specialized, the volumes collected are small, and the *in vivo* methods can be applied only in experimental animals. Nevertheless, the volumes are sufficient for chemical and physical analyses.

METHODS

Micropipetting of Submucosal Glands

This method has been used with cats (4,11,19) but is potentially suitable for any species with tracheal submucosal glands, although it would be difficult to apply to humans *in vivo*. In animals, it can be applied either *in vivo* or *in vitro*.

In Vivo *Method*

The animal is anesthetised and tied supine. The cervical trachea is opened in the ventral midline, the animal breathing through the lower cervical trachea. The cut tracheal cartilages are held firmly with ligatures to minimize movement, and the mucosal surface is gently dried. Water-saturated paraffin oil is placed on the mucosal surface, and duct orifices are identified under a dissecting microscope. This is made possible because of the mucus–oil interface, although in earlier studies the gland ducts and their mucus were identified by staining with dye, such as neutral red (11,19).

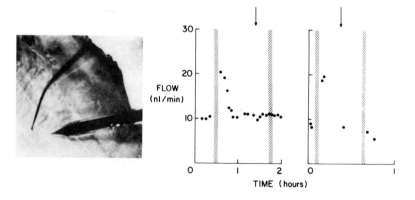

FIG. 1. Photomicrograph of exposed mucosa of cat trachea *in vivo* (left), showing a standard renal micropuncture pipette (lower) and a microsampling pipette (upper) positioned over single gland duct openings (small dots) stained with neutral red. Fluid from a submucosal gland was collected under oil during 1-min periods. A microsampling pipette (found to give more repeatable collections than a micropuncture pipette) was filled with black oil and positioned with a micromanipulator so that the fire-polished tip covered a gland duct opening. In the graphs (middle and right) each point represents a 1-min collection. The left graph shows that phenylephrine (shaded bar) (0.03 mg · kg⁻¹, i.v.) increased flow from a gland; the effect was abolished by pretreatment with phentolamine (at arrow) (0.08 mg · kg⁻¹, i.v.). The right graph shows that electrical stimulation of the cervical vagus nerve (shaded bar) (5 V, 20 Hz, 15 sec) increased flow from the gland. The effect was abolished by pretreatment with atropine sulfate (at arrow) (0.5 mg · kg⁻¹, i.v.). (From ref. 12.)

A glass micropipette containing paraffin oil and with a tip diameter of about 80 to 100 μm is adjusted by a micromanipulator so that its tip surrounds the orifice (Fig. 1). Negative pressure (of undefined size) is applied through the micropipette, and the mucus is withdrawn for 1 to 10 min. At the end of the collection period the tip of the pipette is withdrawn, and a further volume of oil is pulled into it, the collected mucus thus being held in the end of the pipette between the oil seals. The mucus volume is estimated from the length of the mucus segment and the dimensions of the pipette, measured under a microscope.

In Vitro *Method*

The cervical trachea is removed from a newly killed cat (other species do not seem to have been used) and opened along the ventral line, and a portion is mounted in an open Perspex chamber, similar to a modified Ussing chamber (14). The under (submucosal) surface of the dorsal muscular tracheal wall is bathed in warmed physiological solution, and luminal (mucosal) surface is treated for micropipetting as described for the *in vivo* method. Drugs can be applied to the submucosal bathing solution.

Tantalum Dust Hillock Method

This method consists of applying a thin layer of finely powdered tantalum dust to the surface of the trachea and assessing the volume of the near-hemispherical displacements that occur when mucus emerges from the ducts of the submucosal glands and displaces the layer of tantalum upward. The method was first used with the dog trachea *in vivo* (2–4) and has subsequently also been applied to the ferret trachea *in vitro* (1,8).

In Vivo *Method*

The trachea of the anesthetised dog, paralyzed and artificially ventilated, is prepared as described for the cat *in vivo* micropipette method. The opened trachea is viewed through a dissecting microscope, and a thin layer of finely powdered tantalum dust is blown onto the dried epithelial surface (2–4). Submucosal gland secretion is promoted in various ways (see RESULTS), and the number and size of the hillocks produced over the duct orifices are estimated (Fig. 2). This can be done by (a) counting the number of hillocks in the dissecting microscope field at various times and expressing the results as increases in numbers of hillocks, (b) photographing the field at various times, preferably with a Polaroid camera to give a rapid image, and subsequently measuring (from the photograph) the diameters of the hillocks to estimate their volume, assuming them to be hemispheres, or (c) using a videocamera attached to the microscope with a beam splitter, tape recorder, and television monitor. With this last method, the beam splitter allows

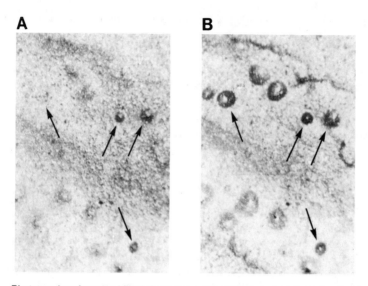

FIG. 2. Photographs of mucus hillock formation under tantalum dust, from the ferret trachea *in vitro.* **A:** Control before electrical field stimulation, showing small hillocks at three of the four arrows. **B:** After 30-sec stimulation, showing enlargement of identified hillocks and production of new hillocks. The arrows are only for identification of some individual hillocks in the photographs. (Modified from ref. 8.)

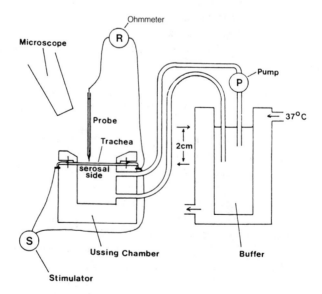

FIG. 3. Diagram of method for assessing mucus secretion by measurement of hillocks under tantalum dust and tissue shrinkage by probing the epithelium between hillocks. (From ref. 8.)

immediate analysis of the diameters of individual hillocks, and the tape recorder allows later detailed analysis of continuous changes of all hillocks.

In Vitro *Method*

Portions of ferret tracheas are mounted in Perspex chambers in a way similar to that described for the *in vitro* micropipetting method (1,8) (Fig. 3). Submucosal gland secretion is induced by drugs applied to the submucosal surface or by electrical field stimulation of the whole tracheal preparation via its metal mounting pins. Rates of secretion are assessed as for the *in vivo* method.

Whole Trachea *In Vitro* Method

This method consists of mounting the whole trachea of a ferret in an organ bath (8,16,21). The trachea remains air filled so undiluted mucus can be collected from it.

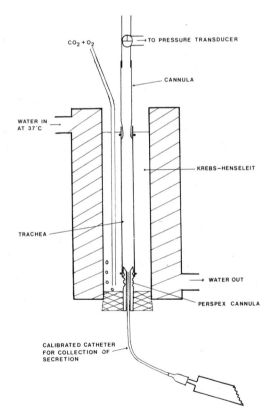

FIG. 4. Diagram of *in vitro* whole trachea preparation.

The ferret is anesthetized, its chest is opened in the midline, and the whole trachea from larynx to carina is removed rapidly. Both ends are cannulated, the laryngeal end with a special Perspex cannula that has a narrow lumen to fit fine catheters for collection of mucus. The trachea is mounted laryngeal end downward so that mucus is carried downward by gravity and by ciliary transport. The organ bath contains gassed Krebs-Henseleit solution, to which drugs can be added (Fig. 4).

Secretions are collected over 15 to 30 min periods into polyethylene catheters that are cut and sealed with bone wax and stored frozen. Volumes of secretion are measured from the difference in weight between the full catheters and those dried after the mucus has been washed out. The secretions can be freeze-dried for subsequent chemical analysis.

RESULTS

Micropipetting Methods

In Vivo

This method was first developed in 1979 (18) and has been fully used by Ueki et al. (1,19,20). They have shown from the effects of vagal block and stimulation that the cholinergic parasympathetic innervation is motor to the cat submucosal glands (19). Intravenous injection of various agonists and antagonists shows that secretion is promoted by cholinoceptor and α-adrenoceptor agonists (12,18,19).

Individual glands have mean secretion rates of about 9 nl·min^{-1}, which are reduced about 40% by vagal blockade (19). Strong neural and pharmacological stimulations approximately double the flow. Collections from a single gland can be maintained for 2 to 4 hr. The volumes of secretion, although small, are suitable for some chemical and rheological analyses (11,20).

In Vitro

This method, also employing the cat, has been used by Quinton (14) to study a range of pharmacological agonists and antagonists. Collections from three to four glands can be added together, and the volumes are suitable for electrolyte and phosphorus and sulfur analyses. Electrical field stimulation to test neural mechanisms should be possible.

Tantalum Hillock Methods

In Vivo

This method has been used for a number of physiological and pharmacological studies with dogs. Electrical stimulation of the superior laryngeal nerve (from the vagus) shows that this is the main motor cholinergic supply to the upper tracheal glands (8,12). Secretion can be reflexly activated from sensory receptors in the lungs and larynx (4,17) and by hypoxia from the peripheral chemoreceptors (2). Resting secretion seems to be variable and to depend on the condition of the animal; in well-ventilated animals, it may be negligible, but it is readily enhanced by underventilation (2).

Pharmacological studies can be performed with drugs given intravenously. To minimize systemic effects, the drugs can be given by close-arterial injection into a branch of the superior thyroid artery that supplies the upper trachea (5,6). The same artery can be perfused, with simultaneous measurements of hillock formation, vascular resistance, and mucosal thickness (8,10).

In Vitro

This method has been used with ferret trachea, with the application of drugs to the solution bathing the submucosal side of the tissue and with electrical field stimulation (1,8). The latter technique confirms other studies showing that submucosal glands have parasympathetic cholinergic and sympathetic α-adrenergic motor supplies but gives no evidence for a peptidergic (NANC) system in this preparation. The pharmacological results confirm the physiological conclusions, and, in addition, a number of inflammatory and neurotransmitters have been tested (1,8).

Whole Trachea *In Vitro* Method

This method was first described in 1983 (16) and has been used mainly with the ferret trachea (9,21,22). Control outputs are usually zero or near zero, and strong secretagogues, such as methacholine, can promote secretions as great as $300 \, \mu l \cdot min^{-1}$. These volumes are suitable for many chemical analyses. Two measurements can be made in addition to mucus secretion: connection of the upper end of the trachea to a pressure recorder allows assessment of changes in smooth muscle tone to be made simultaneously (9), and ion-sensitive and voltage-sensitive electrodes can be inserted in the lower collecting cannula to allow simultaneous measurements of concentrations of hydrogen, sodium, potassium, and calcium ions and of transmural potential difference (7).

This method has been used to assess the effects of many inflammatory and immunological mediators and neurotransmitters and to test and assay drugs thought to act on airway mucus secretion (9,21,22). Changes in the volume of flow as well as in the chemistry of the secretions may be therapeutically important. Assays of lysozyme have been made (22), this substance being a marker for serous cell (as distinct from mucous cell) secretion.

DISCUSSION

The *in vivo* micropipette method is an important advance because it allows quantitation of the secretion flow rate from individual submucosal glands. Thus, both the flows and any subsequent chemical or physical analyses are known to apply to a pure secretion from a single type of tissue. The fluid is not contaminated with epithelial secretions or transudate. The fact that it is *in vivo* makes it appropriate for physiological studies, including the role of innervation and of reflexes. The method demands considerable technical skill, and this may limit its extensive use, for example, for drug screening. There will be serious limits to the range of chemical analyses possible when dealing with nanoliter quantities of secretion. One unexplained feature of the method is the fact that, unlike the other methods of direct collection of secretion, micropipetting shows an appreciable control output of mucus. Possibly the negative pressure that has to be applied to collect secretions into the fine tip of the pipette may distort resting flow, or the mechanical stimulus of the tip of the micropipette might set up a reflex output of mucus. The fact that there is a resting output allows the testing of agents inhibitory to resting mucus secretion, which is not possible with other methods that have zero resting secretion.

The main advantage of the *in vitro* compared with the *in vivo* method of micropipetting is that pharmacological studies can be carried out by applying agents to the submucosal bathing solution. *In vivo,* drugs given intravenously might have systemic effects. The use of close-arterial injection of drugs with this preparation does not seem to have been tried.

The hillock method is also rather complex, especially if videorecording is to be used. If numbers of hillocks are counted to assess flow, this may not correlate well with mucus volume. The assumption that each hillock is a hemisphere is also an approximation but probably does not introduce much error. It is not known if the physical stimulus of the tantalum on the epithelium distorts mucus secretion.

The hillock and the micropipetting methods have many of the same advantages and disadvantages. The main differences are that the hillock method gives a larger total volume change, since many hillocks are measured simultaneously. On the other hand, it has not proved practical to collect secretions from hillocks for chemical or physical analyses. Neither method is suitable for testing drugs applied to the epithelial surface.

The *in vitro* whole tracheal preparation has the advantage that the epithelial surface is exposed to air and is physiological. Also, relatively large volumes of secretion can be collected. Additional measurements, for example, of smooth muscle contraction or of mucus ion concentrations, can be made simultaneously. Solutions or aerosols of drugs can be applied to the epithelial surface. This method has the disadvantage that the secretions may come not only from submucosal glands but also from epithelial cells. In this respect, it is worth noting that the ferret has few goblet (mucous) or serous cells in the tracheal epithelium (15). The preparation has not been applied successfully *in vivo*.

REFERENCES

1. Borson, D. B., Chinn, R. A., Davis, B., and Nadel, J. A. (1980): Adrenergic and cholinergic nerves mediate fluid secretion from tracheal glands of ferrets. *J. Appl. Physiol. Respir. Environ. Exercise Physiol.,* 49:1027–1031.
2. Davis, B., Chinn, R., Gold, J., Popovac, D., Widdicombe, J. G., and Nadel, J. A. (1982): Hypoxemia reflexly increases secretion from tracheal submucosal glands in dogs. *J. Appl. Physiol. Respir. Environ. Exercise Physiol.,* 52:1416–1419.
3. Davis, B., Marin, M., Fischer, S., Graf, J., Widdicombe, J., and Nadel, J. A. (1976): New method for study of canine mucous gland secretion *in vivo:* Cholinergic regulation. *Am. Rev. Respir. Dis.,* 113:257.
4. Davis, B., Roberts, A. M., Coleridge, H. M., and Coleridge, J. C. G. (1982): Reflex tracheal gland secretion evoked by stimulation of bronchial C-fibers in dogs. *J. Appl. Physiol. Respir. Environ. Exercise Physiol.,* 83:985–991.
5. Johnson, H. G., and McNee, M. L. (1983): Secretagogue responses of leukotriene C_4, D_4: Comparison of potency in canine trachea *in vivo. Prostaglandins,* 25:237–243.
6. Johnson, H. G., and McNee, M. L. (1985): Adenosine-induced secretion in the canine trachea: Modification by methylxanthines and adenosine derivatives. *Br. J. Pharmacol.,* 86:63–67.
7. Kyle, H., Robinson, N. P., Ward, J. P. T., and Widdicombe, J. G. (1987): Measurement of mucus [H^+] and other ionic concentrations in the isolated trachea of the ferret. *J. Physiol.* 387:158.
8. Kyle, H., Robinson, N. P., and Widdicombe, J. G. (1987): Mucus secretion by tracheas of ferret and dog. *Eur. J. Respir. Dis.,* 70:14–22.
9. Kyle, H., and Widdicombe, J. G. (1986): The effects of peptides and mediators on mucus secretion rate and smooth muscle tone in the ferret trachea. *Agents Actions,* 22:86–90.
10. Laitinen, L. A., Robinson, N. P., Laitinen, A., and Widdicombe, J. G. (1986): Relationship between tracheal mucosal thickness and vascular resistance in dogs. *J. Appl. Physiol.,* 61:2186–2193.
11. Leikauf, G. D., Ueki, I. F., and Nadel, J. A. (1984): Autonomic regulation of viscoelasticity of cat tracheal gland secretions. *J. Appl. Physiol. Respir. Environ. Exercise Physiol.,* 56:426–430.
12. Nadel, J. A., and Davis, B. (1980): Parasympathetic and sympathetic regulation of secretion from submucosal glands in airways. *Fed. Proc.,* 39:3075–3079.
13. Nadel, J. A., Davis, B., and Phipps, R. J. (1979): Control of mucus secretion and ion transport in airways. *Annu. Rev. Physiol.,* 41:369–381.
14. Quinton, P. M. (1979): Composition and control of secretions from tracheal bronchial submucosal glands. *Nature,* 279:551–552.
15. Robinson, N. P., Venning, L., Kyle, H., and Widdicombe, J. G. (1986): Quantitation of the secretory cells of the ferret tracheobronchial tree. *J. Anat.,* 145:173–188.
16. Robinson, N., Widdicombe, J. G., and Xie, C.-C. (1983): *In vitro* collection of mucus from the ferret trachea. *J. Physiol.,* 340:7–8P.
17. Schultz, H. D., Roberts, A. M., Bratcher, C., Coleridge, H. M., Coleridge, J. C. G., and Davis, B. (1985): Pulmonary C-fibers reflexly increase secretion by tracheal submucosal glands in dogs. *J. Appl. Physiol.,* 58:907–910.
18. Ueki, I., German, V., and Nadel, J. A. (1979): Direct measurement of tracheal mucous gland secretion with micropipettes in cats: Effects of cholinergic and α-adrenergic stimulation. *Clin. Res.,* 27:59A.
19. Ueki, I., German, V. F., and Nadel, J. A. (1980): Micropipette measurement of airway submucosal gland secretion: Autonomic effects. *Am. Rev. Respir. Dis.,* 121:351–357.
20. Ueki, I., and Nadel, J. A. (1981): Differences in total protein concentration in submucosal gland fluid: α-Adrenergic vs. cholinergic. *Fed. Proc.,* 40:622.
21. Webber, S. E., and Widdicombe, J. G. (1987): The effect of vasoactive intestinal peptide on smooth muscle tone and mucus secretion from the ferret trachea. *Br. J. Pharmacol.* 91:139–148.
22. Webber, S. E., and Widdicombe, J. G. (1987): The actions of methacholine, phenylephrine, salbutamol and histamine on mucus secretion from the ferret *in vitro* trachea. *Agents Actions,* 22:82–85.

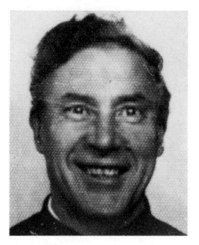

John Guy Widdicombe was born in 1925 in Barnet, England. He received the B.A., B.M., and M.A., respectively, in 1946, 1949, and 1953 in Oxford. He received the D.M. in 1966. Currently he is chairman of the Department of Physiology. His interests include reflex control of respiration, pathophysiology of the respiratory tract, and airway mucus secretion.

2. Physical Methods of Analysis

Methods in Bronchial Mucology,
edited by P. C. Braga and L. Allegra.
Raven Press, Ltd. © 1988.

2.1. BASIC CONCEPTS OF MUCUS RHEOLOGY

2.1.1. Mathematical Description

S. S. Davis

*Department of Pharmacy, University of Nottingham,
Nottingham, United Kingdom*

Rheological Models
  Hooke model
  Newton model
  Maxwell model
  Voigt model
Generalized models

The proper evaluation of the rheology of mucus is essential for a correct understanding of mucociliary clearance, cilial mechanisms, the etiology of disease conditions, biochemical determinants, and the action of pharmacological agents that include mucolytics and mucotropics (7). However, the rheological properties of mucus are complex, and as a result useful parameters that characterize viscous and elastic behavior are not simple to define in mathematical terms, nor are they easy to measure experimentally. Indeed, some have claimed that mucus could be one of the most difficult biological materials to define in biophysical terms. It has even been termed "superelastic" (24).

Before the mid-1960s, the majority of workers studying the rheological properties of respiratory mucus treated the material as a simple liquid and attempted to measure viscosity using a conventional viscometer. Others, realizing the complex nature of the material, preferred a more empirical approach to the assessment of consistency. Interestingly, those attempting to evaluate the properties of respiratory mucus concentrated on viscosity, whereas those dealing with cervical mucus focused their attention on elasticity (Spinbarkeit) (7). In reality, mucus has elements of both viscosity and elasticity, i.e., it is viscoelastic, and methods of evaluation need to reflect this dichotomy. In 1969, Davis and Dippy (9) and Hwang et al. (14), working independently, reported for the first time on the viscoelastic characteristics of respiratory mucus and attempts to measure meaningful physical parameters. Since that time, a number of different methods have been described, and various reports have detailed the practical results of such measurements (3,4,7,15–20, 22,23,25).

Other chapters in this book consider the detailed methodology. The purpose of this chapter is to describe the essential mathematical description of viscoelasticity. The approach used is similar to that employed for the evaluation of the viscoelastic properties of nonbiological polymer systems and employs an analysis based on mechanical models.

RHEOLOGICAL MODELS

The evaluation of rheological parameters appropriate to a viscoelastic material, such as mucus, is best considered by examining the response of a three-dimensional body to applied force (Fig. 1) and the application of two basic mechanical models to describe elastic and viscous behavior (1,12).

Hooke Model

The elastic (or solid) element is represented as a spring and is attributed to Hooke (Fig. 2). The behavior of the spring under applied tensile stress (σ_t) is represented in Figs. 1(left) and 2. On application of the stress, the spring increases in length (extends), and the ratio of the increase to the original length fractional (i.e., extension) is termed the "tensile strain" (γ). If the stress is removed, the spring will return to its original length, i.e., the system recovers. If the stress is

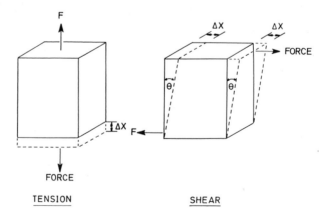

FIG. 1. A solid (elastic object) subjected to tensile and shearing forces.

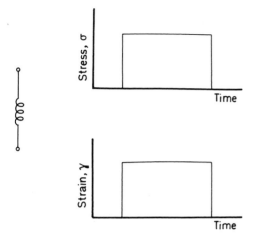

FIG. 2. The Hooke model for elastic behavior.

doubled and the strain increases in direct proportion, the system is defined as being linear. This being so, it is possible to define the behavior of the system by a simple equation:

$$E = \frac{\sigma_t}{\gamma} \qquad [1]$$

where E is the tensile (Young's) modulus. The units are the same as those for stress, i.e., Newton per square meter (Nm^{-2}), since strain is dimensionless. The modulus described in Eq. 1 is for tensile extension.

A type of deformation more relevant to the properties of mucus is that of simple shear. The application of an applied force will result in a deformation, as shown in Fig. 1(right). The shear strain is defined as $\gamma = \tan \theta$ and the shear modulus as:

$$G = \frac{\sigma_s}{\gamma} \qquad [2]$$

E and G are interrelated by the expression:

$$E = 2(1 + \mu)G \qquad [3]$$

where μ is Poisson's ratio. For an incompressible material, $\mu = 0.5$ and, hence, $E = 3G$. For heterogeneous materials, μ can be 0.2 or lower (1).

The shear compliance is the reciprocal of the shear modulus:

$$J = 1/G = \frac{\gamma}{\sigma_s} \qquad [4]$$

and has the units m^2N^{-1}. The modulus of a simple solid can be measured by the application of a tensile (or shearing) stress and then measuring the strain (compliance)

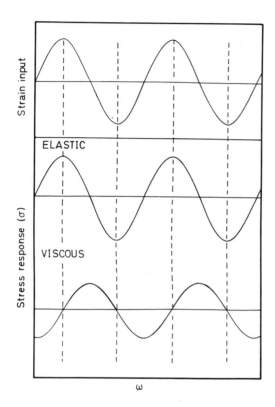

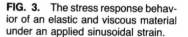

FIG. 3. The stress response behavior of an elastic and viscous material under an applied sinusoidal strain.

response. Alternatively, a constant strain can be induced into the material and the stress relaxation (modulus) determined.

Thus, the behavior of a simple solid can be defined by the modulus or compliance of the material.

A further method of testing can be adopted in which the stress or strain is varied in an oscillatory manner, rather than being applied as a step function (12). The response is studied as a function of angular frequency. Consider the situation where a solid material is contained between two plates. A sinusoidal stress is applied to the bottom plate, and strain response is measured from the upper plate. We would expect, as is indeed the case, the strain response to be directly in phase with the stress (0 degrees phase difference) (Fig. 3). If the stress is written as:

$$\sigma_t = \sigma_0 \cos \omega t \qquad [5]$$

where σ_0 is the maximum stress at the end of each cycle (amplitude), then:

$$\gamma = \frac{\sigma_0}{G} \cos \omega t \qquad [6]$$

Newton Model

The fluid (liquid) element is represented by a dashpot (a piston in a cylinder filled with a liquid) (Fig. 4) and is attributed to Newton. The same stress–strain analysis can be considered as before. While the stress is applied, the piston will more linearly with time until such time as the stress is removed. There is no recovery. A parameter similar to the modulus for the solid can be defined by considering the ratio of the applied stress to the rate of change of strain (i.e., the gradient of the line in strain versus the relation), that is:

$$\eta = \frac{\sigma}{d\gamma/dt} = \frac{\sigma}{\dot{\gamma}} \qquad [7]$$

where for ease of notation, the term $d\gamma/dt$ is written in the usual notation $\dot{\gamma}$. The parameter, η, is the viscosity with units of $Nm^{-2}sec$. The similarity of definition for the solid and liquid can be seen by comparing Eq. 3 and Eq. 7.

A liquid system that conforms to the simple equation is termed Newtonian in nature. If the dashpot is subjected to a stress of x times σ for a time t, the same strain will be produced if the stress σ was applied for x times t (1).

The behavior of the viscous model under oscillatory shearing can also be considered. As already defined by Eq. 7:

$$\frac{d\gamma}{dt} = \frac{\sigma}{\eta} \qquad [8]$$

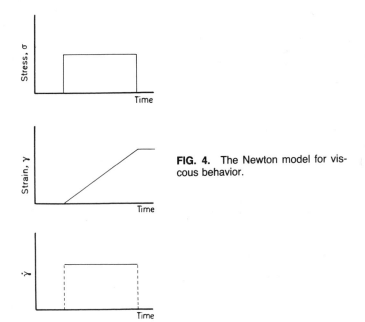

FIG. 4. The Newton model for viscous behavior.

That is, the rate of strain ($d\gamma/dt$) is linearly related to the stress; i.e., the rate of strain will be maximum when the stress is a maximum and minimum when the stress is a minimum. For sinusoidal motion, the maximum rate of change is when it passes through zero amplitude, and the minimum rate of change is when the amplitude is a maximum.

Therefore, undertaking the same experiment described for a solid between two flat plates with a Newtonian liquid, the stress and strain will be out of phase by exactly 90 degrees (Fig. 3). We can write:

$$\frac{d\gamma}{dt} = \frac{\sigma_0}{\eta} \cos \omega t \qquad [9]$$

and then on integration:

$$\gamma t - \gamma_0 = \frac{\sigma_0 \sin \omega t}{\eta \omega} \qquad [10]$$

As will be discussed, a material that is neither elastic nor viscous but has a combination of these properties will have a phase discipline somewhere between the two extremes of 0 degrees (solid) and 90 degrees (liquid). In data analysis, the in phase (solid character) and the out phase (liquid character) are separated in order to characterize the material.

The viscosity can be used to characterize the properties of the pure liquid system in an absolute way. The viscosity is independent of the applied test conditions. In a more practical sense, the system does not change its consistency when subjected to shearing conditions. Newtonian systems are usually simple fluids or suspensions or emulsions containing low quantities (less than 20%) of a dispersed phase. If the system is more concentrated or contains structure (e.g., intertwined polymer chains, particulate aggregates), the system will no longer behave in a simple Newtonian way, and usually the system will demonstrate a reduction in viscosity upon shearing (shear thinning effect). Materials exhibiting fluid flow, whether this be Newtonian or non-Newtonian in character, can be characterized by some suitable form of viscometer.

Mucus is certainly non-Newtonian in its flow characteristics (7–10). However, the material also has significant solidlike (elastic) properties. Consequently, testing mucus as if it were solely liquidlike can lead to invalid results. For example, the elastic properties of the material could cause it to fracture within the measuring apparatus or to be expelled either partly or completely from the measuring surfaces, with the result that the material will appear to be less viscous than it really is.

Mucus can be defined rheologically as a viscoelastic material, i.e., it has characteristics of the solid and the liquid. Its behavior under stress can be best understood by a further extension of the model analysis described previously. By analogy with electronic circuits, it is possible to link the rheological elements in series or in parallel. The spring (that stores energy) is the mechanical analog of the capacitor (that stores current), and the dashpot, where the movement of the piston is resisted by the liquid, is the mechanical analog of the resistor.

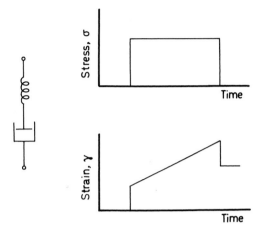

FIG. 5. The Maxwell model.

Maxwell Model

The Maxwell model (Fig. 5) is produced by linking the spring in series with the piston. By performing the same stress–time experiment as described for the Maxwell and Newton models, the effects of the two elements on the strain response are clearly demonstrated. On removal of the stress, the elastic component is recovered but the viscous component is not.

The interrelationship between the elastic and viscous components can be expressed simply by:

$$\eta = \tau G \qquad [11]$$

where the proportionally constant τ has the dimensions of time and is called the relaxation time. The equation for the strain response of the Maxwell unit under constant stress can be obtained by simply combining the Hooke (spring) and Newton (dashpot) in the form of time derivatives (1):

$$\frac{d\gamma}{dt} = \frac{1}{G}\frac{d\sigma}{dt} + \frac{\sigma}{\eta} \qquad [12]$$

Under constant strain, $d\sigma/dt = 0$, and then:

$$\frac{d\gamma}{dt} = \frac{\sigma_0}{\eta} \qquad [13]$$

On integration from time 0 to time t and dividing by applied stress, we can write:

$$\frac{\gamma t}{\sigma} = J_t = J_0 + t/\eta \qquad [14]$$

If, instead of a constant stress a constant applied strain (γ_0) is induced, only the spring element can respond immediately. The dashpot will gradually move (relax) with time, and the stress induced in the system will relax. Since $\dfrac{d\gamma}{dt} = 0$ and $\eta = \tau G$, we can write:

$$\frac{d\sigma}{\sigma} = \frac{-dt}{t} \qquad [15]$$

Integration as before and division by γ_0:

$$G_t = G_0 e^{-t/\tau} \qquad [16]$$

If the Maxwell model is considered in oscillatory shear, there will be contributions from both parts of the model. The relative magnitudes of G and η and the frequency of test will be important. Imagine an experiment conducted at low frequencies (i.e., at time scales longer than the relaxation time τ)—then the viscous element will have time to undergo flow during the oscillatory cycle. Much of the applied energy will be dissipated rather than stored in the elastic element. Therefore, at low frequency the material will demonstrate largely viscous behavior. In contrast, at high frequency (at times shorter than τ) the dashpot has little time to move before the cycle is reversed. Thus, little energy will be dissipated, and the material appears to be largely elastic. Indeed, in viscoelastic analysis the in phase (elastic) component is often termed the ''storage'' component, and the out of phase (viscous) component is termed the ''loss'' component.

A Maxwell unit in oscillatory motion will provide a phase difference somewhere between 0 and 90 degrees (i.e., it is viscoelastic), and from the foregoing it will be realized that the phase difference angle (δ) will be closer to 90 degrees at low frequency (i.e., the system appears more liquidlike), whereas at high frequency δ is closer to 90 degrees (i.e., it is more solidlike). Thus, by examining the properties of a viscoelastic material at different frequencies, it is possible to learn about both parts of the behavior.

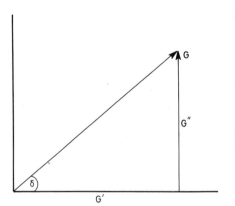

FIG. 6. Vector diagram representation of viscoelastic behavior. (G') Storage (elastic) modulus (stress in phase with strain—real component); (G'') loss (viscous) modulus stress 90 degrees out of phase with strain—imaginary component); (G) complex modulus (viscoelastic material); (σ) phase angle difference.

The resolution of oscillatory data into its separate elastic and viscous parts requires some knowledge of vectors. Space does not permit a detailed treatment here, but Fig. 6 shows a simple vector diagram where the in phase (elastic) and out of phase (viscous) components are depicted with the viscoelastic material lying between the two.

The so-called absolute shear modulus $|G|$, is defined as the magnitude of the stress vector divided by the magnitude of the strain vector (1,12). A derived modulus for a viscoelastic material will be a complex function of the in phase (real part) and out of phase (imaginary part) and is expressed by:

$$G* = G' + iG'' \tag{17}$$

Similarly for compliance:

$$J* = J' - iJ'' \tag{18}$$

where $G*$ and $J*$ are the complex shear modulus and shear compliance, respectively. Parameters with one prime are the storage components and two primes the loss components; i is $\sqrt{-1}$. Note that:

$$\eta' = G'' \tag{19}$$

If the Maxwell model is subjected to a sinusoidal stress, the strain will be out of phase by an angle δ.

We can write:

$$\sigma_{(t)} = \sigma_0 e^{-i\omega t} \tag{20}$$

where σ_0 is the stress amplitude, and then from Eq. 12:

$$\frac{d\gamma_{(t)}}{dt} = \frac{\sigma_0}{G} i\omega e^{-i\omega t} + \frac{\sigma_0}{\eta} e^{-i\omega t} \tag{21}$$

Integration provides:

$$J* = J - \frac{iJ}{t\omega} \tag{22}$$

or in terms of storage and loss:

$$J* = J' - iJ'' \tag{23}$$

Since:

$$J'' = \frac{J}{\tau\omega} - \frac{1}{\eta\omega} \tag{24}$$

Similarly, it can be shown that:

$$G* = \frac{G\tau^2\omega^2}{1 + \omega^2\tau^2} + \frac{i\tau\omega G}{1 + \omega^2\tau^2} \tag{25}$$

$$G* = G' + iG'' \tag{26}$$

Note that the tangent of the angle δ is:

$$\tan \delta = G''/G' \qquad\qquad [27]$$

and also:

$$\tan \delta = \frac{1}{\tau\omega} \qquad\qquad [28]$$

Voigt Model

The model where the elements are linked in parallel is the Voigt or Kelvin model (Fig. 7). The strain response under constant stress is more complex in form, since the movement of the spring is retarded by the viscous dashpot. The higher the viscosity of the liquid in the dashpot element, the greater the retardation.

Under constant stress we can consider both parts of the model with the constraint that the strain must be the same in the two elements and the stress must be the sum of the stresses in the two individual elements. We can write:

$$\frac{d\gamma(t)}{dt} + \frac{\gamma t}{t} = \frac{\sigma_0}{\eta} \qquad\qquad [29]$$

This linear differential equation can be integrated to yield (1):

$$J_t = J(1 - e^{-t/\tau}) \qquad\qquad [30]$$

where J is the total compliance at infinite time and τ is the retardation time, defined in an analogous way to the relaxation time for the Maxwell unit as $\eta/G = \tau$.

On removal of the stress, the system recovers completely, since in this model the spring can cause the piston to return to its original position in the dashpot. As for the Maxwell model, it is a simple matter to undertake an experiment to measure strain response under applied stress and to determine the values of G and η by graphic or computer procedures.

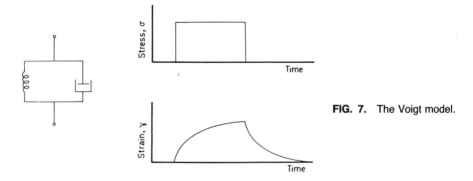

FIG. 7. The Voigt model.

The application of constraint strain conditions and the conduct of a stress relaxation experiment is not appropriate for the Voigt model. The application of sinusoidal stress and strain provides similar results to those for the Maxwell system.

GENERALIZED MODELS

Complex materials such as mucus do not conform to either the simple Maxwell or Kelvin models, and more complex models are required to describe viscoelastic behavior. The generalized models for viscoelastic behavior are shown in Fig. 8. These consist of a number of Maxwell elements connected in parallel (Maxwell-Wiechert model) or a Voigt model connected in series (Voigt-Kelvin model) (1). The models can be modified so that they can reflect contributions from uncoupled elements.

The Maxwell-Wiechert model is a useful representation for a complex viscoelastic material subjected to constant strain and undergoing stress relaxation. The equation is rewritten in a modified form:

$$G_t = \sum_{i=1}^{n} G_i e^{-t/\tau i} \qquad [31]$$

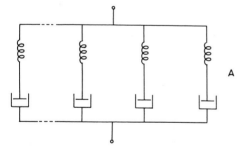

A

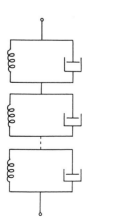

B

FIG. 8. Generalized viscoelastic models. **A:** Maxwell-Wiechert model. **B:** Voigt-Kelvin model.

where the total response is made up from the individual contributions from the various n elements.

In a sinusoidal experiment, the appropriate equation is:

$$G' = \sum_{i=1}^{n} \frac{G_i\omega^2\tau_i^2}{1 + \omega^2\tau_i^2} \qquad [32]$$

$$G'' = \sum_{i=1}^{n} \frac{G_i\omega\tau_i}{1 + \omega^2\tau_i^2} \qquad [33]$$

The Voigt-Kelvin model is best examined in terms of constant stress conditions, and the derived strain response will be:

$$J_t = \sum_{i=1}^{n} J_i(1 - e^{-t/\tau_i}) \qquad [34]$$

Experimental studies on respiratory mucus subjected to constant stress (creep tests) show that such a Voigt-Kelvin analysis can be instructive and that the full viscoelastic model is one that has uncoupled spring and dashpot elements (Fig. 9), i.e., the addition of one Maxwell unit to the generalized Voigt-Kelvin model. The full equation for the compliance at any time t is then:

$$J_t = J_0 + \sum_{i=1}^{n} J_i(1 - e^{-t/\tau_i}) + t/\eta_0 \qquad [35]$$

In order to gain some understanding of underlying processes, the different regions of the strain response can be associated tentatively with molecular structures in

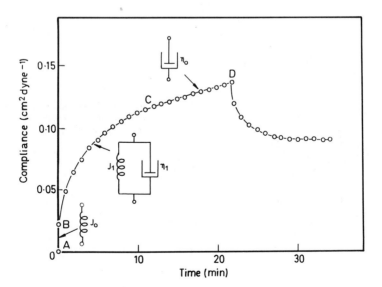

FIG. 9. Creep curve for respiratory mucus.

the system being tested (7). Thus, in Fig. 9, the region A–B can be associated with elastic permanent links within a system, e.g., crosslinked structures, and the Voigt-Kelvin region (B–C) can be associated with secondary bonds that require time for their modification under applied stress. These could include entanglements or hydrogen or hydrophobic bonds. The viscous region C–D is related to the properties of the viscous matrix of the material.

As expected, a biological material such as mucus will not be well characterized by just a single viscoelastic element and one retardation time (6,18) but may have structures that provide a whole spectrum of such times. When a large number of Maxwell or Voigt elem. nts is necessary to characterize a material, a continuous distribution spectrum of relaxation or retardation times is an alternative to the mechanical model (discrete viscoelastic analysis) approach (12). For example, in the case of the generalized Voigt-Kelvin model, an infinite number of retardation times is considered, as defined by the retardation spectrum L in the form:

$$J_t = \int_{-\infty}^{\infty} L_{(t)}(1 - e^{-t/\tau})d \ln \tau + t/\eta_0 \qquad [36]$$

L has the nature of a distribution function with the dimensions of compliance. The spectrum over a wide range of time could provide information at the molecular level. For example, a maximum in a derived retardation spectrum may give an indication of a concentration of retardation processes.

In viscoelastic testing, usually it can be instructive to obtain information over a wide time scale in order to gain detailed insight into responsible processes at a molecular level. In a sinusoidal experiment at low frequency, the response is largely a viscous one, since there is adequate time for loss of stored energy, whereas at high frequency, a largely elastic response is attained (Fig. 9). The exact manner in which the viscoelastic parameters change with frequency is indicative of, for example, the amount of crosslinking between (bio)polymer chains and the state of polymer entanglements (18,19).

For respiratory mucus, such data can then be used to follow the effects of disease conditions and the action of drugs or for correlation with biochemical estimates. The two most popular methods for analyzing the viscoelastic properties of mucus are the transient (creep) tests conducted under constant stress conditions and the determination of the compliance values or some form of dynamic (oscillatory) experiment (7). The data from these two approaches can be combined in order to cover as wide a time scale as possible. Transient data can be transformed to dynamic data (the usual procedure) and vice versa (less often applied) (12). At the extremes, it is to be expected that at very low frequency:

$$\eta'(dyn) \to \eta_0(creep)$$

and at high frequency:

$$G'(dyn) \to G_0(creep)$$

Transformation methods (both exact and approximate) can be found in the literature (12). The calculation of J' and J'' from creep compliance data can be performed by the Fourier sine and cosine transformations. In our work, we have preferred to use numerical formulae outlined by Ferry (12). These require creep compliance data obtained on a logarithmic time scale. The simplest formula is:

$$J'(\omega)nJ_t - 0.86 [J(2t) - J(t)] \tag{37}$$

and a more exact version is:

$$\begin{aligned} J'(\omega) \sim J(t) &- 0.0007[J(32t) - J(16t)] - 0.0185[J(16t) - J(8t)] \\ &+ 0.197[J(8t) - J(4t)] - 0.778[J(4t) - J(2t)] \\ &- 0.181[J(t) - J(t/2)] - 0.049[J(t/4) - J(t/8)] \end{aligned} \tag{38}$$

Similarly,

$$J''(\omega) \sim 2.12 [J(t) - J(t/2)] \tag{39}$$

or a more exact form:

$$\begin{aligned} J''(\omega) \sim &-0.470[J(4t) - J(2t)] + 1.674[J(2t) - J(t)] + 0.198[J(t) - J(t/2)] \\ &+ 0.620[J(t/2) - J(t/4)] + 0.012[J(t/4) - J(t/8)] \\ &+ 0.172[J(t/8) - J(t/16)] + 0.043[J(t/32) - J(t/64)] \\ &+ 0.012[J(t/128) - J(t/256)] \end{aligned} \tag{40}$$

where $\omega(\text{rad sec}^{-1}) = 1/t$ sec.

The calculation used values of the creep compliance that are spaced equally on a logarithmic time scale so that the ratio between successive times is a factor of 2. The value of $J(t)$ required for calculations at a given value of t can be read directly from the experimental creep curve (or recorded in digital form using a logarithmic clock) (i.e., $J(t)$ at the times, $t/256$, $t/128$ . . . through to t itself, $2 \times t$, $4 \times t$ sec]. Further details can be found in references 2, 11, and 12.

If discrete spectral analyses have been conducted, we can write:

$$J'(\omega) = J_0 + \sum_{i=1}^{n} J_i/(1 + \omega^2\tau_i^2) \tag{41}$$

and:

$$J''(\omega) = \sum_{i=1}^{n} J_i\omega\tau_i(1 + \omega^2\tau_i^2) + t/\eta_0 \tag{42}$$

Values for G', G'', and η' can be obtained from:

$$G' = \frac{J'}{(J'^2 + J''^2)} \tag{43}$$

and:

$$G'' = \frac{J''}{(J'^2 + J''^2)} \tag{44}$$

Figure 10 shows a dynamic response plot for respiratory mucus where creep data were converted to oscillatory data by numerical methods (6). The data cover

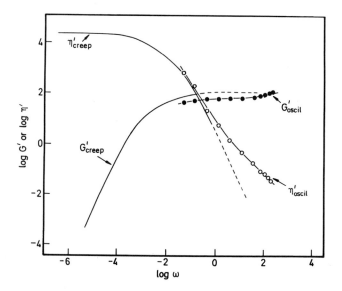

FIG. 10. Combined dynamic and transient (creep) data for respiratory mucus.

an eight-unit frequency (time) scale. The agreement between the two sets of data is good.

Once again the different regions of the curve can be discussed in terms of molecular mechanisms (Fig. 11). At high frequency, the motions of the constituent molecules are restricted to backbone bone stretching and vibration as well as

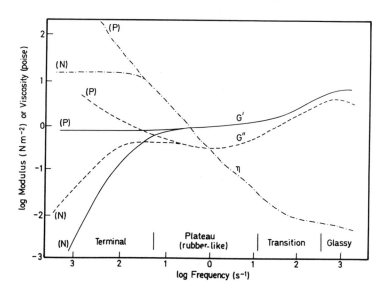

FIG. 11. The response of a viscoelastic material in dynamic (oscillatory) testing. (P) Permanently crosslinked; (N) noncrosslinked material. (After ref. 22).

some motion of side chains in relation to the backbone. Elastic behavior dominates at low frequency. For a nonpermanently crosslinked system, such as respiratory mucus (the terminal zone), rearrangement of large segments of the backbone and slippage of molecules past one another can occur and viscous behavior dominates, η' levels off and approaches η_0 found in creep studies. G' falls rapidly and becomes less than G''. A system that conforms to a definite mechanical model should exhibit a direct proportionality between G' and ω at low frequency when η' is constant (slope of 1 on a double log plot). Conversely, in this terminal zone, G' is proportional to $\omega^2 t^2$, which gives a theoretical slope of 2 on a double log plot (12). A permanently crosslinked system shows a different behavior, particularly in that η' does not level off and G' remains constant at low frequency (22).

At intermediate frequencies, there is a plateau zone where the material exhibits rubberlike behavior. Here, conformation rearrangement of chain backbones with different degrees of molecular cooperation will occur (23). Derived data for respiratory mucus support the view that mucoprotein chains are partially entangled at coupling points between molecules and molecular segments, such that the material behaves as if it is partially crosslinked (9,14). A spectrum of relaxation times centered at about 100 sec has been used to characterize this region (14). The modulus G' can be related to the concentration of mucin in the mucus sample and the molecular weight characteristics (7).

In all the foregoing discussions, it has been assumed that the materials have behaved in a linear manner and that the theories of linear viscoelasticity can be applied. Linearity can be assessed experimentally by the superposition concept. Theories of nonlinear viscoelastic behavior have been developed, but these are highly complex mathematically (13,21).

REFERENCES

1. Aklonis, J. J., and MacKnight, W. J. (1983): *Introduction to Polymer Viscoelasticity.* 2nd ed. Wiley, New York.
2. Barry, B. W. (1974): Rheology of pharmaceutical and cosmetic semisolids. *Adv. Pharm. Sci.,* 4:1–72.
3. Chen, T. M., and Dulfano, M. J. (1976): Physical properties of sputum VI: Physical-chemical factors in sputum rheology. *Biorheology,* 13:211–218.
4. Chen, T. M., and Dulfano, M. J. (1978): Mucus viscoelasticity and mucociliary transport rates. *J. Lab. Clin. Invest.,* 91:422–431.
5. Cox, A., Jabbal-Gill, I., Marriott, C., and Davis, S. S. (1982): Effects of *S*-carboxymethylcysteine on the biophysical and biochemical properties of mucus on chronic bronchitics. In: *Mucus in Health and Disease II,* edited by E. Chantler, J. Elder, and M. Elstein, pp. 423–429. Plenum Press, London.
6. Davis, S. S. (1973): Techniques for the measurement of the rheological properties of sputum. *Bull. Physiopathol. Resp.,* 9:47–90.
7. Davis, S. S. (1980): In: *Cough and Expectoration,* edited by E. Berglund, B. S. Nilsson, B. Mossberg, and B. Blake, pp. 141–152. Munksgaard, Copenhagen.
8. Davis, S. S., and Deverell, L. C. (1977): Rheological factors in mucociliary clearance. *Mod. Probl. Pediatr.,* 19:207–217.
9. Davis, S. S., and Dippy, J. E. (1969): The rheological properties of sputum. *Biorheology,* 6:11–21.

10. Dippy, J. E., and Davis, S. S. (1969): Rheological assessment of mucolytic agents on sputum of chronic bronchitics. *Thorax,* 24:707–713.

11. Eccleston, G. M., Barry, B. W., and Davis, S. S. (1973): Correlation of viscoelastic functions for pharmaceutical semisolids. Comparison of creep and oscillatory tests for oil-in-water creams stabilised by mixed emulsifiers. *J. Pharm. Sci.,* 62;1954–1961.

12. Ferry, T. D. (1980): *Viscoelastic Properties of Polymers,* 3rd ed. Wiley, New York.

13. Findley, W. N., Lai, J. J., and Onaran, K. (1976): *Creep Relaxation of Nonlinear Viscoelastic Materials.* North Holland, Amsterdam.

14. Hwang, S. H., Litt, M., and Forsman, W. C. (1969): Rheological properties of mucus. *Rheol. Acta,* 8:438–448.

15. Khan, M. A., Wolf, D. P., and Litt, M. (1976): Effect of mucolytic agents on the rheological properties of tracheal mucus. *Biochim. Biophys. Acta,* 444:369–373.

16. King, M., Gilboa, A., Meyer, F. A., and Silberberg, A. (1974): On the transport of mucus and its rheologic simulants in ciliated systems. *Am. Rev. Respir. Dis.,* 110:740–745.

17. King, M., and Macklem, P. T. (1977): Rheological properties of microliter quantities of normal mucus. *J. Appl. Physiol.,* 42:797–802.

18. Litt, M. (1970): Mucus rheology. *Arch. Intern. Med.,* 126:417–423.

19. Litt, M., Khan, M. A., Charkin, L. W., Wardell, J. R., and Christian, P. (1974): The viscoelasticity of fractionated canine tracheal mucus. *Biorheology,* 11:111–117.

20. Litt, M., Khan, M. A., and Wolf, D. P. (1976): Mucus rheology: Relation to structure and function. *Biorheology,* 13:37–48.

21. Lockett, F. J. (1972): *Nonlinear Viscoelastic Solids.* Academic Press, London.

22. Lojdahl, C. G., and Odeblad, E. (1980): Biophysical variables relating to viscoelastic properties of mucus secretions with special reference to NMR methods for viscosity measurement. In: *Cough and Expectoration,* edited by E. Berglund, B. S. Nilsson, B. Mossberg, and B. Blake, pp. 113–127. Munksgaard, Copenhagen.

23. Lutz, R. J., Litt, M., and Charkin, L. W. (1973): Physical–chemical factors in mucus rheology. In: *Rheology of Biological Systems,* edited by H. L. Gabelnick and M. Litt, pp. 119–157. Charles C Thomas, Springfield, IL.

24. Philippoff, W., Han, C. D., Barnett, B., and Dulfano, M. J. (1970): A method for determining the viscoelastic properties of biological fluids. *Biorheology,* 7:55–67.

25. Puchelle, E., and Zahm, J. M. (1974): Role de l'effectbout sur le mesure de la visco-elasticite de l'expectoration determinee a l'aide d'un rheometre rotatif a cylindres coaxieux. *Biorheology,* 11:323–330.

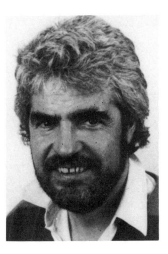

Stanley Stewart Davis was born in Leamington, U.K., in 1942. He received B. Pharm., Ph. D., and D. SC. degrees, respectively, in 1964, 1967, and 1981, all from London University. He is Lord Trent Professor of Pharmacy at Nottingham University. sity. Fields of interest include design and evaluation of drug delivery systems.

Methods in Bronchial Mucology,
edited by P. C. Braga and L. Allegra.
Raven Press, Ltd. © 1988.

2.1.2. Models of Mucus Structure

A. Silberberg

Department of Polymer Research, Weizmann Institute of Science, Rehovot, Israel

The structure of mucus glycoprotein
Mucus structure
The organization of the mucus gel
The peptide-carbohydrate bond (lectin) hypothesis
Discussion

The conditions under which sizable quantities of mucus can be collected from the lung are under practically all circumstances rather severely nonphysiological (15). Most often, the subjects are ill and are oversecreting for that reason or the mucosae are exposed and, despite all care, are in a condition of overstimulation and stress. Almost all the information we possess is on lung mucus produced at nonphysiological rates, since in cases of normally functioning respiratory epithelia, there may be practically no mucus present at all (3,15). Hence, neither the concentration nor the composition of respiratory mucus as collected for analysis need be typical of the mucus that is secreted, in only small quantities, under normal, mildly stimulatory conditions, i.e., in a healthy lung breathing only mildly polluted air. Even in normally functioning lungs, however, mucus collects cellular debris, airborne materials, and a large variety of other substances. The potential contents of pathological mucus, therefore, are extremely varied. They represent almost a biochemical index of what can occur in the lung (6,14,15). Nevertheless, the analysis of pathological lung mucus, like that of mucus from almost any other source, shows the presence of one dominant component, a highly characteristic structural glycoprotein (1,5–7,11–13,15,19,20).

This glycoprotein is distinguished by a very high sugar content and a very large molecular size (1,4–6,8,12,15,19,20). In mucus normally, it is present as a network that may be crosslinked throughout or merely very heavily entangled. In order to study mucus, the network has to be solubilized, which can be achieved by mild stirring, after which the glycoprotein is separated from the solubilized product by size exclusion chromatography (1) or, more effectively, by density gradient centrifugation (1,3–6,10,12,13).

In purifying the mucus glycoprotein, many other mucus components, including a large number of proteins, are separated (1,3–6,13,15,20). *A priori,* there is no reason to think that these mucus components are functionally unimportant or that they represent merely material the mucus was intended to sweep up or components that aid mucus in this task, e.g., enzymes, bactericidal agents (14), and such solubilizing materials as lipids and surfactants. Could there not, therefore, be other materials involved with mucus structure?

There are two main reasons to concentrate on the heavily glycosylated glycoprotein that we have indicated: (a) The production of such a material, built up of what seem to be 500 kilodaltons (kD) molecular subunits, characterizes all secretory epithelia. The subunit may vary in sugar composition (5,20) but seems in all cases to have nearly the same protein chain, ∼700 amino acids long. (b) The material exists in mucus as a network but, when mildly broken down, disentangled mechanically or chemically, and purified, yields a product that forms a gel that when reconstituted at equivalent concentrations mimics mucus in its rheological response (15). It is thus reasonable to assume that most, if not all, structural features of mucus can be associated with this macromolecule and that differences in concentration and possibly sugar composition give rise to the differences in rheology that the varied functions of mucus require. It is one of the most exciting aspects of mucus research that this glycoprotein subunit as derived from the many different organs and places where mucus has a role shows essentially the same chemical composition, organization, and basic size (1,4–6,10,11,13,15,20).

THE STRUCTURE OF MUCUS GLYCOPROTEIN

Figure 1 illustrates the structural principle of the basic subunit of mucus glycoprotein. A single protein backbone chain is involved, which is partly glycosylated and partly bare (nonglycosylated), i.e., partly covered with a tightly packed array of short (about 10 sugar units long) side chains, and partly not covered (regions B and A,A', respectively). The bare protein regions are either at both ends (A and A') (Fig. 1a) or only at one end (A) (Fig. 1b). The bottlebrush structure of Fig. 1b is the one usually cited.

The amino acid composition is unusual (Fig. 1). Almost half the amino acids in the glycosylated region (B) are either threonine or serine, either of which can be linked by an O-glycosidic bond to *N*-acetylgalactosamine. This is always the innermost sugar of the side chain. The bare protein regions are rich in aspartate and contain a very large number (about 13–16) of cysteine units capable of forming covalent —S—S— bonds with each other or with other cysteines on other chains (intramolecular or intermolecular bonds, respectively).

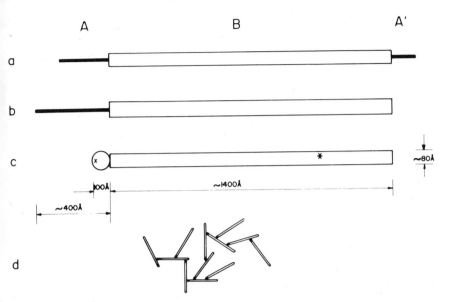

FIG. 1. Basic structural subunit of mucus glycoprotein. MW ~ 500 kD; A, A' = Bare protein backbone, B = Glycopeptide [Carlstedt et al. (4) refer to region B as the "T-domain"].

	A,A'	B
Number of amino acids	240–300	400–500
Threonine and serine	30–37	200–250
Cysteine	13–16	1–2
Aspartic acid	36–40	8–10
Number of sugar moieties	0	1600–2000
Number of side chains	0	160–200

a: Subunit structure capable of forming networks by intersubunit protein-to-protein disulfide bonds. **b:** The bottlebrush model for the subunit. **c:** The lectin model for the subunit. The rare sugar sequence (*) to which the lectin X can link could occur zero times, once, twice, and so on among the sugar side chains of the subunit. **d:** Network formed by the lectin in a case where there is slightly more than one recognized site per subunit.

Such a large number of bonding sites in the same portion of chain should be seen as an indication that the protein is meant to be folded in a highly specific way and that a particular conformation is to be stabilized by intramolecular bonding. Assuming that all —S—S— bonds are intramolecular, the bare peptide region will be collapsed into a globular structure and the appearance of the molecule will resemble Fig. 1c. We can then imagine that the bare protein, by being specifically folded, has generated a very effective binding site for a specific sugar or sugar sequence. This would make the bare peptide of the basic mucus glycoprotein subunit a lectin. As is well known, a lectin-sugar bond is generally extremely strong and specific and has all the stability of a covalent link (2). The composition of the side chains and the sequence in which the sugars appear in it are thus of considerable interest.

In order to understand how sugar composition and sequence are controlled, one has to appreciate the manner in which the sugars are added to the protein backbone (5,15,17). This occurs in the Golgi apparatus of the mucus-producing cell. The sugars are added by a set of glycosyltransferases that transfer the sugar for which they are specific to the growing chain. The first sugar in the chain, as stated, is N-acetylgalactosamine. It is attached to an available hydroxyl group of serine or threonine. There is generally an excess of serine and threonine over the number actually used to produce a tight coat of side chains. One may assume that this excess is present to facilitate the growth of side chains until no more can be added for steric reasons. Addition of sugars follows two principles, the availability of sugar-loaded glycosyltransferases and the addition rules of "what can follow what," i.e., the rules of chemical spelling. Not every sugar will permit every other sugar to be added, but some sugars will permit a choice. In some cases, there is only one site to which another sugar can add; in other cases, two sugars can be added (branching). The choice of which sugar among those permitted will actually be added is made by availability, so that a great deal of variability can exist in the sugar coat even though one pattern and one sequence probably will dominate. The addition of fucose or a neuraminic acid terminates the chain so that there also will be considerable variety in chain length. Mucus glycoproteins exhibit what has been called "microheterogeneity" (5). Since there are some 160 to 200 side chains on the subunit of Fig. 1, the composition of the sugar coat, even within each subunit, will closely reflect the conditions obtaining in the Golgi apparatus at the time of synthesis.

Although the average composition may thus be the same, considerable differences will have been built in among the large number of side chains of the subunit. It is reasonable to assume that practically all the "words" that the Golgi apparatus knows how to spell will have been expressed along the mucus glycoprotein backbone with some finite probability, i.e., at some frequency. This is expected to include the sugar sequence recognized by the lectin, a rather rare occurrence. Among the sugar sequences there will be those that serve in the attachment and elimination of different organelles. There could even be sequences that are recognized only by potential invaders, e.g., bacteria, of which the animal could not have had a priori knowledge. The sugar coat of mucus might be intended as an all purpose biochemical screen, conveniently studded with a compendium of binding sites able to act as decoy targets for all manner of biopolymers and microorganisms (14).

The glycoprotein subunit when completed is concentrated and packed into granules formed from the membrane surrounding the Golgi complex. The mechanism of packing and the actual concentration in the storage vesicles is not fully known. The granules constitute the reservoir from which mucus is secreted. It is conceivable that if reducing conditions prevail in the granules, no disulfide bonds are formed until the granular contents are exteriorized through the cell's plasma membrane. During exteriorization, the lipid membrane of the granule is shed and partly combined into the plasma membrane. The stimulus initiating secretion does not affect al mucus-producing cells equally. Cells in crypts are triggered by cholinergic agents, and mucus-producing surface cells are activated by proteinases, but a whole spectrum of agents modulates secretion (15). The granular contents fuse rapidly, and no seams suggestive of the granular history are visible in macroscopic blobs of mucus. It is not known what crosslinks are formed and what rearrangements take place during secretion.

Along with secretion, mucus apparently swells and spreads over the epithelium. It is not clear what limits swelling and thus determines the concentration and with it the structure and the rheological character. The source of the water that dilutes the secreted mucus glycoprotein down to physiological concentration is not known, although obviously, it is locally derived. According to Verdugo, a blob of mucus secreted by the cell swells by a factor of 10^3 (15). The granule would thus have to contain almost pure glycoprotein for the final concentration to be 1 mg/ml at least. In Verdugo's *in vitro* case, swelling is controlled, but it remains unclear by what means it is limited physiologically.

The physiological role of mucus in clearance requires that its properties be rheologically matched to optimize the transfer of momentum from the beating cilia on the epithelium to the mucus layer and from there to the mucus-carried debris (9,18,20). When mucus is too concentrated or when it is too dilute, there is less than optimal matching and a decline in transport velocity is experienced (9). It is essential, moreover, that just the right thickness layer of interciliary fluid surround the cilia. The depth of this layer controls the extent to which the ciliary tip penetrates the overlying mucus during the active stroke of the cilium. Here too there is an optimum. Since periciliary fluid is a source of water that would certainly be used by the freshly secreted mucus if it must swell, a compensatory secretion of a serous fluid would be required to make up lost volume and to ensure that cilia are always immersed to just the right depth. We have speculated that it is the contact between an applied load and a quiescent epithelium that stimulates secretion and causes ciliary activity to follow (21). A local, temporary loss of periciliary fluid as the granular contents are secreted could thus be the factor that activates quiescent cilia.

As the swollen, swelling mucus is transported over the epithelium, its state, i.e., its structure, may become stabilized. On the other hand, there is evidence also that it may deteriorate spontaneously (10). Any particular amount of mucus may thus have only a transient span over the epithelium (21). Rheologically, mucus will be transported only when it has the character of an incipient gel (9), but enzymes or other mechanisms may cause it to break down. It is not unreasonable to think that the glycoprotein network of an expended mucus patch might be chemically attacked, go into solution, and become reabsorbed by the epithelium. On frog palate epithelium, it has been shown that mucus is present only when the epithelium has been challenged (21). Under abnormal, overstimulatory conditions, therefore, mucus could accumulate, interfere with function, and become a burden on the system, although it would be then collectable in macroscopic amounts. In other words, a continuous mucus blanket may arise in the lung only under pathological conditions. Under normal unchallenged conditions, there is essentially no mucus present, and the cilia are at rest. Whether stimulus first produces mucus release and ciliary movement is the response to this, as we have speculated (21), or vice versa is not really known.

Contrary to what is seen with nascent mucus, mucus as collected tends not to swell and does not dissolve when exposed to excess water or saline. Even when mucus samples are dehydrated, they do not tend to swell back to their original volume. Can resident mucus, therefore, be in equilibrium with the excess water surrounding the cilia? Does swelling maintain the incipient gel character of mucus at which it functions optimally in clearance by cilia? Perhaps this is not necessary. If we are correct in thinking that fresh mucus is always secreted before cilia are set in motion, only the thin, freshly secreted layer that is in immediate contact with cilia would need to be adjusted to be optimal.

MUCUS STRUCTURE

In order to characterize the chemical and molecular properties of mucus, it must be dissolved. Dissolution can be achieved in a number of ways:

1. Mild mechanical agitation
2. Proteolytic digestion
3. Reduction of disulfide bonds
4. Thermal digestion

Mechanical Agitation

Stirring under mild conditions will solubilize mucus (1,4,11,12,20). It is not clear if this breaks a number of strategic bonds or merely disentangles large macromolecules, or both. The molecular weight of the first breakdown product that gives a solution is 31,000 to 40,000 kD (1,4,11,12,15,20). It is this molecule that generally represents the starting material for further diminutions in size. It is important to have protease inhibitors present during solubilization and during the purification stages that follow (4,5).

Proteolytic Digestion

The region B in Fig. 1 is so heavily glycosylated that it is inaccessible to enzymes and is protected from degradation. Hence, when mucus is exposed to proteases, only the regions A and A' are digested, and a product results that is essentially the glycosylated region. Carlstedt et al. refer to this region as the "T-domain" (4). It is a unifying feature of all mucus glycoproteins that essentially the same kind of end-product results after total proteolysis. Excessive exposure to enzyme does eventually, of course, produce some breakdown of the B region as well, but in general terms the presence of a relatively stiff, glycosylated cylindrical repeat unit, a block involving 400 to 500 amino acids about 1,400 Å long and 50 to 100 Å thick, is fairly well established. As already stressed, about half of the 400 to 500 amino acids in this block are serine or threonine, one sixth is proline, and one sixth is valine and alanine. The presence of proline in the backbone and all the sugar side chains it carries tend to make B a rather stiff rod. At about 500 kD, such a rod has a mass per unit length of about 0.28 kD/Å, much higher than the DNA double helix or even the collagen triple helix (20).

Dissolution by proteases clearly establishes the bare peptide as an essential partner in the crosslink. From this evidence, however, it is not known if the crosslink is between two such bare peptide regions or, as we propose, between the bare peptide and carbohydrate binding site.

Reduction of Disulfide Bonds

Reduction of the —S—S— bond to —SH tends to liberate the 500 kD basic subunit. Various reagents can be used, but the reaction does not go to completion under all conditions (1,4–6,11,12). It is our belief that incomplete reduction is the only reason that molecular residues in excess of 500 kD are found in many cases.

Meyer (12), for example, discusses a 4,000 kD unit (possibly eight 500 kD subunits?) that is formed after digestion in 0.1 M dithiothreitol/6 M guanidinium hydrochloride, conditions under which close to 100% of the —S—S— bonds can be shown to be reduced. About 130 cysteines are involved with eight subunits, but only seven cysteines are required to link these eight subunits into one molecule by intermolecular —S—S— bonds. Hence 94% of the disulfide bonds could be reduced and a 4,000 kD unit could still result if 1 strategic intermolecular link of almost 20 was particularly resistant. In other words, even if chemically the reduction seems to be complete, there are many cysteines per basic subunit, and only one intermolecular bond is required to build a basic subunit into the network. Subunits of molecular weights larger than 500 kD could easily exist, although chemically all the bonds have apparently been reduced (1,4,5,11,12).

The alternative explanation—that we are dealing here with an extra-long protein chain—is very hard to believe. In the case of the basic subunit, we are talking about a protein of about 700 amino acids with a molecular weight close to 100 kD, comparable approximately to the single strand of collagen. It would be most unusual if instead of such a long, rather stiff protein chain, a chain several multiples of 100 kD in weight was being synthesized by the cell.

There is the possibility that a linker protein may be involved in the case of some mucus secretions (1). Such a protein could act in addition to or be the sole link between some of the mucus glycoprotein subunits and so create a bond resistant to disulfide bond reduction.

Disulfide crosslinks, if the bonds are interchain rather than intrachain, would have to be between an A and an A′ region (Fig. 1). If the structure were that shown in Fig. 1b the bonds could only cluster the subunits into spherical aggregates and not build long chains of them. Structure Fig. 1a is thus necessary. Long chains involving A—A, A′—A′, or A—A′ —S—S— bonds are then easily built up. Some of these could be bonds that are stronger and more resistant than others, and total breakdown might be achieved only under the most severe reducing conditions. The same argument could be applied only to the breakdown of intramolecular —S—S— bonds, which fold the bare peptide into a lectin (Fig. 1c). Here, too, we could visualize bonds of different strength. The carbohydrate substrate would help to stabilize the folded bare peptide and could act to do so more effectively in some situations than in others. An explanation for the incomplete breakdown of the mucus glycoprotein network, under some reducing conditions, could thus be advanced in both cases.

Thermal Digestion

It was observed by Meyer (10) that mucus degraded spontaneously, without stirring and without any chemical or biological agent being added. The rate of degradation was higher if the temperature was higher. Experiments performed over the entire accessible temperature range (0°C–100°C) showed that a unique activation energy was involved that was independent of solvent properties, such as ionic strength or hydrogen bond breaking power. Monomolecular breakdown of some essential bond seems to occur. The units formed by this process tend to be about 500 kD in molecular weight, although smaller sized units are formed in the course of time. This again suggests that the dominant thermally labile bond is in the bare peptide region. The activation energy, 22.3 kCal/mol, associated with the degradation process fits rather well the known energy of activation for the hydrolysis of a peptide bond next to aspartic acid, a known preferred locus for protein hydrolysis. The bare peptide region is very high in aspartate and is thus the statistically favored site of attack, although this will not be exclusively the case. The results are consistent with this conclusion but cannot clarify if breakdown was achieved by intermolecular A—A, A′—A′, or A—A′ bonds being bypassed or if the hydrolysis broke up the lectin of Fig. 1c.

THE ORGANIZATION OF THE MUCUS GEL

It is known that the sperm have to traverse a cervical isthmus filled with mucus before entering the vagina. It was thus believed that mucus, cervical mucus at any rate, is sufficiently coarsely grained so that sperm can penetrate its meshes with ease (15). In apparent support of this idea, mucus, as seen in routine preparations for the scanning electron microscope, showed rather wide open spaces and thick fibrous bundles. However, when samples were prepared using extremely fast freezing techniques, a very delicately structured network appeared, a network showing a level of dispersion that was consistent with the measurements of permeation rate of suspending medium through the gel (20). The permeation constant is a very sensitive way to assess pore dimensions, which were shown to be small, consistent with the crosslink model and the structure seen after fast freeze-drying (16). Since reasonably pure mucus is optically clear, any heterogeneities are smaller than the wavelength of light. At the concentrations involved, the pore size found indicated that the strands are mainly chains of single subunits with some crosslinking (branching) occurring along the tree. Recent theoretical work (19) based on the lectin model shows that rather high molecular weight, randomly coiled, and slightly branched molecules are to be expected.

THE PEPTIDE-CARBOHYDRATE BOND (LECTIN) HYPOTHESIS

Is it easily imagined that the bare peptide chain, A, will fold and be stabilized by a large number of strategic —S—S— bonds. In this manner, both a highly specific and a very resistant binding site could be formed. Such lectin, protein-to-carbohydrate, binding sites in mammalian systems have now been established in several cases, including some slightly related to mucus (2,14). In mucus, the binding site would be a sugar or a sugar sequence, which is so rare that only once among the roughly 2,000 sugar moieties of the basic subunit would the right sugar or sugar combination occur. One or more binding sites per subunit, on the average, would lead to the formation of an infinite network (19). If the binding site occurred somewhat less frequently, very large but limited size, predominantly linear aggregates would form. Although each basic subunit has its lectin combining site, there is, in this case, an insufficient number of recognized sites for a complete network to arise. On the other hand, if there is slightly more than one recognized sugar site per subunit, there is a strong tendency to build infinite, strongly collapsed gels (Fig. 1d). The system is thus very delicately balanced. The mechanisms in the Golgi complex that produce the variability in the sugar side chain composition and size would thus be in exquisite control of the kind of mucus that is stored and secreted by the cell.

It should be stressed, however, that there is as yet no direct biochemical proof of the lectin bond hypothesis in mucus. Such a proof would, for example, involve the dissolution of mucus by the addition of an oligosugar containing the recognized sequence in sufficiently large amounts.

DISCUSSION

Mucus from all sources involves a heavily glycosylated structural subunit that almost certainly has the character of the rod shown in Fig. 1c. A large number of cysteines occur in the bare protein region A. This may thus be folded and stabilized by intramolecular disulfide bonds. The network required for the rheological functioning of mucus is build up of these units. As the crosslink, either a direct intermolecular disulfide bond or a dissulfide bond stabilized lectin protein-to-sugar bond, is involved. There may be two levels of crosslinking. Bonds entered into in nascent mucus may be labile, so that the mucus blob swells easily. In the course of time, the links become more stable and will no longer exchange with ease. The mucus gel network is probably not infinite but only very effectively entangled. In cases of normally functioning respiratory epithelia, it may even be transient. Anything that destroys the bare peptide region will dissolve the network. There are no side-to-side associations of the individual glycoprotein strands into thicker fibers, and there are few branches. The lectin hypothesis would give the cell very easy control over the structural and rheological properties of the secreted product. No direct proof of the lectin hypothesis exists, however, and a more conventional model, involving intermolecular —S—S— bonds is possible.

The mucus glycoprotein molecules, in mildly solubilized mucus, has been called "the first unit into solution." There is little systematic uniformity in this product (8). We have called the unit in Fig. 1 the "basic subunit." Other subunits, which may be preparational artifacts, lie between these extremes. It is obvious that chemical breaks, less clean than those envisaged, could produce any combination of cuts. It is generally agreed that proteolysis yields the B region. This is called the "T-domain" by Carlstedt et al. (4). In our view, the basic subunit is that of Fig. 1. We believe it to contain the protein chain as it is genetically encoded and synthesized by the cell.

REFERENCES

1. Allen, A. (1981): Structure and function of gastrointestinal mucus. In: *Physiology of the Gastrointestinal Tract*, edited by L. R. Johnson, pp. 617–639. Raven Press, New York.
2. Beyer, E. C., and Barondes, S. H. (1982): Secretion of endogenous lectin by chicken intestinal goblet cells. *J Cell Biol*, 92:28–33.
3. Bhaskar, K. R., O'Sullivan, D. D., Seltzer, J., Rossing, T. H., Drazen, J. H., and Reid, L. M. (1985): Density gradient study of bronchial mucus aspirates from healthy volunteers (smokers and nonsmokers) and from patients with tracheostomy. *Exp Lung Res*, 9:289–308.
4. Carlstedt, I., Lindgren, H., and Sheehan, J. K. (1983): The macromolecular structure of human cervical-mucus glycoproteins. *Biochem J*, 213:427–435.
5. Carlstedt, I., Sheehan, J. K., Cosfield, A. P., and Gallagher, J. T. (1985): Mucus glycoproteins: A gel of a problem. *Essays Biochem*, 20:40–76.
6. Creeth, J. M. (1978): Constituents of mucus and their separation. *Br Med Bull*, 34:17–24.
7. Gibbons, R. A., and Roberts, G. P. (1963): Some aspects of the structure of macromolecular constituents of epithelial mucus. *Ann NY Acad Sci*, 106:218–232.
8. Harding, S. E. (1984): An analysis of the heterogeneity of mucus. No evidence for a self association. *Biochem J*, 219:1061–1064.
9. King, M., Gilboa, A., Meyer, F. A., and Silberberg, A. (1974): On the transport of mucus and its rheological simulants in ciliated systems. *Am Rev Respir Dis*, 110:740–745.
10. Meyer, F. A. (1976): Mucus structure: Relation to biological transport function. *Biorheology*, 13:49–58.
11. Meyer, F. A. (1977): Comparison of structural glycoproteins from mucus of different sources. *Biochem Biophys Acta*, 493:272–282.
12. Meyer, F. A. (1983): Polymeric structure of a high-molecular-weight glycoprotein from bovine cervical mucus. *Biochem J*, 215:701–704.

13. Meyer, F. A., Eliezer, N., Silberberg, A., Vered, J., Sharon, N., and Sade, J. (1973): An approach to the biochemical basis for the transport function of epithelial mucus. *Bull Physiopathol Respir*, 9:259–272.
14. Murray, P. A., Levine, M. J., Tabak, L. A., and Reddy, M. S. (1982): Specificity of salivary-bacterial interactions: II. Evidence for a lectin on *Streptococcus sanguis* with specificity for a NeuAcα2–3 Galβ1–3GalNAc sequence. *Biochem Biophys Res Commun*, 106:390–396.
15. Nugent, J., and O'Connor, M., eds. (1984): *Mucus and Mucosa. Ciba Foundation Symposium 109*. Pitman, London.
16. Parish, G. R., Beeson, M. F., Brown, D. T., and Marriott, C. (1982): A freezing artefact associated with the preparation of mucus for examination using the scanning electron microscope. In: *Mucus in Health and Disease. II*, edited by E. N. Chantler, J. B. Elder, and M. Elstein, pp. 297–300. Plenum Press, New York.
17. Phelps, C. F. (1978): Biosynthesis of mucus glycoprotein. *Br Med Bull*, 34:43–48.
18. Sade, J., Eliezer, N., Silberberg, A., and Nevo, A. C. (1970): The role of mucus in the transport by cilia. *Am Rev Respir Dis*, 102:48–52.
19. Silberberg, A. (1987): A model for mucus glycoprotein assembly. *Biorheology* (in press).
20. Silberberg, A., and Meyer, F. A. (1982): Structure and function of mucus. In: *Mucus in Health and Disease. II*, edited by E. N. Chantler, J. B. Elder, and M. Elstein, pp. 53–74. Plenum Press, New York.
21. Spungin, B., and Silberberg, A. (1984): Stimulation of mucus secretion, ciliary activity and transport in frog palate epithelium. *Am J Physiol* 247:C299–C308.

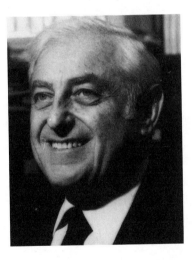

Alexander Silberberg was born in 1923 in Vienna, Austria. He was graduated in 1944 with a B.Sc. (Eng) degree in Chemical Engineering and, in 1952, received the Ph.D. degree. Currently, he is Professor in the Weizmann Institute of Science, Israel. He is Editor-in-Chief of *Biorheology*. His interests include macromolecular physics and chemistry, biorheology, and molecular physiology.

Methods in Bronchial Mucology,
edited by P. C. Braga and L. Allegra.
Raven Press, Ltd. © 1988.

2.2. DYNAMIC METHODS IN VISCOELASTICITY ASSESSMENT

2.2.1. Sinusoidal Oscillations Method

P. C. Braga

Department of Pharmacology, University of Milan, Milan, Italy

---

Method
    Coaxial cylinder assembly
    Driving mechanism
    Measuring devices
Comments

Physicochemical studies of bronchial mucus have shown that different kinds of proteins and glycoproteins are the main polymeric constituents of mucus, which is a mixture of randomly coiled entangled macromolecules crosslinked by disulfide bridge bonds and further joined by hydrogen, electrostatic, and hydrophobic bonds, with water, ions, and lipids, all arranged in a three-dimensional gel network (Fig. 1). This material is produced by and even mobilized in the airways, that is, it flows, so from a physical point of view, rheology is the branch of physics that we must apply to investigate the physical properties of bronchial mucus.

Because of its complex biochemical and polymeric nature, bronchial mucus has a number of nonlinear and time-dependent flow properties. Rheologically, it is a complex non-Newtonian viscoelastic material. This means that in its response to stress it behaves neither as a solid nor as a liquid but as some combination of the two. Quantitative measures of its viscoelasticity can be obtained with different kinds of instruments that measure two basic parameters of the flow of a material: stress and strains. Stress is the force per unit area causing a deformation, and strain is the amount of deformation.

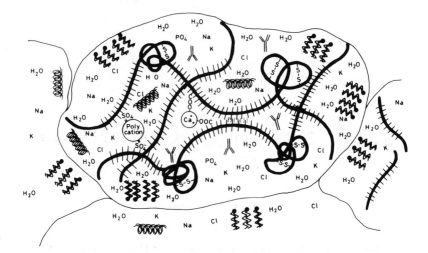

FIG. 1. Schematic representation of a drop of mucus with randomly coiled entangled macro-molecules.

Proper investigation of the viscoelasticity of a bronchial mucus sample is not easy, not only because its behavior is not linear but also because there are technical difficulties, such as inhomogeneity and/or contamination of the mucus, insufficient amounts collected, and interference in the process of measuring (because testing in a rheometer disturbs the original structure). Moreover, there is considerable variation in the measurements of samples obtained from different patients and from the same patient at different times (days).

To try to overcome these problems, several different technical approaches have been used, the limiting factor being the creativity of the investigator (1,2). At present, the most common tests are the creep test, the relaxation test, and the oscillation test. In this chapter, the forced oscillation technique is examined.

METHOD

Techniques for the evaluation of the viscoelastic properties of polymers can be divided into two main groups: those that consider longer time scales (transient tests) and those that consider shorter time scales (dynamic tests) (2). In rheological investigations of the behavior of a polymer in solution, oscillatory techniques (dynamic tests) frequently are used, and since the mucus layer flows because of cilia oscillatory movements, an oscillatory test at a shear rate with a frequency comparable to that of the cilia would seem to be appropriate (7,8).

Coaxial Cylinder Assembly

The instrument for dynamic testing of bronchial mucus is a rotational rheometer with coaxial concentric cylinders (Couette type), which is the same as the one used for transient tests (Fig. 2). The basic mechanical structure of this instrument consists of an outer cylinder (cup) with the function of a reservoir of prefixed volume, into which is introduced the amount of mucus to be investigated, and an inner cylinder (bob), which is suspended coaxially by a calibrated torsion wire. The annular gap between the two cylinders must be as close as possible to 0.1 cm, which corresponds to the maximum linearity of measure. The resonance frequency of the whole system must have a value that does not interfer with measurements of mucus. These requirements call for a high degree of precision in the construction and alignment of the cylinders and in their movements.

When the sample is in the cup, the bob is very slowly lowered into position to minimize shear degradation. The cup must be thermostatically controlled, and a very small quantity of light paraffin oil can be used to cover the sample to prevent evaporation of water in long studies. This is the coaxial cylinder assembly. In an elastoviscometer, there are two other components: the driving mechanism and the measuring devices.

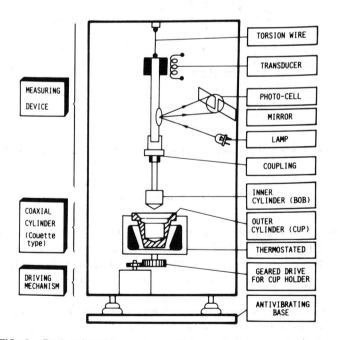

FIG. 2. Basic schematic arrangement of a general purpose rheometer.

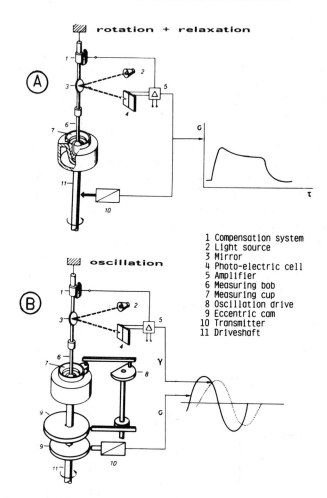

1 Compensation system
2 Light source
3 Mirror
4 Photo-electric cell
5 Amplifier
6 Measuring bob
7 Measuring cup
8 Oscillation drive
9 Eccentric cam
10 Transmitter
11 Driveshaft

FIG. 3. Geometry of the measuring systems: **A:** Rotational + relaxation. **B:** Oscillatory.

Driving Mechanism

The driving mechanism of the cup is designed to obtain cup oscillation with definite frequency and fixed small amplitude. The motor driving the cup can be wired, for instance, to a sine voltage so that the cup, instead of rotating at constant speed, as in the rotational mode, oscillates periodically in a sinusoidal movement (mechanical eccentrics are also used).

If the speed of the external cylinder varies sinusoidally with time, the mucus sample transmits to the inner cylinder a sinusoidal movement with the same frequency but with a phase difference and an amplitude that depend on the rheological features (dynamic mechanical properties) of the material under study.

Measuring Devices

The measuring device that is usually adopted to measure the movement transmitted to the bob is a torsion wire (beryllium–copper). The torque on the bob is measured as the deflection or twist of the torsion wire from which the bob is suspended. Magnetic devices also have been used. Angular movements of the bob about its vertical axis can be observed with the aid of an optical lever (light beam–mirror–scale) or a differential transformer or other system (Fig. 3).

This is the basic description of a forced oscillation rheometer, which is very similar to that used for rotational studies except for the movements of the driving mechanism. Viscoelasticity investigation of natural or synthetic polymers has been performed routinely for many years in several industrial fields, and many technical solutions with different kinds of refinements have been proposed (4,5,11,12).

COMMENTS

Many of these devices are laboratory instruments, but there are also commercial rheometers for viscoelastic measurement. These high-priced rheometers are designed for general purposes, primarily for industrial applications, but can generally be used also for mucus (see Appendix). A mechanical model for elasticity can be idealized as a spring with a dashpot for viscosity. Complex biopolymeric fluids combine both springlike and viscouslike properties in their viscoelastic behavior. This can be represented schematically by a Maxwell or a Voigt element or by a combination of the two (Fig. 4).

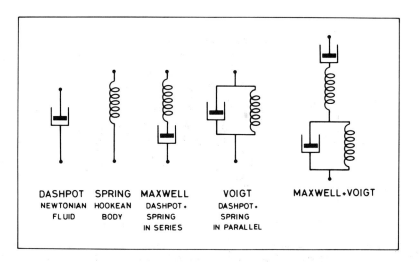

FIG. 4. Mechanical analogs of different rheological systems.

In the resting state, before measure, the sample of mucus placed in the gap between the two cylinders has random distribution and orientation of its viscoelastic elements (Fig. 5A). After movement has been applied, there is a bending, stretching, slippage, and reorientation of the viscoelastic elements, and the resulting displacement is measured (Fig. 5B). If the material is purely elastic, the strain is in phase with the stress. If it is purely viscous, the strain is 90 degrees out of phase with the stress (10). If the material is linearly viscoelastic, the strain will vary sinusoidally also, but the phase shift versus stress will depend on the degree of viscoelasticity (Fig. 6). These measurements can be visualized in a two-channel graphic recorder. An alternative is to plot the shear stress versus the strain on an XY plotter. The resulting plot is a so-called Lissajous figure, and in the case of a viscoelastic fluid an elliptical figure is obtained (Fig. 6). The rheological behavior

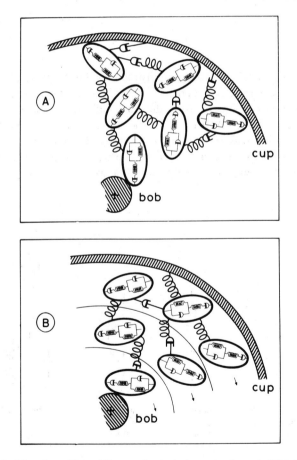

FIG. 5. Model of the disposition of the mechanical elements characterizing the viscoelastic behavior of mucus. **A:** Random disposition of the viscoelastic elements in quiet status. **B:** Orientation of the viscoelastic elements following laminar flow during cup rotation.

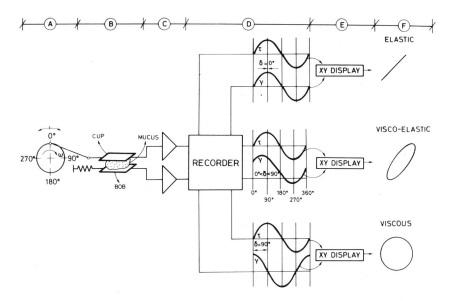

FIG. 6. Schematic procedure to record the phase difference between stress and strain and the corresponding Lissajous figures that characterize elastic, viscoelastic, and viscous behavior. (A) Oscillatory movements; (B) rheometer; (C) amplifiers; (D) recorder; (E) XY display; (F) Lissajous figures.

of the bronchial mucus under different pathological conditions or before or after a treatment will be characterized by different shapes of the ellipse. The mathematical resolution of the elliptical figure (see chap. 2.3.3.) gives a measure of the viscosity and the elasticity.

The equation of state for a linear elastic liquid undergoing forced sinusoidal oscillations of small amplitude can be written as:

$$\sigma = 2 \eta^* \dot{\gamma}$$

in which σ is the shear stress, $\dot{\gamma}$ is the shear rate, and η^* is known as the "complex dynamic viscosity," which is a function of the frequency of oscillation $\omega (\text{rad} \cdot \text{sec}^{-1})$ and is usually complex (3).

It is usual to express η^* as:

$$\eta^* = \eta' - i \frac{G'}{\omega}$$

in which η' is the dynamic viscosity, G' the dynamic rigidity, and $i = \sqrt{-1}$. For a purely viscous liquid, η' is constant and G' is zero. G' is also known as the "storage modulus" and is a measure of the energy that is elastically stored and can be released on cessation of the deforming stress. The loss modulus G'' = $\omega \eta'$ is a measure of the energy dissipated or lost as heat per cycle (3,5).

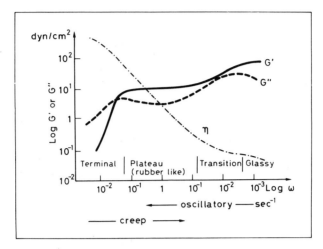

FIG. 7. Typical viscoelastic curves of high molecular weight polymer solution. Creep and oscillatory test regions of application are indicated.

Another useful viscoelastic parameter is $\tan \delta = \dfrac{G''}{G'} \left(= \dfrac{\eta'\omega}{G'} \right)$, which is of potential value for relating the rheological properties of mucus to mucociliary clearance (6).

One of the advantages of the oscillatory technique is that the parameters G'' (or $\eta'\omega$), G', and η' can be obtained in a short time at different frequencies of oscillation and the corresponding results can be presented as a diagram (Fig. 7) illustrating the complete spectrum of response (9). On the other hand, the most valuable information for viscoelastic measurements is obtained at small strains and low frequencies at which, with some limitations, the structure of the mucus is maintained. Large strains and high shear rates tend to disrupt the intrinsic elastic network structure of mucus.

REFERENCES

1. Aiache, J. M., Pradelle, J., and Molina, C. (1970): La rheologie des expectorations. Materiels et methodes. *Poumon Coeur*, 16:35–49.
2. Davis, S. S. (1980): Practical applications of viscoelasticity measurement. *Eur. J. Respir. Dis.*, 61 [Suppl. 110]:141–156.
3. Davis, S. S., and Dippy, J. E. (1969): The rheological properties of sputum. *Biorheology*, 6:11–21.
4. Eirich, F. R. (1958): *Rheology, Theory and Applications*, Vol. II. Academic Press, New York.
5. Ferry, J. D. (1980): *Viscoelastic Properties of Polymers*. Wiley, New York.
6. King, M. (1980): Relationship between mucus viscoelasticity and ciliary transport in guaran gel/frog palate model system. *Biorheology*, 17:249–250.
7. Litt, M., Khan, M. A., Chakrin, L. W., Wardell, J. R., and Christian, P. (1974): The viscoelasticity of fractionated canine tracheal mucus. *Biorheology*, 11:111–117.

8. Litt, M., Khan, M. A., and Wolf, D. P. (1976): Mucus rheology. Relation to structure and function. *Biorheology,* 13:37–48.
9. Lofdahl, C. G., and Odeblad, E. (1980) Biophysical variables relating to visco-elastic properties of mucus secretions, with special reference to NMR-methods for viscosity measurements. *Eur. J. Respir. Dis.,* 61 [Suppl. 110]:113–127.
10. Lutz, R. J., Litt, M., and Chakrin, L. W. (1973): Physical-chemical factors in mucus rheology. In: *Rheology of Biological Systems,* edited by H. L. Gabelnick and M. Litt, pp. 119–157. Charles C Thomas, Springfield, IL.
11. Tanner, I. R. (1985): *Engineering Rheology.* Oxford Engineering Science Series No. 14, Clarendon Press, Oxford.
12. Walters, A. (1975): *Rheometry.* Chapman and Hall, London.

APPENDIX—INSTRUMENTS

Carri-Med Ltd. Interpet House, Vincent Lane Dorking, Surrey, RH43YX, England
Contraves A.G., Schaffhauserstrasse 580, Postfach CH-8052, Zurich, Switzerland
Haake GmbH, Dieselstrasse 6, D-7500 Karlsruhe 41, Germany
Rheo-Tech International Ltd, 120–122 Woodgrange Road, Forest Gate, London E7OEW, England
Sangamo Transducers Rheology Division, North Bersted, Bognor Regis, W. Sussex PO22 9BS, England
Sefam, Rue du Bois de la Sivrite, Parc d'Activités de Brabois, 54500 Vandoeure-les-Nancy, France

Methods in Bronchial Mucology,
edited by P. C. Braga and L. Allegra.
Raven Press, Ltd. © 1988.

2.2.2. Magnetic Microrheometer

M. King

Pulmonary Defense Group, University of Alberta, Edmonton, Canada

---

Method and Material
   Description of apparatus
   Theory
   Measuring technique
   Correction factors
Results
Discussion

The magnetic rheometer is an alternative type of dynamic viscoelastometer that is suited to the study of respiratory tract secretions. It was originally developed in the laboratory of Litt (12) and subsequently adapted and modified by several others, including this author (10). It works on the following principle: A sample of mucus, into which has been inserted a small steel ball, is placed between the poles of an electromagnet. The ball is then oscillated within the mucus by creating an oscillating field gradient with the magnet. The amplitude of oscillation and the current in the magnetic coil are used to determine viscosity and elasticity at different driving frequencies.

METHOD AND MATERIAL

Description of Apparatus

The magnetic microrheometer, as developed in the author's laboratory, is illustrated schematically in Fig. 1. An electromagnet is created by winding three coils, one of about 600 turns and two of about 400 turns each (14-gauge, coated wire),

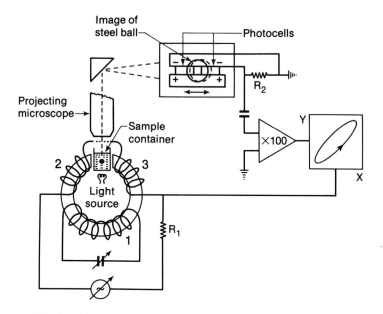

FIG. 1. Schematic representation of the magnetic microrheometer.

on a steel toroid from which a 2.5-mm sector has been removed. The magnet is mounted on the stage of a microscope and connected with both a DC power supply (coil 1) and an AC power amplifier (coils 2 and 3), driven by a sine-wave generator. The microscope is equipped with long working distance (11 mm) objectives, to accommodate the magnet, and a projecting prism.

The mucus sample is placed in a rectangular, clear-bottomed container that sits in the toroid gap. The sample containers are fashioned from Plexiglas and glass, bonded by epoxy resin (Fig. 2). Thin coverslip glass is used to form the

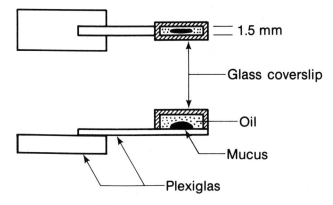

FIG. 2. Fabrication of sample containers for the magnetic rheometer.

side walls of the containers in order to conserve space. The mucus sample is placed in the sample container as illustrated and layered with light paraffin oil [viscosity < 1 poise (P), saturated with water] to minimize evaporation. A small steel ball (diameter 50–150 μm) is inserted in the mucus, and the sample container is then placed between the poles of the electromagnet. The image of the ball is magnified and projected onto a pair of photocells, which generate a signal that is transmitted to an oscilloscope. Measurements normally are carried out at room temperature.

Magnetic rheometers developed in other laboratories (3,12,14) differ somewhat in details of design, but all operate on the same physical principles.

Theory

In the magnetic rheometer technique, the small steel ball inserted in the sample of mucus acts as a rheological probe. It is set in motion by applying an oscillating magnetic force. The forces opposing the motion of the ball are the viscous and elastic forces exerted by the medium and inertial forces.

The magnetic driving force F_m is generated by passing a direct current I_d through coil 1 and an alternating current I_a through coils 2 and 3. The latter coils are connected in series with their polarities such that, in each half-cycle, the field generated by one coil opposes and the other reinforces the constant field B induced by the direct current. This creates an oscillating field gradient ∇B proportional to the alternating current, provided that the magnitude of I_a is somewhat smaller than that of I_d.

The force per unit volume F_m/V_{ball} acting on a particle in a magnetic field is proportional to $M \cdot \nabla B$, where M is the induced magnetic moment. For a small particle that does not significantly distort the field, M is proportional to B, which in the central plane of the gap is determined by I_d alone, which is constant. Thus for any given value of I_d:

$$F_m/V_{ball} \cdot \nabla B \cdot I_a \qquad [1]$$

or:

$$F_m = K_1 \cdot I_a \cdot r_{ball}^3 \qquad [2]$$

where K_1 is a constant.

This sinusoidally oscillating magnetic force can be described in complex notation as:

$$F_m = F_0 e^{i\omega t} = F_0(\cos \omega t + i \cdot \sin \omega t) \qquad [3]$$

where ω is the angular frequency in rad/sec and $i = \sqrt{-1}$. The sinusoidal displacement of the particle about its resting position, which lags the applied force by δ radians, can similarly be written as:

$$X = X_0 e^{i(\omega t - \delta)} \qquad [4]$$

The magnetic driving force (normal to gravity) is opposed by two types of forces: viscous drag and inertial forces (of the ball and of the fluid). For steady flow, the viscous drag F_v on a sphere of radius r is given by Stokes law:

$$F_v = 6\pi\eta r\dot{X} \tag{5}$$

where $\dot{X} = dX/dt$ is the velocity of the sphere and η is the viscosity of the medium. For a ball oscillating in a viscoelastic medium, it has been shown (2) that F_v and $\dot{X}$ in the Stokes law equation can be replaced by their Fourier transforms, and η can be replaced by η^*, the complex dynamic viscosity, provided that the fluid inertia is small. η^* has a component η' in phase with $\dot{X}$ and a component η'' out of phase with $\dot{X}$ (and hence in phase with X). In complex notation:

$$\eta^* = \eta' - i\eta'' \tag{6}$$

For the case where the ball inertia can also be neglected (low frequencies and small ball diameters), the Fourier transform approach leads to the relationship:

$$\eta^* = -F_0 i e^{i\delta}/6\pi r\omega X_0 = (F_0/6\pi r\omega X_0) \cdot (\sin\delta - i \cdot \cos\delta) \tag{7}$$

Thus, by comparison with Eq. 6:

$$\eta' = F_0 \sin\delta/6\pi r\omega X_0 \tag{8}$$

and:

$$\eta'' = F_0 \cos\delta/6\pi r\omega X_0 \tag{9}$$

The latter parameter η'', which is in phase with the displacement, is more commonly expressed in terms of the shear storage modulus (dynamic elasticity) G', given by the following relationship:

$$G' = \omega\eta'' \tag{10}$$

Hence:

$$G' = F_0 \cos\delta/6\pi r X_0 \tag{11}$$

Thus, to determine the dynamic mechanical properties (G' and η') at any given frequency, it is only necessary to determine F_0, X_0, and δ.

Measuring Technique

X_0 is determined in the following way: The image of the sphere is magnified and projected onto a screen, as indicated in Fig. 1, such that it partially covers each of a matched pair of rectangular (1×2 cm) silicon solar cells. As the shadow of the ball moves back and forth at low amplitude, the illuminated area of one photocell increases while the illuminated area of the other decreases, and vice versa. For the resistance range selected ($R_2 = 1\ K\Omega$), the photocell current I_p is proportional to the area illuminated. Because the photocells are connected differentially, the current generated across R_2 is proportional to the displacement of the ball as it oscillates about an equilibrium value provided that the maximum displacement of the image does not exceed the length of the photocell. The differential connection tends to minimize the effects of variations in line voltage and background light intensity (4). The alternating component of the photocell current thus provides a direct and continuous measure of the displacement X, dependent only on the magnification factor Mag, the length of the photocell L_{cell}, and the total current generated in the absence of the ball image I_{cal}.

Mag is the nominal microscope magnification adjusted for two minor correction factors, the postmagnification by the prism (normally 1–1.5) and the distortion of the image by the oil covering the mucus (the lens effect, normally 0.7–0.9). I_{cal} is the calibration factor that accounts for variations in the optical density of mucus; it can be obtained by manually moving the prism to illuminate maximally each of the photocells in turn. The resulting difference in current level then corresponds to a displacement of the image equal to length of a photocell. All of these geometric factors can be lumped together as the following:

$$X_0 = (L_{cell} \cdot I_p)/(Mag \cdot I_{cal}) = K_2 I_p \qquad [12]$$

The driving force F_m is proportional to the alternating current flowing in coils 2 and 3; it is monitored across a 1-ohm series load R_1. The constant K_1 relating F_m to $r^3 I_a$ in Eq. 2 can be determined by calibration with a Newtonian liquid of known viscosity (i.e., where $\delta \equiv \pi/2$, $G' = 0$, and $\eta' = \eta_N$). This was accomplished using an oil of $\eta_N = 1,010$ P at 25°C. Thus, from Eqs. 8 and 2:

$$\eta_N = K_1 r^3 (I_a)_0 / 6\pi r \omega X_0 \qquad [13]$$

or:

$$K_1 = 6\pi\omega X_0 \eta_N / r^2 (I_a)_0 \qquad [14]$$

This form of calibration is not entirely straightforward, since a ball suspended in a nonelastic medium falls under the influence of gravity at a constant rate out of the field of view of the microscope. The rate of fall is minimized by using a high-viscosity oil and small ball radius, but this results in very low amplitudes of vibration. For this reason, the calibration was verified (10) for samples of a polysaccharide gel (crosslinked guaran) of similar rheological properties to mucus by comparison with the results obtained with the mechanical spectrometer (Rheometrics, Inc.). This independent comparison gave a satisfactory fit for both G^* (within 10–20%) and δ (within 2 degrees).

The phase lag between ball displacement and driving force is determined from the shape of the ellipse that results when X is plotted against F_m on an oscilloscope or an X–Y recorder (at lower frequencies). As illustrated in Fig. 3, $\delta = $ arc sin $\Delta X/X = $ arc sin $\Delta Y/Y$. Thus from the values of F_0, X_0, and δ at any given frequency, G' and η' are directly determinable from Eqs. 11 and 8, respectively. Alternatively, the results can be expressed as G^* and tan δ, which are rather more independent of each other (5).

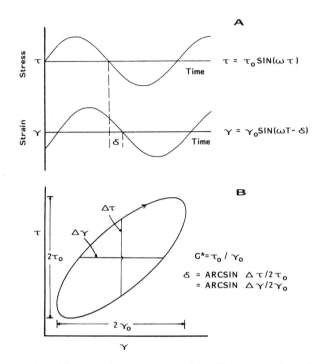

FIG. 3. Computation of the viscoelastic parameters G* and δ from recordings of stress (magnet current) and strain (photocell current).

The magnetic rheometer can also be used to measure the steady-shear viscosity $\eta_{ss'}$, which can be estimated from the nonrecoverable displacement ΔX after the application of a constant magnetic force for a fixed period of time t (creep experiment, Fig. 4). This is accomplished by applying a direct current I_d' to coils 2 and 3 in place of the alternating current normally used. By analogy with Eq. 13, η_{ss} is given by:

$$\eta_{ss} = K_1 r^2 I_d' t / 6\pi(\Delta X) \qquad [15]$$

This steady-shear viscosity can be identified with $\eta_{0'}$ the low-frequency or low-shear limiting viscosity, provided that the maximum displacements and shear rates during the transient testing are kept low.

Correction Factors

Stokes law (Eq. 5) was derived for a ball moving in an infinite medium. A ball moving in a finite (bounded) medium will be subject to a higher resistive force than that predicted by the Stokes equation because of the resistance of the walls of the container. Two types of wall effects are considered: end effects, a

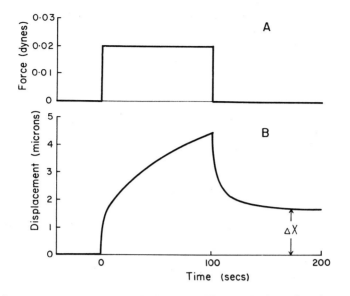

FIG. 4. Creep experiment with magnetic rheometer. The steady-shear viscosity, η_{ss}, is computed from the nonrecoverable displacement, ΔX, according to Eq. 15.

ball moving toward or away from a surface, and edge effects, a ball moving parallel to a surface. End effects are accounted for in the following manner:

$$F_v = (F_v)_{\text{Stokes}} \; [1+1.145 \text{x}(2\text{r/w})+3.0 \text{x}(2\text{r/w})^2]^2 \qquad [16]$$

where w is the width of the sample container. For the containers normally used, w = 1.5 mm; thus, for a ball diameter of 100 μm, the correction is about 18%.

Edge effects are taken into account by a second equation:

$$F_v = (F_v)_{\text{Stokes}}(1+0.502\text{xr/h})\cdot(1-0.502\text{xr/d}) \qquad [17]$$

where h is the distance from the center of the sphere to the bottom surface of the container, and d is the distance to the upper surface of the sample. In most cases, these two factors are offsetting.

It must be remembered that the correction factors for both types of deviations from Stokes law were derived for steady motion in a Newtonian fluid. Their applicability in the oscillatory testing of viscoelastic media has not been established. However, their use can be justified, at least in part, by the fact that the same range of container, sample, and ball sizes used in the testing of mucus were used in the calibration with crosslinked guaran, and thus the magnitude of the correction factor was the same for both calibrant and sample.

No corrections are made for the possible effects of a nonlinear viscoelastic response because the amplitudes of vibration normally employed are very small, generally of the order of 5 μm or 5% of the diameter of the ball. These amplitudes, at a frequency of 10 rad/sec, correspond to maximum (Newtonian) shear rates of less than 0.1 sec. Also, no correction is made for the effect of fluid inertia. Hwang et al. (2) estimated that deviations from the simple Fourier transformation of Stokes law at 10 rad/sec due to fluid inertia are of the order of 1%. Since the inertial effect increases with frequency, this would provide some limitation of the method at higher frequencies.

RESULTS

An example of the rheological data obtained for samples of normal respiratory tract mucus is shown in Fig. 5, which shows G' and η' plotted against ω on a logarithmic scale. In this frequency range η' decreases rapidly with increasing frequency (logarithmic slope 0.7–0.9), whereas G' increases only slowly (logarithmic slope 0.1–0.2). This rheological behavior is typical of crosslinked gels. If G^* and tan δ had been chosen as the independent variables, the magnitude and frequency dependence of G^* would have been very similar to G', while tan δ would have increased from about 0.2 to 0.4 at 1 rad/sec to about 0.7 to 1.0 at 100 rad/sec.

Magnetic rheometry has been used to characterize mucus in a variety of studies. Of particular note are investigations relating the viscoelastic properties of mucus with mucociliary clearance rates. In this category, one should mention the work of Giordano et al., who correlated *in vivo* tracheal clearance in dogs with the

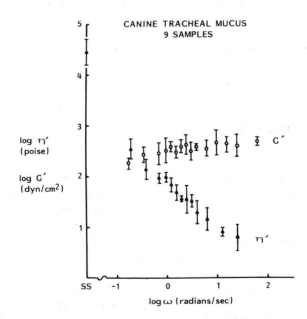

FIG. 5. Dynamic viscoelastic data (G' and η' as a function of ω) of canine tracheal mucus. Steady-shear viscosity from creep experiment is also shown. (From ref. 10.)

viscoelasticity of mucus collected from a tracheal pouch preparation (1). The same group also related the clearance of mucus on the isolated frog palate mucosa with the rheology of reconstituted canine tracheal pouch mucus (15). In the author's laboratory, we have related frog palate clearance to mucus viscoelasticity in several studies involving pharmacological manipulation of tracheal mucus (5,8,9,11). We have also used the magnetic rheometer to characterize the viscoelastic properties of mucus simulants in model studies of mucus clearance (6,7).

Recently, Sakakura used magnetic rheometry to study the viscoelastic properties of nasal secretions and middle ear effusions (13,14). The rheometer used in these studies is of special note in that the oscillating magnetic field gradient is applied in the vertical direction. The effect of gravity on the steel ball, which becomes significant with weakly crosslinked gels, is balanced by applying a DC bias to the AC creating the oscillating field gradient. This modification enables the determination of the viscoelastic properties of very weakly crosslinked samples and, in the latter-mentioned study (14), enabled the authors to determine values of G' down to about 1 dyn/cm^2.

DISCUSSION

The magnetic microrheometer is ideally suited for the study of the viscoelastic properties of normal respiratory tract mucus. It works best with samples that are moderately clear and of intermediate viscoelasticity. However, with care and with certain adaptations, it can be readily used for sputum, with its wider variability of rheological properties and greater opacity.

Indications

This is ideally suited for use with small samples of mucus from normal or paranormal sources, such as from healthy animals and humans and from patients in whom hypersecretion is not a particular feature. It works easily with samples of 1 to 10 μl, quantities that are readily obtained by bronchoscopy by means of a cytology brush.

Contraindications

The magnetic microrheometer is not ideal with opaque sputum samples, particularly those of high viscoelastic modulus. Since it is inherently a low-amplitude dynamic viscoelastometer, it probably does not give information that relates directly to high-amplitude events, such as cough clearance. On the other hand, since the amplitude of vibration (1–10 μm) and the frequency range are comparable to those of beating cilia, it appears to be an ideal instrument to describe rheological properties that relate to mucociliary clearance (1,5).

Helpful Hints

One of the greatest difficulties encountered in using the magnetic rheometer is in introducing the steel ball into the sample of mucus. This requires both patience and practice. One method is to employ a pick or sharpened wire that can be magnetized temporarily by touching a permanent magnet to it. By pulling the ball into the mucus farther than one wants it to go, holding it, and then releasing the magnet and letting the ball recoil partially, one can generally manipulate the ball into its desired position.

Limitations

Sample Size

In principle, the magnetic rheometer has no sample size limitation. As long as one maintains a reasonable ratio of ball size to sample size, the end/edge effects do not grow disproportionately large as the sample size decreases. In practice, the rheometer works comfortably with sample sizes in the range of 1 to 10 µl in its usual format. It could be readily miniaturized to 100 nl and probably further by simply reducing the size of the ball and the width of the magnet gap. Samples larger than about 10 µl have no particular advantage and are potentially troublesome because of the difficulty in transmitting light through thick layers of mucus. With large samples of mucus, such as with sputum samples, one should normally take smaller aliquots to get around the problem of optical transmission. In this case, one must then consider the sampling problems associated with interaliquot variability.

Sample Rheology

One of the requirements of the magnetic rheometer is that the ball be supported by the medium in a stable position. For weakly crosslinked samples (low G*), this presents a problem, because when the ball is placed in the sample of mucus, it will more or less rapidly fall to the bottom of the sample container, where (a) its image will go out of focus and (b) the displacement amplitude will be too low because of the edge effect. This problem can be remedied by turning the magnetic rheometer on its side and oscillating the ball in the vertical direction. By applying an appropriate bias voltage to the AC coil, one can balance the ball against the force of gravity (14).

Optical Density

The lack of optical clarity of purulent sputum samples, particularly those of high viscoelastic modulus, represents a major limitation to the usefulness of the magnetic rheometer. It is important to limit extraneous sources of light from the rheometer photocells in these cases to maximize the differentiation between ball image and background.

REFERENCES

1. Giordano, A. M., Holsclaw, D., and Litt, M. (1978): Mucus rheology and mucociliary clearance: Normal physiologic state. *Am. Rev. Respir. Dis.*, 118:245–254.
2. Hwang, S. H., Litt, M., and Forsman, W. C. (1969): Rheological properties of mucus. *Rheol. Acta*, 8:438–448.
3. James, S. L., and Marriott, C. (1982): A modified oscillating sphere magnetic microrheometer for use with biological secretions. *J. Phys. [E] Sci. Instr.*, 15:179–180.
4. King, M. (1977): The effect of mucus cross-linking on the clearance of mucus. *Mod. Probl. Paediatr.*, 19:182–189.
5. King, M. (1979): Interrelation between mechanical properties of mucus and mucociliary transport. Effect of pharmacologic interventions. *Biorheology*, 16:57–68.
6. King, M. (1980): Relationship between mucus viscoelasticity and ciliary transport in guaran gel/ frog palate model system. *Biorheology*, 17:249–254.
7. King, M., Brock, G., and Lundell, C. (1985): Clearance of mucus by simulated cough. *J. Appl. Physiol.*, 58:1776–1782.
8. King, M., Cohen, C., and Viires, N. (1979): Influence of vagal tone on rheology and transportability of canine tracheal mucus. *Am. Rev. Respir. Dis.*, 120:1215–1219.
9. King, M., Engel, L. A., and Macklem, P. T. (1979): Effect of pentobarbital anesthesia on rheology and transport of canine tracheal mucus. *J. Appl. Physiol.*, 46:504–509.
10. King, M., and Macklem, P. T. (1977): The rheological properties of microliter quantities of normal mucus. *J. Appl. Physiol.*, 42:797–802.
11. King, M., and Viires, N. (1979): Effect of methacholine chloride on rheology and transport of canine tracheal mucus. *J. Appl. Physiol.*, 47:26–31.
12. Lutz, R. J., Litt, M., and Chakrin, L. W. (1973): Physical-chemical factors in mucus rheology. In: *Rheology of Biological Systems*, edited by H. L. Gabelnick and M. Litt, pp. 119–157. Charles C. Thomas, Springfield IL.
13. Majima, Y., Sakakura, Y., Hirata, K., and Ukai, K. (1986): Viscoelastic measurement of nasal mucus and its clinical application [Abstract]. *Biorheology*, 23:253.
14. Sakakura, Y., Majima, Y., Hirata, K., Takeuchi, K., and Ukai, K. (1986): The significance of rheological properties of middle ear effusions in mucociliary transport [Abstract]. *Biorheology*, 23:254.
15. Shih, C. K., Litt, M., Khan, M. A., and Wolf, D. P. (1977): Effect of nondialyzable solids concentration and viscoelasticity on ciliary transport of tracheal mucus. *Am. Rev. Respir. Dis.*, 115:989–995.

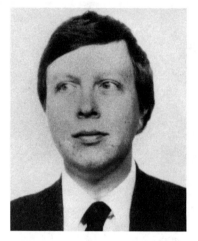

Malcolm King was born in Ohsweken, Ontario, Canada, in 1947. He received the B.Sc. (chemistry) in 1968 from MacMaster University, Hamilton, Canada, and the Ph.D. in 1973 from McGill University Montreal, Canada. He is currently Associate Research Professor in the Department of Medicine, University of Alberta, Edmonton, Canada. His interests are mucus rheology, mucociliary clearance, cough, and two-phase flow.

Methods in Bronchial Mucology,
edited by P. C. Braga and L. Allegra.
Raven Press, Ltd. © 1988.

2.2.3. Mathematical Analysis of Dynamic Measures

*P. C. Braga, **L. Allegra, and †M. King

*Department of Pharmacology, University of Milan, Milan, Italy, **Institute of Respiratory Diseases, University of Milan School of Medicine, Milan, Italy, and †Pulmonary Defense Group, University of Alberta, Edmonton, Canada.*

Mathematical calculation

The forced oscillation technique applied to a concentric cylinder rheometer provides two signal outputs. One output (stress) is from the motor, which drives the oscillating movements of the outer cylinder (cup). The second output (strain) is from the couple-measuring system connected with the inner cylinder (bob), recording the corresponding oscillation, which will depend on the physicochemical properties of the material being studied.

The forced oscillation technique also can be applied to microliter quantities of mucus to investigate its rheological behavior, using an alternating magnetic field acting on a miniature ferromagnetic ball with a specific microrheometer arrangement (1,2).

MATHEMATICAL CALCULATION

The resulting plots for both the magnetic and coaxial cylinder setups record two sine waves (Fig. 1A), one for strain and one for stress. The phase angle and the angular amplitude ratio between the two sine waves can be analyzed to give

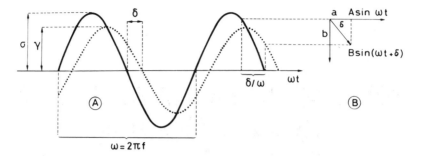

FIG. 1. **A:** Time dependence of the shear stress (σ) and shear (γ) during a low-frequency dynamic test. **B:** Vector treatment of sinusoidal deformation. a and b are the in phase and out of phase components of the output signal with respect to the input waveform.

the various η and G' terms that indicate the values for viscosity or elasticity of the material.

For liquids, the angular amplitude ratio is the ratio of the displacement of the inner cylinder to that of the outer cylinder, and δ is the phase angle by which the inner cylinder lags behind the outer cylinder. A sine or cosine function can be treated as a rotating vector, with one revolution of the vector being equivalent to a full cycle (6).

Typical relations between stress and strain are shown in Fig. 1A. The phase angle δ is given by the law of cosines (4). The harmonic motion from the motor (cup) varies periodically, with a frequency ω (rad/sec) according to the law, represented by A sin ωt. The other harmonic motion from the measuring system (bob) is B sin ($\omega t + \delta$) (Fig. 1B). Two correlation functions are calculated simultaneously, one to calculate the in phase component, a, and the other the out-of-phase component, b. These two components, a and b, in rheological terms can be referred to the elastic and viscous components of the material being tested (7).

A different kind of approach is to feed into the xy axes of an oscilloscope or of an xy-plotter the output signals from an oscillatory test, from cup and bob or from magnet and photocell (magnified by two identical amplifiers). Since there is a phase lag between force and displacement due to the viscoelasticity of the mucus, a so-called Lissajous figure is obtained (Fig. 2).

For a phase-angle difference of $\delta = 0$ degrees, i.e., when the two sinusoids are in phase, a straight line is obtained. With phase differences of 0 degrees $< \delta < 90$ degrees, various shaped elliptical figures appear. With a phase difference of $\delta = 90$ degrees, a circle is produced (3,5). The rheological behavior of bronchial mucus in different pathological conditions or before and after treatment is then characterized by the shape of the ellipse. Since the ellipse is the resultant of the relationship between a component in phase with the shear strain (elasticity) and a component in phase with the shear rate (viscosity), it is possible to quantify this relationship by calculating the phase shift and the amplitude ratio, to obtain η

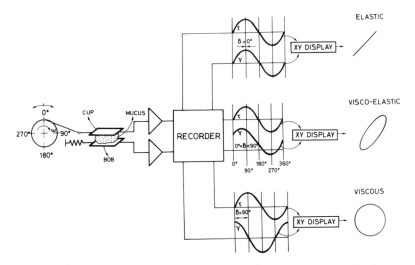

FIG. 2. Lissajous figures from materials with different rheological behavior.

and G'. For an elliptical figure, δ (the phase shift) can be obtained with the equation:

$$\delta = \text{arc cos}\ \frac{a}{b}$$

which gives a and b in mm (Fig. 3A).

Applying the Maxwell relations for viscoelastic fluid, we have:

$$\eta = \frac{1}{\sin \delta} \cdot c \cdot U \qquad (\text{mPa} \cdot \text{s})$$

$$G' = \frac{1}{\cos \delta} \cdot c \cdot U \cdot \omega \quad (\text{mPa})$$

in which c is in mm; $U = \frac{\tau}{D}$; $\omega = 2\pi\upsilon$; υ = frequency of oscillation.

$$\tau = \frac{1 + \left(\dfrac{R_a}{R_i}\right)^2}{2 \cdot \left(\dfrac{R_a}{R_i}\right)^2} \cdot \frac{M_{max}}{2\pi h R_i^2 C_i}$$

where R_a = cup radius; R_i = bob radius; $M_{max} = 6 \cdot 10^{-6}$ Nm; h = bob length; C_i = Din Norms correction parameter.

$$D = \frac{D_0 \cdot \omega_{osc}}{\omega}$$

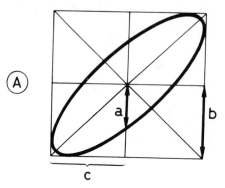

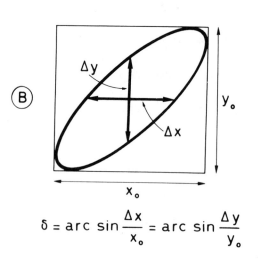

FIG. 3. **A:** Graphic method to obtain δ for coaxial cylinder equipment. **B:** Graphic method to obtain δ for micro-rheometer equipment.

$$\delta = \arc \sin \frac{\Delta x}{x_o} = \arc \sin \frac{\Delta y}{y_o}$$

where:

$$D_0 = \omega \frac{1 + \left(\dfrac{R_a}{R_i}\right)^2}{\left(\dfrac{R_a}{R_i}\right)^2 - 1}$$

where $\omega = 2\pi\upsilon$; $\omega_{osc} = 2\pi\upsilon a$; a = degree of oscillation.

A variation of this method can be applied to the microrheometer data as another graphic solution of the ellipse (Fig. 3B). This relationship for determining δ is analogous to that of coaxial cylinders. The following equations are solved from the specific parameters of the microrheometer:

$$\eta = G^* \frac{\sin \delta}{\omega}$$

$$G^* = \frac{K_1}{K_2} \cdot \frac{r^2}{6\pi} \cdot \frac{x_0}{y_0}$$

$$G' = G^* \cos \delta$$

in which K_1 and K_2 are constants determined by calibration. The solution of these equations is time consuming, but by using a digitizer to introduce the points of the ellipse into a computer programmed to solve these equations, the graphic method is very rapid and results can be obtained in 1 or 2 min.

REFERENCES

1. Denton, R., Hwang, S. H., Litt, M., Forsman, W. C., and Miller, C. E. (1968): Viscoelasticity of mucus. *Am. Rev. Respir. Dis.,* 98:380–389.
2. King, M., and Macklem, P. T. (1977): Rheological properties of microliter quantities of normal mucus. *J. Appl. Physiol.,* 42:797–802.
3. Lammiman, K. A., and Robert, J. E. (1961): Notes on the measurement of visco-elasticity in materials of high viscosity. *Lab. Pract.,* 10:816–824.
4. Markovitz, H., Yavorsky, P. M., Harper, R. C., Zapas, L. J., and De Witt, T. W. (1952): Instrument for measuring dynamic viscosities and rigidities. *Rev. Sci. Instr.,* 23:430–437.
5. Tee, T. T., and Dealy, J. M. (1975): Nonlinear viscoelasticity of polymer melts. *Trans. Soc. Rheol.,* 19:595–615.
6. Van Wazer, J. R., Lyons, J. W., Kim, K. Y., and Colwell, R. E. (1963): *Viscosity and Flow Measurement,* pp. 342–344. Interscience, New York.
7. Watson, J. D. (1969): The measurement of frequency response characteristics applied to oscillatory testing in rheology. *Rheol. Acta,* 8:201–205.

Methods in Bronchial Mucology,
edited by P. C. Braga and L. Allegra.
Raven Press, Ltd. © 1988.

2.3. NONDYNAMIC METHODS IN VISCOELASTICITY ASSESSMENT

2.3.1. Creep Test at Constant Stress

E. Puchelle and J. M. Zahm

INSERM U314, Faculté de Medecine, 51095 Reims, France

In the creep test a constant stress is applied to the sample, and the resultant strain response is recorded against time (creep curve). A typical creep curve for respiratory mucus is shown in Fig. 1 (1).

The strain is divided by the applied stress and is expressed as compliance. We can observe various regions of creep behavior. The compliance J_0 is due to the gel–like network of the mucus (instantaneous elastic response, like a spring).

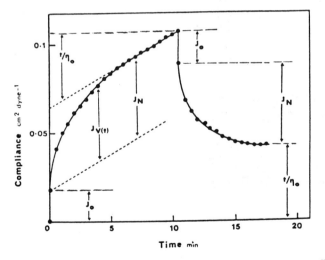

FIG. 1. A creep curve for a typical sputum sample. (J_o) Instantaneous compliance; ($J_{v(t)}$) distance from the lower dotted line to the curve; (J_N) total distance from the lower dotted line line to the curve; (η_o) viscosity at steady state. (From ref. 1.)

91

The compliance J_N is associated with the retarded elastic response of the system (represented by spring and a dashpot in parallel). This curve region can be characterized by a retardation time T_i, which is defined as $J_i \times N_i$, where J_i is the compliance of the spring and N_i is the viscosity of the dashpot. After a definite time, the creep curve becomes linear, and this region is characterized by the viscosity term η_o.

If the stress is removed, both compliances J_o and J_N completely recover. The compliance at a given time t can be represented by the following equation:

$$J(t) = J_o + \Sigma J_i (1 - e^{t/T_i}) + t/\eta_o$$

which corresponds to a Maxwell unit in series with Voigt units.

The creep test can be performed with controlled stress rheometers equipped with either a concentric cylinder geometry or a cone-plate geometry, such as the CS Rheometer (Carri-Med) or the Rotovisko RV 100 (Haake).

REFERENCE

1. Davis, S. S. (1973): In: *Rheology of Bronchial Secretions and Respiratory Functions,* edited by E. Puchelle. pp. 47–90. Masson et Cie, Paris.

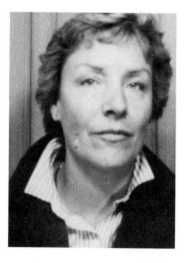

Edith Puchelle was born in 1943 and received the Ph.D. degree in 1976. She is Director of Research of the INSERM Unity 314. Her research interests include mucus rheology and biochemistry, mucociliary transport, and airway epithelial cell culture.

Methods in Bronchial Mucology,
edited by P. C. Braga and L. Allegra.
Raven Press, Ltd. © 1988.

2.3.2. Capillary Type Viscometer

C. S. Kim

*Aerosol Research Laboratory, Harry Pearlman Biomedical Research Institute,
Mount Sinai Medical Center, Miami Beach, Florida 33140*

Methods and Materials
    Theoretical considerations
    Flow through a double capillary
    Capillary viscometer system
    Correction factors
    Experimental procedure
    Materials
Results
Discussion

The viscoelastic properties of respiratory secretions are important determinants of airway mucociliary transport (1,3) as well as clearance of excessive secretions by two-phase flow mechanisms, such as cough (7,8). Therefore, various techniques have been used to assess the viscoelastic properties of airway secretions (2,11). Among them, the capillary type viscometer is of particular interest because of its simplicity in system construction and data interpretation (6,12). Furthermore, the method uses a very small sample volume, which is essential for analyzing respiratory secretions.

METHODS AND MATERIALS

Theoretical Considerations

When a fluid flows through a circular tube, viscosity of the fluid (η) is defined by the equation:

$$\tau_w = \eta\dot{\gamma} \tag{1}$$

where τ_w is the wall shear stress and $\dot{\gamma}$ is the shear rate. Under fully developed laminar flow conditions, viscosity of Newtonian fluids can be expressed according to the Poiseuille equation as:

$$\eta = \pi r^4 \Delta P/8lQ \tag{2}$$

where r is the tube radius, l the length of the tube, ΔP the pressure drop across the length of the tube, and Q the volumetric flow rate. Here, the shear stress (τ_w) and shear rate ($\dot{\gamma}$) are expressed as:

$$\tau_w = r\Delta P/2l \tag{3}$$

$$\dot{\gamma} = 4Q/\pi r^3 \tag{4}$$

and η is a constant independent of shear stress or shear rate and thus can be determined by measuring ΔP and Q in the tube of known dimensions. For non-Newtonian fluids, the law of viscosity is complicated, the shear stress being nonlinear with the shear rate. However, for simplicity, the same functional form as Eq. 1 is usually used, with η replaced by η_a, the apparent viscosity. The η_a is then no longer a constant but a function of shear rate.

For elastic fluids, the shear elastic modulus (G) may be determined according to Philipoff (12) by the equation:

$$G = \tau_w/S_R \tag{5}$$

where S_R is the recoverable shear strain, which is related to the elastically recoiled volume (V) of the fluids as:

$$S_R = 4V/\pi r^3 \tag{6}$$

The shear elastic modulus may thus be obtained by measuring two parameters, the applied pressure to the fluid and the recoiled volume of the fluid after releasing the pressure.

Flow Through a Double Capillary

When a fluid is pulled through a single capillary with a fixed vacuum pressure, the flow does not reach a steady-state condition because the effective tube length increases as the fluid advances through the capillary. This problem, however, can be overcome by pulling the fluid through a small-bore capillary and subsequently into a large-bore capillary connected in series. Since the pressure drop in the tube is inversely proportional to the fourth power of the tube radius, in the double capillary configuration, most of the pressure drop occurs across the small-bore capillary. Therefore, Eq. 2 can be applied to the small-bore capillary along with a small correction for a pressure drop occurring in the large-bore capillary and for other nonuniform flow effects.

Capillary Viscometer System

A double capillary of a particular design consists of a precision bore stainless steel capillary of 0.029 cm in radius and 0.5 cm in length (cut accurately and burr free by manufacturer, Pepper and Sons, Inc., New Hyde Park, NY) and a glass capillary of 0.059 cm in radius and approximately 2.0 cm in length (cut precision 100 μl micropipette; Clay Adams, Parsippany, NJ) (see Appendix). The two capillaries are connected in series using polyethylene microtubing sleeves. In practice, the large-bore glass capillary is also connected to the entrance tip of the small-bore capillary for the purpose of sample holding. Therefore, the capillary assembly in fact consists of three capillaries. The sample-holding capillary retains a sufficient amount of sample to allow uninterrupted flow of the sample into the measuring capillary during the measurement period while also protecting the sample from being exposed to air.

The capillary assembly is connected to a three-way valve via flexible extension tubing. The three-way valve is subsequently connected to a vacuum control unit consisting of a precision vacuum gauge, vacuum regulator, and microvacuum release valve. A microscope, equipped with a micrometer eyepiece with 100 linear divisions, each representing 0.001 cm under a magnification of ×100, is used to observe the movement of the meniscus in the large-bore capillary. A schematic diagram of the system is shown in Fig. 1.

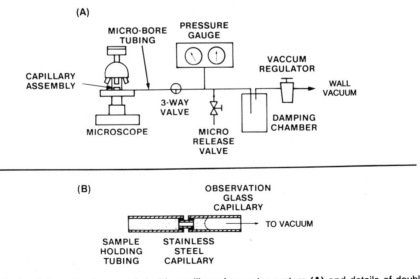

FIG. 1. Schematic diagram of double capillary viscometer system **(A)** and details of double capillary assembly **(B)**.

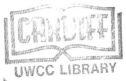

Correction Factors

Because of the serial arrangement of the capillary tubes, the actual pressure drop across the small-bore capillary is lower than the pressure drop across the entire capillary assembly:

$$\Delta P_S = \Delta P_D - \Delta P_L \qquad [7]$$

where the subscripts S, L, and D refer to small, large, and double capillaries, respectively. Assuming that flows in both small- and large-bore capillaries are steady, and equating values based on each of the capillaries, the following relationship will be obtained:

$$\Delta P_L = \Delta P_S (L/l)(r/R)^4 \qquad [8]$$

and subsequently:

$$\Delta P_S = \Delta P_D/(1 + B) \qquad [9]$$

where:

$$B = (L/l)(r/R)^4 \qquad [10]$$

Here, R and L are the radius and the length of the large-bore capillary, and r and l are those of the small-bore capillary. The effect of small pressure drops in the large-bore capillary can thus be minimized by properly choosing the dimensions of the capillaries. In our present capillary system, the pressure loss in the glass capillaries consists of 19% of the total pressure drop as calculated from Eq. 9.

Further corrections may be needed because Eq. 2 for the viscosity calculation is based on a fully developed laminar flow in a circular tube, and this flow condition is not usually met in a short tube, particularly near the entrance and exit of the tube. When a fluid flows into a tube, a certain entrance length is required before the flow becomes fully developed. In laminar flow, the entrance length (Le) for Newtonian fluid can be determined by the equation, $Le = dR_e/20$, where d is the tube diameter and R_e is the Reynolds number (5). For non-Newtonian fluid, Le may be two to three times longer than that of Newtonian fluid (4). This entrance effect, however, is practically negligible in capillary flow because R_e is usually in the range of 10^{-4} to 10^{-3}. The inertia effect, which might occur due to a converging flow at the tube entrance, is also negligible at this low R_e. When a fluid moves out from a small-bore capillary to a large-bore tube, the flow stream lines diverge near the exit of the tube, resulting in a decrease of flow velocity. This has an effect equivalent to increasing the tube length by $\Delta l = \alpha r$, where the value of α has been experimentally determined in the range between 0.57 and 0.82 for Newtonian fluids (11). Since viscoelastic fluids exhibit a characteristic swelling at the exit of the tube (4), this may result in a more pronounced exit effect in viscoelastic fluids. The effect, however, can be minimized by using a tube with a large ratio of l/r. In our system (the ratio $l/r = 17.2$), this may cause a 3 to 5% error in the measured ΔP.

The surface tension may also affect the movement of sample fluid in the capillary. The total surface tension force (F) applied to the fluid is F = πd cos 0, where F is the surface tension and 0 is the contact angle. However, this force is usually in the range of 10^{-2} cm H_2O, which is negligible when compared with the experimental pressure range of 1 to 30 cm H_2O. In our double-capillary system, this effect is eliminated because the meniscus formed in the sample holding tube directly opposes the one in the observation tube.

Adding all of these corrections and expressing them as a single correction factor f, which is to be multiplied by the measured pressure drop, the value of f used in this study was 0.80.

Experimental Procedure

The sample to be measured is drawn slowly into the sample holding tube by using a small syringe (1–5 ml) until the tube is completely filled with the sample fluid. The capillary assembly is then placed on the stage of the microscope so that the exit portion of the stainless steel capillary together with the entrance portion of the observation glass capillary are positioned at focus. The desired negative pressure is applied to the capillary assembly by turning the three-way valve. The sample fluid is then pulled through the small-bore stainless steel capillary and subsequently into the large-bore glass capillary. If the sample fluid emerges into the glass capillary too slowly or too fast, the level of pressure is reset by adjusting a vacuum regulator and a microvacuum release valve so that the fluid moves in a slow and steady motion.

The linear scale of the eyepiece micrometer is aligned on the axis of the glass capillary, and advancing movement of the frontal meniscus is timed over 0.1 mm distance with a precision stopwatch. The timing distance, however, can be changed depending on the speed of fluid movement; a longer distance for a fast movement, and vice versa. After the timing, the negative pressure applied is released by opening the three-way valve and the recoil distance (X) of the sample meniscus is measured along the capillary axis. The same procedure is repeated with different pressures covering a desired range of shear stress and shear rate. With each of the pressure settings, both the timing and recoil measurements are repeated at least three times.

Volumetric flow rate (Q) of the sample fluid during steady movement is determined by dividing the product of the cross-sectional area of the glass capillary and the axial distance of movement by the time elapsed. The shear stress and the shear rate applied to the sample in the small-bore capillary are then calculated by using Eqs. 3 and 4. In using Eq. 3, the measured ΔP is multiplied by an appropriate correction factor, f, which was discussed in the preceding section. Subsequently, the apparent viscosity is determined from Eqs. 1 or 2. In determining the recoiled volume (V), the following equation can be used:

$$V = \pi R^2 kX \qquad [11]$$

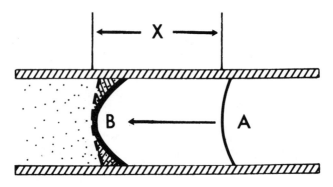

FIG. 2. A schematic diagram showing a difference in meniscus shape before **(A)** and after **(B)** the release of the applied vacuum. The recoiled volume may be overestimated by the amount indicated by the hatched area.

where X is the central distance between the menisci before and after the release of the applied pressure and k is the correction factor compensating the volume difference caused by differences in meniscus shape (Fig. 2). The value of k is usually determined experimentally by comparing photographic pictures of the menisci taken before and after the recoil. Equation 6 can then be reexpressed as:

$$S_R = (4X/r)k(R/r)^2 \qquad [12]$$

In determining the shear elastic modulus (G), Eq. 5 may not be used directly because S_R does not always vary linearly with τ_w. Therefore, G is determined graphically by the initial slope of S_R versus τ_w curves (Fig. 3).

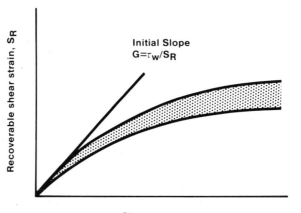

FIG. 3. A graphic method for determining the shear elastic modulus. The stippled area represents a curve pattern of the actual data.

Materials

Many biological and nonbiological fluids have been tested with the double capillary viscometer (1,3,6,7,9,12), including expectorated or suctioned human respiratory mucus, lower airway secretions from human or animal, egg white, polymer solutions including polyisobutylene, polyethylene oxide, and carboxymethyl cellulose, and standard viscosity silicone oils. The standard viscosity oils and polymer solutions of known viscoelastic properties are particularly useful in validating the performance of a viscometer.

RESULTS

Results of viscosity measurement with Newtonian oils are shown in Fig. 4. The measured viscosity values were within ±10% of the standards over a viscosity range of 40 to 3,000 poise (P) at 23°C, which indicates an excellent performance of the capillary viscometer in measuring viscosity. For non-Newtonian polymer solutions, the capillary viscometer correctly responded to the pseudoplasticity of polyethylene oxide solutions by showing a decrease of viscosity with increasing shear rate (Fig. 5). It is noticed that the slope of the curves, which is an indicator of non-Newtonian behavior, is higher with solutions with higher molecular weight. In Fig. 6, it is shown that human sputum has a pseudoplastic nature, and its viscosity ranges from 100 to a few hundred P at a shear rate of 0.5 sec^{-1} at 23°C. A considerable variation in viscosity among samples is also evident. In Fig. 7, the recoverable shear strain of three different viscoelastic samples, including

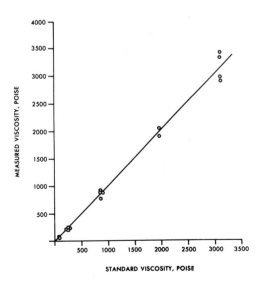

FIG. 4. Viscosity values of standard viscosity oils measured by the double capillary viscometer as compared with standard values.

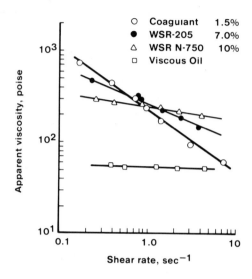

FIG. 5. Apparent viscosity as a function of shear rate for three different polyethylene oxide (Polyox) solutions and a standard viscosity oil. Approximate molecular weight of the Polyox is 3×10^5 for WSR N-750, 6×10^5 for WSR-205, and 5×10^6 for coagulant.

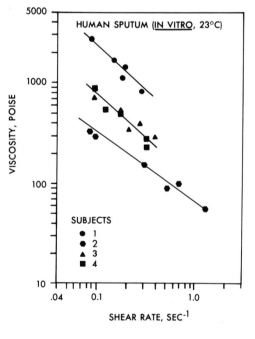

FIG. 6. Apparent viscosity of human sputum as a function of shear rate. Sputum samples were obtained from four patients with chronic bronchitis by using a suction catheter.

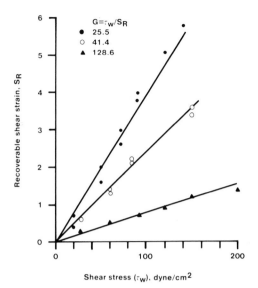

FIG. 7. Shear elastic recoil values of three different samples as a function of shear stress. (○) Human sputum; (●) Polyox coagulant 1% solution in water; (▲) polyisobutylene 3% in decaline.

human sputum, is seen as a linear function of shear stress. The linear relationship, however, may not be warranted if the shear stress is extended to higher values (Fig. 3).

DISCUSSION

Several methods are used currently to examine the rheological properties of respiratory secretions (2,11), and the choice of any particular method may depend on such factors as sample size, cost, accuracy, and type of data obtainable. The cone-and-plate type viscometer offers the convenience of changing shear rates over a wide range. However, the method uses high shear rates that tend to break down the sample structure, thereby altering its rheologic properties (2). The method does not offer elasticity measurement of the sample. The Weissenberg rheogoniometer provides comprehensive rheological data, but the method is complicated and data interpretation is laborious without a computer (2). The double capillary method is a simple method that requires only a small sample volume (~20 μl) (6). It measures both viscosity and elasticity as a function of shear rate. Since the respiratory secretions are often available only in small quantities, the capillary method becomes particularly important in analyzing these types of samples. Furthermore, shear rates utilized in the method (0.01–10 sec^{-1}) are comparable to those expected *in vivo,* and sample destruction, which may occur at a high shear rate, will not occur in this method. The data interpretation is straightforward and based on simple fluid mechanical principles.

The double capillary method, however, has many potential and practical problems, too. Since the dimension of the capillary is very small, the capillary tube tends to become clogged if the sample fluid contains clumps, fibers, or other aggregates. The small sample volume may cause a measurement variation within the same sample, particularly in the case of heterogeneous samples, such as human sputum (3,10,13). In some samples with low viscosity and high water content, vaporization of the sample fluid may occur because of heat generated by the focused light beam during the measurement. This tends to distort the shape of the meniscus of the sample in the observation capillary. A subsequent condensation of the vapor on the wall of the capillary can also change the surface condition of the capillary and result in an inconsistent sample movement. A cold light source in the microscope may be helpful in this case.

Because of the difference in the meniscus shape of samples before and after releasing the applied vacuum, the recoiled volume tends to be overestimated, as illustrated in Fig. 2. The magnitude of the difference varies with the capillary dimensions, the level of applied pressure, and the type of sample fluid. However, the difference is usually negligible at low pressure levels, and even at high pressure levels, errors in the volume estimation remain less than 20% (12). In practice, a unilateral correction factor $k = 0.90$ may be used for convenience in the entire pressure range (1–30 cm H_2O), which is usually encountered in measuring the respiratory sputum (6). The volume measurement error may, therefore, be kept within $\pm 10\%$. For samples with low elasticity (i.e., $G > 500$ dynes/cm^2), an accurate measurement of elasticity is difficult because of a limited reading accuracy of micrometer scale for such a small change in recoil distance.

The major disadvantage of the capillary viscometer is that the shear rate in the capillary tube is not uniform, varying from zero at the tube axis to a maximum at the tube wall. Therefore, the apparent viscosity of non-Newtonian fluids will vary accordingly along the tube radius. The viscosity value determined by using the total flow rate at the applied pressure is thus likely to be weighed in favor of the lowest viscosity existing within the tube cross-section area. The rheological data obtained with the capillary method may, therefore, not be adequate for a theoretical analysis of the sample. However, its simplicity and relative ease in use make the method particularly valuable in assessing changes in rheological properties of bronchial secretions in disease or in relation to pharmacological treatment.

REFERENCES

1. Chen, T. N., and Dulfano, M. J. (1978): Mucus viscoelasticity and mucociliary transport rate. *J. Lab. Clin. Med.*, 91:23–431.
2. Davis, S. S. (1973): Techniques for the measurement of the rheological properties of sputum. *Bull. Eur. Physiopathol. Respir.*, 9:47–90.
3. Dulfano, M. J., and Adler, K. B. (1975): Physical properties of sputum. VII. Rheological properties and mucociliary transport. *Am. Rev. Respir. Dis.*, 112:341–347.

4. Fredrickson, A. G. (1964): *Principles and Application of Rheology,* p. 200. Prentice-Hall, Engle-wood Cliffs, NJ.
5. Kays, W. M. (1966): *Convective Heat and Mass Transfer,* p. 63, McGraw-Hill, New York.
6. Kim, C. S., Berkly, B. B., Abraham, W. M., and Wanner, A. (1982): A micro double capillary method for rheologic measurements of lower airway secretions. *Bull. Eur. Physiopathol. Respir.,* 18:915–927.
7. Kim, C. S., Greene, M. A., Sankaran, S., and Sackner, M. A. (1986): Mucus transport in the airways by two-phase gas-liquid flow mechanism: Continuous flow model. *J. Appl. Physiol.,* 60:908–917.
8. King, M., Brock, G., and Lindell, C. (1985): Clearance of mucus by simulated cough. *J. Appl. Physiol.,* 56:426–430.
9. Leikauf, G. D., Ueki, I. F., and Nadel, J. A. (1984): Autonomic regulation of viscoelasticity of cat tracheal gland secretions. *J. Appl. Physiol.,* 56:426–430.
10. Lutz, R. J., Litt, M., and Charkin, L. (1973): Physical-chemical factors in mucus rheology. In: *Rheology of Biological System,* edited by H. L. Gabelnick and M. Litt, pp. 119–157. Charles C Thomas, Springfield, IL.
11. Oka, S. (1960): Principals of rheometry. In: *Rheology, Vol. 3,* edited by F. R. Eirich, pp. 17–82. Academic Press, New York.
12. Philipoff, W., Han, C. D., Barnett, B., and Dulfano, M. J. (1970): A method for determining the viscoelastic properties of biological fluids. *Biorheology,* 7:55–67.
13. Powell, R. L., Aharonson, E. F., Schwarz, W. H., Proctor, D. F., Adams, G. K., and Reasor, M. (1974): Rheological behavior of normal tracheobronchial mucus of canines. *J. Appl. Physiol.,* 37:447–451.

APPENDIX

Pepper & Sons, Inc., 300 Denton Avenue, New Hyde Park, NY 11040 (Stainless Steel Capillary)

Clay Adams, Parsippany, NJ 07054 (Glass micropipette [Accu-Fill 90, Micropet])

Dwyer Instruments, Inc., Michigan City, IN 46360 (Magnehelic Pressure Gage)

Union Carbide Corp., Specialty Chemicals Division, Danbury, CT 06817 (Polyethylene Oxide [Polyox])

Brookfield Engineering Laboratories, Inc., 240 Cushing Street, Stoughton, MA 02072 (Standard Viscosity Silicone Oils)

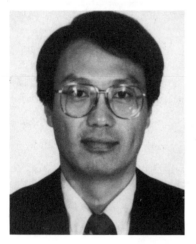

Chong S. Kim was born in Korea in 1945. He received the Ph.D. in mechanical engineering in 1978 from the University of Minnesota, Minneapolis. He is Director of the Aerosol Research Laboratory, Division of Pulmonary Disease, Mount Sinai Medical Center in Miami Beach. Fields of interest are aerosol production, delivery, and deposition, and mucus transport and fluid dynamics in the airways.

Methods in Bronchial Mucology,
edited by P. C. Braga and L. Allegra.
Raven Press, Ltd. © 1988.

2.3.3. Nuclear Magnetic Resonance

E. E. Odeblad

Department of Medical Biophysics, University of Umeå, Umeå, Sweden

---

Basic physics
Elementary theory
Recording nuclear magnetic resonance
Chemical shift and spin–spin coupling
Level populations and relaxation times
Measurable parameters of NMR signals
    Measurement of T_1 and T_2
    Factors influencing T_1 and T_2
    Factors affecting aqueous shift in biological material
Magnetic resonance tomography
Experimental studies on bronchial mucus
    Preliminary studies on bronchial secretion (sputum)
Comments

BASIC PHYSICS

An atomic nucleus is characterized by several fundamental properties, including proton number (charge), neutron number, and nuclear radius. For the understanding and application of nuclear magnetic resonance (NMR), other nuclear properties are, however, more important, notably the nuclear spin, I.h, the nuclear magnetic moment, μ, and sometimes the nuclear electric quadrupole moment, Q.e. (Fig. 1).

The nuclear spin is quantized, so that the spin quantum number, I, can only take integer or half-integer values, i.e., 0, ½, 1, ³⁄₂, and so on. The symbol h denotes the Planck constant, $6.625 \cdot 10^{-34}$ joule sec. Commonly (but not correctly) the nuclear spin quantum number is called "nuclear spin."

Nuclei with spin zero have no magnetic moment. Biologically important nuclei of this kind are ^{12}C, ^{16}O, ^{32}S, ^{40}Ca, and several others. Nuclei with spin ½ have a magnetic moment, e.g., ^{1}H (the proton), ^{13}C, ^{15}N, ^{19}F, ^{31}P, and the radioactive ^{3}H (tritium). Nuclei with spin 1 have, in addition to the magnetic moment, an electric quadrupole moment. This is also the case with nuclei with spin ³⁄₂ or higher. Examples of such nuclei are ^{2}H (deuterium), ^{14}N, ^{17}O, ^{23}Na, ^{39}K, and the two stable chlorine isotopes. A very important effect of a quadrupole moment is that it shortens the time that a nucleus stays in any given orientation in the magnetic field, with a broadening of the magnetic resonance line as a consequence.

The spin can be said to be a spinning or rotation of the nucleus around an axis, the direction of the spin vector. The magnetic moment can be understood if we look at the nucleus as a tiny bar magnet. The electric quadrupole moment can be explained as a nonspherical shape of the nuclear charge, either prolate (cigarlike) or oblate (disk-shaped). Figure 1 gives an illustration of the most important nuclear properties in NMR.

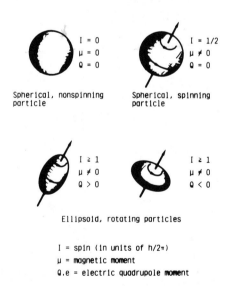

NUCLEAR MOMENTS FOR CHARGED NUCLEI

I = 0 μ = 0 Q = 0	I = 1/2 μ ≠ 0 Q = 0
Spherical, nonspinning particle	Spherical, spinning particle
I ≥ 1 μ ≠ 0 Q > 0	I ≥ 1 μ ≠ 0 Q < 0

Ellipsoid, rotating particles

I = spin (in units of h/2π)
μ = magnetic moment
Q.e = electric quadrupole moment

FIG. 1. Pictorial representation of spin, magnetic moment, and electric quadrupole moment in different kinds of atomic nuclei.

ELEMENTARY THEORY

NMR is based on absorption of radiofrequency energy by nuclear spins in a magnetic field. In such a field (Fig. 2), the nuclear spins cannot be oriented at random but only in fixed directions with respect to the magnetic field vector. Each of these permitted spin orientations has a certain potential energy, and consequently there is an energy difference, ΔE, between two adjacent spin directions. According to Planck's equation, the frequency, f, associated with ΔE is given by:

$$\Delta E = h \cdot f \qquad [1]$$

But the energy difference ΔE is also related to the gross magnetic field, B, the nuclear magnetic moment, μ, and the spin quantum number, I, by the equation:

$$\Delta E = \frac{\mu \cdot B}{I} \qquad [2]$$

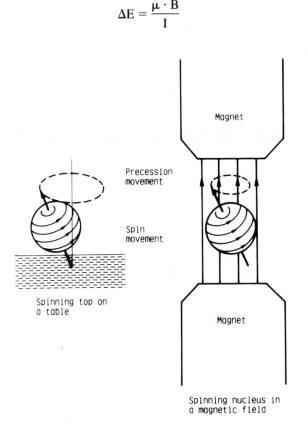

Magnet

Precession
movement

Spin
movement

Spinning top on
a table

Magnet

Spinning nucleus in
a magnetic field

FIG. 2. Analogy between a spinning top on the table in the gravitational field and a spinning nucleus in a magnetic field. Note the difference between the spin movement and the precession movement. In the case of a magnetic nucleus spinning in a magnetic field, the precession corresponds to the NMR frequency or Larmor frequency, given by Eq. 3.

Equalizing these two equations we obtain for the magnetic resonance frequency, f_r (Fig. 2):

$$f_r = \frac{\mu \cdot B}{I \cdot h} \tag{3}$$

This frequency is also called the Larmor frequency or precession frequency.

The number of allowed nuclear orientations is given by the simple formula $2 \cdot I + 1$. Nuclei with spin ½, therefore, have two allowed orientations, spin 1 has three, and spin ³⁄₂ has four allowed orientations in the magnetic field. The two allowed spin orientations for a spin ½ nucleus, e.g., the proton, are shown in Fig. 3.

Recording NMR

A sample containing magnetic nuclei is placed in a magnetic field (Fig. 4). The magnetic field can be varied by allowing current of varying strength to flow in the magnet coils. This magnet current is normally varied only slowly. The sample is surrounded by a smaller coil, the detector coil, and a radiofrequency (RF) current flows in this coil. With pure water as the sample and a radiofrequency of 10 mHz supplied by a stable radiofrequency generator, increasing the magnet current from low to high values allows the magnetic field (B) to increase slowly from nearly zero. When the magnetic field finally passes through 0.23 tesla (B_r), there occurs a transitory absorption of radiofrequency energy in the sample due to flipping of nuclear spins from low-energy to high-energy orientation in the magnetic field. By inserting the sample coil in an electronic bridge and allowing

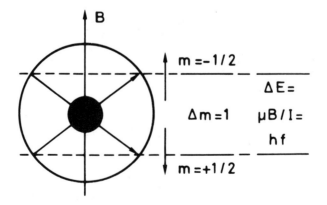

FIG. 3. Two allowed nuclear spin orientations in a magnetic field, B, for a nucleus with spin = ½. The corresponding two magnetic quantum numbers and the corresponding two energy levels are shown. The corresponding difference, Δm, of the quantum number and the energy difference, ΔE, for the energy are also shown. The conditions for the NMR phenomenon to occur are that Δm = 1 and that the ΔE is supplied by the appropriate radiofrequency (see Eq. 1).

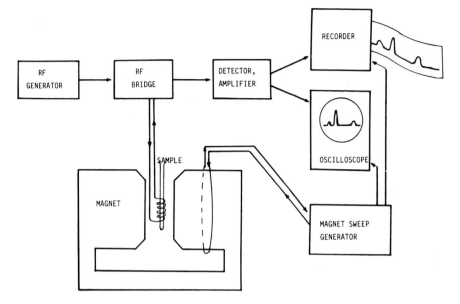

FIG. 4. Basic principle of an NMR experiment.

the bridge output to be recorded on paper, a permanent display of this magnetic resonance signal can be obtained.

Physically, the NMR signal is equivalent to a change in the magnetic susceptibility of the sample. The susceptibility, X, has several components, a diamagnetic, an electron paramagnetic, and a nuclear part, the latter denoted X_n. The susceptibility, in addition, has a real and an imaginary part, and in NMR absorption, the imaginary part, X_n'', changes. The coordinate axis in Fig. 5, showing an NMR signal, is therefore $\Delta X_n''$. The abscissa is magnetic field B. Using Eq. 3, the field can be transformed to a frequency scale (Fig. 5).

Using a sample containing ethanol, disodium phosphate, lithium iodide, and sodium fluoride, all dissolved in heavy water (D_2O), gives the magnetic resonance spectrum, up to about 1.6 tesla magnetic field, shown in Fig. 6 (top). The various signals come out well separated from each other in the spectrum. Study of the region around the ^1H (proton) signal in successively increasing magnification and resolution reveals a broad, somewhat asymmetrical NMR signal. Adjusting the homogeneity of the magnetic field provides a new kind of information, in that the signal is divided into three partial signals. We have recorded the chemical shift (Fig. 6).

CHEMICAL SHIFT AND SPIN–SPIN COUPLING

A closer study of the proton spectrum reveals that three signals mainly derive from the three types of protons in the ethanol molecule, the hydroxyl, the methylene,

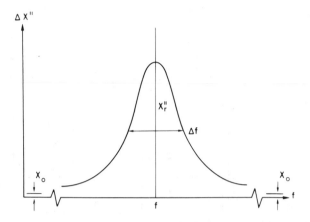

FIG. 5. The essential features of a magnetic resonance line. The ordinate is the change in sample magnetic susceptibility. The abscissa is a frequency scale, which could easily be transformed to a magnetic field scale, using Eq. 3.

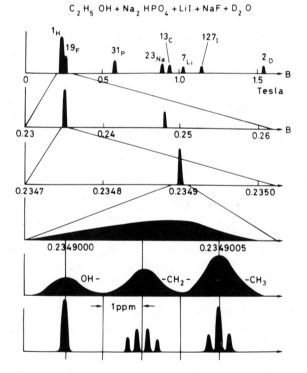

FIG. 6. The complete NMR spectrum at 10 mHz for a sample containing ethanol, disodium phosphate, lithium iodide, sodium fluoride, and heavy water. The proton resonance region is successively magnified until the chemical shift and the spin–spin coupling become visible.

and the methyl groups. Expressed in a relative scale, in parts per million (ppm), their separation is rather small. The OH and CH_3 peaks are only about 4.5 ppm from each other.

The chemical shift depends on different electron densities around the nuclei in different chemical bondings. The methyl protons are more shielded than the hydroxyl protons; therefore, we have to impose a slightly higher magnetic field to overcome this shielding and get the resonance. On an absolute shielding scale, the hydroxyl protons are shielded to about 26 ppm and the methyl protons to about 30.5 ppm. The difference of 4.5 ppm is visible in the spectrum.

If the resolution is increased still more, e.g., by spinning or rotating the sample with an air turbine, a new effect is seen, the spin–spin coupling. The methyl signal is split into three with the proportions $1:2:1$ because of the various combinations of spin orientations in the adjacent methylene group.

Level Populations and Relaxation Times

It was stated earlier that the proton can be present in one of two possible orientations in a magnetic field and also that each direction is associated with a certain energy, i.e., it corresponds to an energy level. Accordingly, in a magnetic field, the proton is present in one of the two possible energy levels. Also, the NMR signal originates from transitions from the low-energy level to the high-energy magnetic level, often denoted the m $= -\frac{1}{2}$ and m $= +\frac{1}{2}$ level, respectively (m = magnetic quantum).

The largest NMR signal would be obtained if originally all protons occupied the lower level. However, this is far from the reality. The difference in number (population) between the levels is very small and depends on the motion, which has average energy k_T (k is the Boltzman constant, and T is temperature in degrees Kelvin). The magnetic level energy is of the order of μH, a much smaller quantity than k_T. Therefore, the excess nuclei in the lower level are only of the order or $2\mu B/k_T$. In the example given of proton resonance at 10 mHz, i.e., 0.23 tesla, the difference in level population is only about 1.6 of 1 million nuclei. At 200 mHz, the difference is 20 times larger, 32 of 1 million nuclei. This in itself makes the NMR signal much larger at higher magnetic fields.

If a sample is suddenly inserted into a magnetic field, it takes some time for this level difference (and NMR signal) to reach its final magnitude. The time constant for this process is T_1, or spin–lattice relaxation time, because it depends on how rapidly the nuclei exchange their magnetic energy with the surroundings. Within the total assembly of nuclear moments, any two nuclei can also mutually exchange their spin directions and magnetic energy. The time constant for this process is T_2, or spin–spin relaxation time. Other names are longitudinal relaxation time for T_1 and transversal relaxation time for T_2.

MEASURABLE PARAMETERS OF NMR SIGNALS

Any arbitrary NMR signal can be characterized by several parameters:

1. The frequency, f_r, at which the center of the signal is located. Using Eq. 3, f_r can be equivalently expressed as the resonance field, B_r.

2. The amplitude or the maximum amplitude of the signal. This can, of course, be given in microvolts or some other electronic measure, but the most original parameter is a change in the radiofrequency susceptibility (imaginary part, or $\Delta X''$).

3. Signal area $\int \Delta X''$ df. This is proportional to the number of nuclei taking part in the resonance process and is often proportional to the number of corresponding nuclei in the sample or the amount of substance in the sample.

4. The signal width, Δf (Fig. 5). Theoretically, the signal shape should be a Lorentz curve (can usually be verified experimentally). The inverse parameter or, more correctly, $1/\pi\Delta f$ (if Δf is the line width av half-maximum height) is a measure of the lifetime of a nuclear spin orientation. This depends on both T_1 and T_2 and is approximately given by:

$$f = \frac{1}{T_1} + \frac{1}{T_2} \qquad [4]$$

In liquids, T_1 and T_2 are often of approximately the same magnitude (Fig. 7). In biological samples, T_2 is often shorter than T_1 (Fig. 7), and this is especially the case in solid matter, in which, therefore, T_2 governs the line width.

5. Accordingly, T_1 is one important parameter of the NMR line.

6. T_2 is also an important property of the signal.

Measurement of T_1 and T_2

T_1 can be determined by killing the signal by a strong RF pulse (saturation pulse, S, Fig. 8) and measuring the growth or return of the ordinary signal by a series of test signals (T, Fig. 8). More elaborate signal sequences have been developed for measuring T_1 and T_2. The reader is referred to the standard literature for details. Sometimes, two or more components of T_1 and T_2 can be observed in the regrowth sequence (Fig. 9).

Factors Influencing T_1 and T_2

Both T_1 and T_2 are very sensitive to the relative movements of the nuclei in relation to the surrounding molecules and atoms. This is due to the presence of near-resonance and near-zero components in the motion spectra of the surrounding molecules. Figure 10 provides a tentative explanation. The motion spectra for

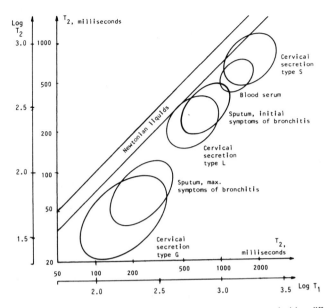

FIG. 7. The T_1–T_2 diagram for representing the various areas occupied by different types of samples. The values for the three cervical mucus types are from ref. 8, the value for blood serum are from the author's unpublished work, and the values for the two sputum types are from the present work. All data are normalized to 60 mHz NMR frequency.

small, medium-sized, and large molecules are schematically shown, and the spectral intensities at near-resonance and near-zero frequencies are given. The correlation time is also indicated for the small molecule species, and it is easily understood that the correlation time is longer for the medium-sized and much shorter for the very large molecules. Because liquids with large molecules usually are more viscous,

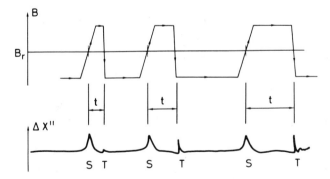

FIG. 8. The saturation pulse (S) method for measuring the spin–lattice relaxation time T_1. Successive saturation pulses with a series of corresponding test pulses (T) are given, and the test signal amplitude is analyzed as a function of time t between S and T. An example is shown in Fig. 9.

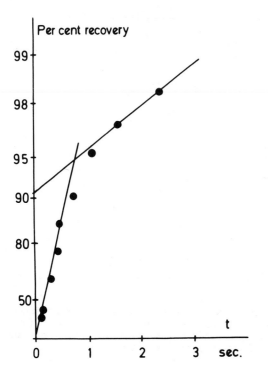

FIG. 9. Increase of test pulse (T) amplitude on a logarithmic scale for analyzing the relaxation time. In this case, two components with T_1 (approximately) 0.2 sec and 1.4 sec were obtained.

T_1 and T_2 become shorter with increasing viscosity. Note that in Fig. 10, the inverse of T_1 and T_2, i.e., the corresponding relaxation rates R_1 and R_2 are also given.

However, the resonance frequency influences the magnitudes in a complicated fashion, especially that of T_1 but also that of T_2 (Fig. 11).

Factors Affecting Aqueous Shift in Biological Material

The degree of hydrogen bonding of water in biological tissues is influenced by the ions and organic substance present. Hydrogen bonding removes part of the electron cloud surrounding the proton taking part in this bond. Therefore, increased hydrogen bonding displaces the water line (aqueous line) toward a lower magnetic field. Normally, about 50% of the water molecules take part in hydrogen bonding, but this figure can increase or decrease several percent in biological material. Decrease in the percentage of hydrogen bonding displaces the aqueous proton line toward a higher magnetic field. The effects are within 0.1 to 0.2 ppm, and very sensitive techniques have been developed in our laboratory to measure these small shifts. The sample is inserted in an outer tube containing a suitable standard (Figs. 12 and 13). This standard should have two distinct NMR lines, one on each side of the sample and with precisely known chemical shift.

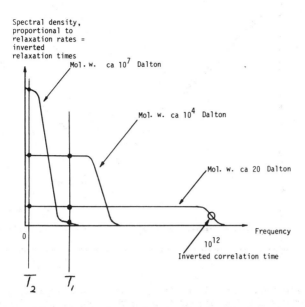

FIG. 10. Diagram of the approximate spectral density of molecular movements for small, medium-sized, and large molecules in a biological sample. The frequencies corresponding to T_1 and T_2 are approximately indicated. This pictorial representation explains crudely the behavior of T_1 and T_2 for molecules of various sizes. The correlation time is indicated for the small molecule spectrum curve and is the inverse frequency at the middle of the declining spectral region.

MAGNETIC RESONANCE TOMOGRAPHY

In NMR tomography [magnetic resonance tomography (MRT) or magnetic resonance imaging (MRI)], NMR signals are picked up from living tissue in such a way that they can be localized. A typical method for obtaining an MRT picture is illustrated in Fig. 14. The gross magnetic field is not homogeneous but has a gradient. Somewhere in this gradient, the field has the resonance value B_r, as given by Eq. 3, at the frequency used. NMR phenomena are now proceeding in a tissue slice located at the field B_r. This slice can be excited by a strong RF pulse, such as the S pulse of Fig. 8. With the aid of auxiliary coils (not shown in Fig. 14) the slice can be tilted, e.g., 90 degrees. The resonance signals now picked up by the RF coils come only from a tissue pillar in the intersection between the original and the tilted slices. By adjusting the magnet current in the auxiliary coils, various tissue pillars can be examined. Feeding the signals into a computer provides a pictorial representation showing the distribution of the NMR activity.

MRT can be designed either to depict the density distribution of the nucleus studied (usually protons) or to give a picture of the T_1 or T_2 distribution over the slice. This can be attained by appropriate RF pulse sequences and computer programs. Usually, the proton density pictures give very sparse information, but T_1

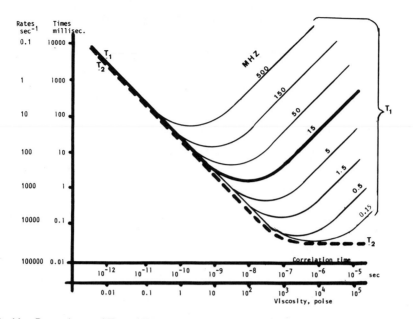

FIG. 11. Dependence of T_1 and T_2 on correlation time and viscosity of aqueous solutions is shown. The corresponding viscosity values are given on the abscissa. The inverse of the time, i.e., the relaxation rates are shown on the ordinate scale. Note that T_1 is dependent on the NMR resonance frequency (and therefore depends on the strength of the magnetic field). The data refer to proton resonances.

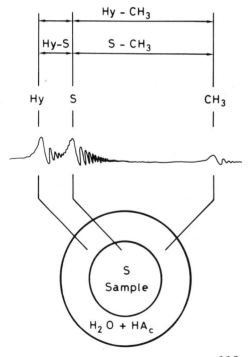

FIG. 12. Principle for determination of the precision shift of the aqueous line in biological material. The sample is in the inner tube. A calibration substance is in the outer tube. See Fig. 13 for further explanation.

116

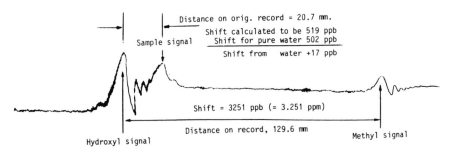

FIG. 13. Example of precision measurement of aqueous signal shift in a sputum sample (Sample signal). The calibration substance is a precisely made solution of acetic acid (40.00 ml) and distilled water (60.00 ml), contained in the outer tube. An important feature of this choice of calibration substance is that the determination of shift is rather insensitive to temperature variations in the region 18 to 38°C.

records often give very high-contrast pictures that are useful for diagnosis of tumors and inflammations.

MRT can also be modified to measure bloodstream velocity and, to some extent, chemical shifts. Since an MRT picture usually requires 5 to 30 min of time, moving organs, such as heart and lungs, can be studied in a meaningful way only by gating the information by electrocardiogram or respiratory movements to reduce the effective time of the NMR imaging.

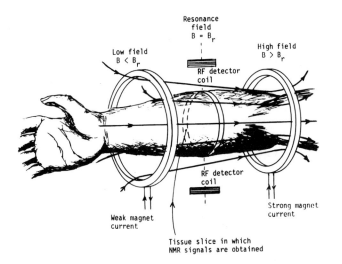

FIG. 14. Method of MRT or MRI. The part of the body to be examined is inserted into a magnetic field, which can be adjusted in various ways. The drawing shows how a field gradient is applied so that only a narrow tissue slice responds to the NMR frequency. After application of an RF pulse of type S (Fig. 8), several test pulses are used after the field gradient has been adjusted so that only small parts of the slice respond. The test pulses (corresponding to T of Fig. 8) are fed into a computer, which reconstructs a picture (tomogram or image) of the slice.

EXPERIMENTAL STUDIES ON BRONCHIAL MUCUS

For NMR purposes, the structure and components of mucus can be described as follows (Fig. 15).

The solvent is water, which always comprises the main part (85–98% w/w) of the mucus. In water, about one half of the molecules are free, and one half are part of hydrogen-bonded and very short-lived units of type $(H_2O)_n$, with $n = 2$, 3, with occasionally higher values.

Solutes of different types include (a) such ions as Na^+, Cl^-, K^+, and others,

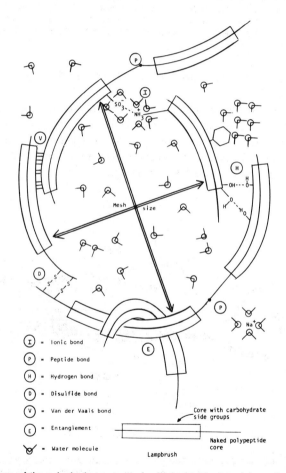

FIG. 15. Diagram of the principal structure of a biological hydrogel (e.g., bronchial mucus). Mucin units (or subunits) occur, each being a polypeptide chain with side groups of a carbohydrate nature, so that a lampbrushlike structure results. These units interact to form a network. The meshes of this network contain water and solutes, as described in text. Note that the viscosity of the liquid phase gives the most important contribution to T_1 and T_2. The mechanical properties of the network phase have yet to be investigated with other methods.

which are surrounded by hydration shells that break down part of the hydrogen bonds of water, (b) nonionic small molecules, such as glucose, that are surrounded by hydrogen-bonded hydration shells and, therefore, increase the net degree of hydrogen bonding in water, (c) small molecules, such as amino acids and oligopeptides that have a rather small effect on the net hydrogen bonding in water, and (d) soluble macromolecules, such as proteins and RNA, that hydrate water by more or less different mechanisms.

The gelforming substances or mucin usually consist of a protein or polypeptide core with different carbohydrate side groups, arranged in a lampbrush fashion. Part of the polypeptide core is naked and can form peptide or disulfide bonds with other lampbrushes (Fig. 15). The carbohydrate-like side groups can also form ionic, van der Vaals, or hydrogen bonds with other lampbrushes. In this way, meshes are formed in the mucus. The lampbrushes can also entangle. All these factors contribute to the three-dimensional network of mucin in mucus. Ionic bonds can partially break down water structure, and some carbohydrate groups can partially increase the normal water hydrogen-bonded structure (as indicated in Fig. 15).

In spite of the great potential value of NMR in studying mucus secretions, the number of studies on bronchial mucus are few. On the basis of our experience in studying the cyclic variations and molecular structure of cervical mucus, it was proposed in 1974 that studies should be performed in a similar way with bronchial secretions (5). A study was conducted on the effect of mucolytics on sputum viscosity in chronic asthma (3). The results from NMR were, however, essentially noninformative, since no differences in the control group were obtained. On the basis of extended studies on the cervical mucus, a new plea for the use of NMR in mucology was made in 1980 (4), and a section on NMR was included in a lecture on biophysical properties of biological fluids (9). High-resolution ^{13}C-NMR spectra of mucus, notably dog tracheal mucus, also have been reported (1), and high-resolution proton spectra of the three cervical mucus types have been published (7).

The various possibilities for NMR studies on bronchial secretion are:

1. Studies on the aqueous proton signal in bronchial mucus *in vitro*
   a. Precision shift
   b. T_1 (spin–lattice relaxation time)
   c. T_2 (spin–spin relaxation time)
2. Studies on the high-resolution spectra (^{1}H, ^{13}C, and ^{17}O) of the mucin in bronchial mucus
3. *In vivo* studies with NMR tomography. This presents obvious difficulties because of the very thin film of mucus normally covering the respiratory airway and because of the respiratory movements. It is hoped that in the future these difficulties will be overcome.

In the following section, preliminary studies relating to points 1a, b, and c are reported.

Preliminary Studies on Bronchial Secretion (Sputum)

For measurements on precision shift and T_1 on sputum in acute bronchitis, sputa were collected during various phases in five cases of acute bronchitis. Sputum was immediately separated mechanically from saliva and inserted into a small glass tube (0.5 mm inner diameter). The tube was inserted into an outer tube of 1.4 mm inner diameter containing a mixture of acetic acid and distilled water (40 ml analytic grade acetic acid and 60 ml distilled water). This system is shown in principle in Fig. 12 and in detail in Fig. 13. The separation of the calibration signals was carefully measured by an interference method to be separated by 3.251 ppm (=3,251 ppb). If the tubes are of the same dimensions as used in this study, the water signal is 502 ppb to the right of the hydroxyl peak (Fig. 13). The shift of the sample aqueous peak could be measured from pure water with an accuracy of ±3 ppb (SE). The bridge and the magnet used are shown in Fig. 16. For measurement of T_1 the sample tube was removed, wound with a thin (0.15 mm) copper wire (Fig. 17), and measured with a pulse method (saturation recovery). The error in T_1 was about 8%. The sample was subjected to Raman spectroscopy for measurement of bound water in mucus (6). The results (Table 1) indicated that the amount of free water in sputum decreased up to the time of maximum symptoms (coughing and expectoration of a viscid mucus) and then slowly returned to normal.

These results stimulated continued work, and new studies were undertaken to measure T_1 and the amount of mucin (using Rayleigh scattering). The results

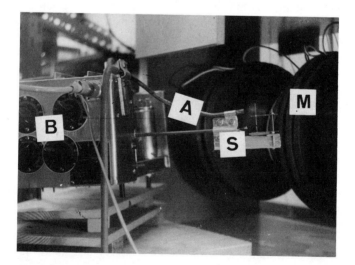

FIG. 16. Central parts of the NMR spectrometer for measuring small quantities of mucus. The sample is just ready to be introduced into the magnetic field. (M) Magnet; (S) sample holder with 1.8 mm outer diameter glass tube with sample and calibration substance; (A) air tube for the air turbine to spin the sample; (B) bridge unit.

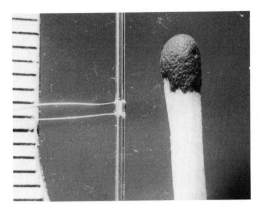

FIG. 17. Sample tube (0.5 mm inside diameter, 0.7 mm outside diameter) with an RF coil wound around it with 0.15 mm copper wire. The sample is ready for measurement of T_1 and T_2. A millimeter scale (left) and a match serve to show the dimensions of the sample. The smallest samples investigated weighed about 1 mg.

from one series of measurements three times a week on sputum from one subject are shown in Fig. 18. T_1 (presented as $R_1 = 1/T_1$) showed a similar course but did not parallel the mucin content, which had its maximum before the T_1 minimum.

In a third series, sputum was collected and separated and subjected to T_1 and T_2 measurements in the initial phase and the maximum symptom phase in 10 cases of acute bronchitis. The results are shown in Table 2, in which T_1 and T_2 are expressed in milliseconds, and their 10 logarithms were taken. The values are given for the corresponding encircled areas in Fig. 7.

COMMENTS

The application of different NMR techniques to bronchial secretion may help to characterize some of its biophysical and biochemical properties. However, NMR preferably would be used in conjunction with other methods. Since NMR methods

TABLE 1. *Comparison of results of Raman spectroscopy and NMR on sputum in cases of acute bronchitis*

Case identification	Day of disease	Proportion bound to free water from Raman spectra	$1/T_1$ for protons (sec^{-1})	Shift, ppb from H_2O
B.S.	4	6.5	0.6	+ 4
A.A.	6	19	1.4	+11
B.S.	9	26	3.7	+32
K.H.	15	71	5.5	+46
K.H.	22	35	2.7	+35
S.L.	25	14	2.2	+19
K.S.	34	9.7	1.8	+17

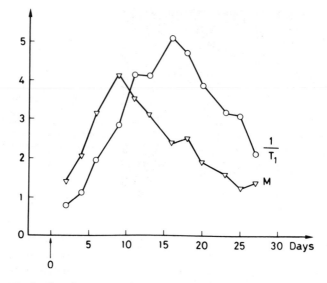

FIG. 18. Diagram showing the course of acute bronchitis as visualized by the amount of mucus in percent (w/w) ($\triangle$) and the nuclear magnetic relaxation rate, $R_1 = 1/T_1$) in sec^{-1} ($\bigcirc$). Day 0, indicated by an arrow, is the beginning of symptoms of bronchitis. Maximum period or symptoms (cough, expectoration, feeling sick and tired) occurred during days 11 to 16. The mucus contents, determined by Rayleigh scattering, reached a maximum on day 9, and the relaxation rate, probably reflecting the percentage of water hydrated on mucus, had its maximum on day 16.

are essentially nondestructive, after finishing an NMR analysis, the sample could easily be subjected to other studies.

Of particular interest would be to use the NMR imaging techniques in various conditions of abnormal bronchial secretion. This will, however, probably require refinements of the present day *in vivo* techniques. It is essential for the investigator to understand fully the physical and biological basis of NMR to maximize use of

TABLE 2. *Measurements of* T_1 *and* T_2 *in the initial phase and the time of maximum symptoms in 10 instances of acute bronchitis; proton resonance on fresh, separated sputum samples*

Phase of the disease	Log T_1			Log T_2		
	Mean[a]	±SD	±SE	Mean	±SD	±SE
Initial phase	2.91	0.22	0.07	2.48	0.23	0.08
Maximum symptoms	2.35	0.27	0.09	1.84	0.29	0.10
Difference	0.56		0.12	0.64		0.13
Significance	$p < 0.001$			$p < 0.001$		

[a] Values given as logarithms of relaxation times in milliseconds.

the method and draw the correct conclusions. The reader is referred to standard textbooks on this subject (2).

REFERENCES

1. Barrett-Bee, K., Bedford, G., and Loftus, P. (1982): The use of high-resolution carbon-13 NMR in the study of mucus. *Adv. Exp. Med. Biol.,* 144:109–111.
2. Beall, P. T., Amtey, S. R., and Kasturi, S. R. (1984): *NMR Data Handbook for Bio-Medical Applications.* Pergamon Press, Elmsford, NY.
3. Heilborn, H., Pegelow, K. O., and Odeblad, E. (1976): Effect of bromhexine and guaiphenesine on clinical state, ventilatory capacity and sputum viscosity in chronic asthma. *Scand. J. Respir. Dis.,* 37:88–96.
4. Löfdahl, C.-G., and Odeblad, E. (1980): Biophysical variables relating to viscoelastic properties of mucus secretions, with special reference to NMR methods for viscosity measurement. *Eur. J. Respir. Dis. (Suppl.),* 110:113–127.
5. Odeblad, E. (1974): Measurement of sputum viscosity with the NMR method. *Scand. J. Respir. Dis. (Suppl.),* 90:37–40.
6. Odeblad, E. (Aug. 16, 1982): Preliminary Investigations on bronchial secretions with the aid of Raman spectroscopy. Seminar given at UCSF Medical Center, San Francisco.
7. Odeblad, E., et al. (1983): The biophysical properties of the cervical–vaginal secretions. *Int. Rev. Natl. Fam. Planning,* 7:1–56.
8. Odeblad, E., Ingelman-Sundberg, A., Åsberg, K., Höglund, A., and Strandberg-Bergström, L. (1984): Proton magnetic relaxation times T_1 and T_2 for normal types of cervical secretions. *Acta Obstet. Gynecol. Scand.,* 63:667–668.
9. Odeblad, E., Strandberg-Bergström, L., and Åsberg, K. (1987): *Biophysical Properties of Biological Fluids. Middle Ear Research with Special Reference to Connective Tissue and Middle Ear Effusion,* pp. 59–77. University of Umeå Printing Press.

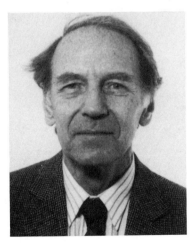

Erik Emanuel Odeblad was born in Kristinehamn, Sweden, in 1922. He received the M.D. degree in 1952 in Stockholm, Sweden, and the Ph.D. in 1966 in Uppsala, Sweden. He is Professor of Medical Biophysics, University of Umeå, Sweden. Fields of interest include biophysics, NMR, fertility, and family planning.

Methods in Bronchial Mucology,
edited by P. C. Braga and L. Allegra.
Raven Press, Ltd. © 1988.

2.3.4. Two-Phase Gas–Liquid Flow

S. W. Clarke

*Department of Thoracic Medicine, The Royal Free Hospital,
London, United Kingdom*

Two-phase gas–liquid flow is commonplace in engineering processes, occurring in boiler tubes, distillation columns, plastic processing and chemical reactors (9). More recently, its relevance to flow in the human tracheobronchial tree has been recognized (2,3,5–7). However, most forms of two-phase flow are so complex that work done in the field has been empirical and esoteric.

The normal human bronchial tree is lined by a thin (about 5 μm) layer of liquid, which in endobronchial disease, such as chronic bronchitis, may be considerably increased (up to 10 μm) and changed in viscosity and elasticity (12). The effects of this liquid layer have hitherto been investigated relatively little. However, the situation lends itself to two-phase gas–liquid flow, and this has become a topic of increasing interest. Previously, it was assumed that bronchial secretions would increase airflow resistance only in proportion to the degree of airway narrowing produced, but this hypothesis is no longer tenable.

Visual studies of two-phase flow in glass tubes have shown that several different patterns of flow may occur (Fig. 1). At low gas flow rates, bubbles of gas may be dispersed in the liquid (bubble flow). As the gas flow rate is increased, the bubbles become larger and fill most of the tube cross-section. These gas slugs alternate with volumes of liquid and are displaced toward the top of the tube during horizontal tube flow (slug flow). As the gas flow rate is increased further, these slugs emerge randomly until in the horizontal tube the liquid may occupy the lower part of the tube with a fairly smooth surface—stratified flow—which gives way to marked surface roll waves termed ''wavy flow'' at even faster flow rates. At the highest gas flow rates, the liquid is dispersed into a film surrounding the lumen of the tube, the surface of which is covered by a dense array of small waves that may cause the surface to appear smoother than it really is, since there is extreme agitation of the liquid. This is annular flow. The difference between the gas and liquid velocities becomes great and the liquid hold up much higher than would be expected on the basis of the relative flow rates (9).

In such circumstances, the presence of the liquid phase influences the pressure drop in the gas stream greatly. This is particularly so with wave formation that results in a marked increase in pressure drop in the gas phase. This high pressure loss probably results both from energy losses in the liquid due to gas–liquid interaction and from energy losses in the gas due to liquid surface roughness, as a consequence of surface interaction. It has been suggested that viscous energy loss in the liquid must be the main cause of the pressure drop. For extreme levels of gas flow, the liquid waves are entrained and blown through the tube in the form of droplets—mist flow. The liquid viscosity and shear elasticity will modify the flow pattern and pressure gradient. Elastic forces in the liquid may tend to inhibit wave formation and reduce energy loss in the liquid.

Much of the earlier work on two-phase flow dealt with liquids of relatively

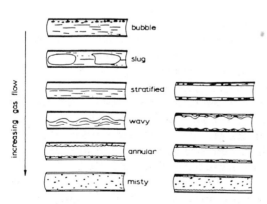

FIG. 1. Diagrammatic representation of the effect of increasing gas flow through liquid-filled tubes (left) and liquid-lined tubes (right).

FLOW PATTERNS IN TWO PHASE GAS-LIQUID FLOW

low viscosity, whereas sputum often has much higher apparent viscosity coupled with marked elasticity and a nonhomogeneous structure (2).

METHODS AND MATERIALS

Model Tubes

The majority of studies that are directly relevant to medicine and, in particular, to flow in the human lung have been performed using smooth glass (or Plexiglas) tubes of dimensions similar to those in the human tracheobronchial tree. Glass was chosen principally because it is transparent and allows visual appraisal of gas–liquid flow interaction, it is smooth, thus causing no boundary layer problems, and it is both easy and cheap to make. Where a lateral pressure drop is to be measured, a simple porthole is easily inserted. The adult human trachea and main bronchi have been simulated with tubes of 1.7 cm internal diameters (id) and 12.0 cm length (l) for the trachea, id 1.2 cm and l 4.8 cm for the mainstem bronchi, and i.d. 0.8 cm and l 1.9 cm for the second bronchial division—dimensions all taken from or similar to Weibel's model (13).

Most studies have been performed with the tubes positioned horizontally. This enabled the liquid to be instilled into the tube without runing out under the influence of gravity, although it would tend to pool along the lower wall depending on its viscoelasticity and layer thickness. In other studies, the tube models were positioned vertically, either with a static fluid layer or with a continual feed liquid flow mechanism at the bottom, with the layer carried upward by continuous upward airflow (6). This latter way is a novel simulation of the conditions within the tracheobronchial tree in upright humans.

Flow

There are several means of generating airflow. An electric fan motor connected to a smoothing chamber leading to an inflow tube at least 50 diameters in length is used to create laminar flow conditions at low flow rates. Alternatively, a compressed air supply with a suitable smoothing arrangement can be used with a modified Harvard pump for phasic flow, which may be required to simulate respiration (7). Any pressure drop can be measured with sensitive transducers, and the airflow can be measured with a Fleisch pneumotachograph or other suitable device. It may be convenient to plot pressure versus flow on an X-Y plotter. These curves may be recorded with each tube dry and then repeated with the tube lined by a liquid film of known thickness (e.g., 0.5, 1.0, and 2.0 mm) and viscoelasticity, distributed in an annular fashion (2). Rudimentary rigid branching tubes lined with sputum also have been used (2,4).

Cough

Mucus transport by cough has been simulated by blowing Newtonian* and non-Newtonian liquids out of a straight tube by a turbulent gas flow from a rigid 10 liter tank pressurized by either nitrogen or helium to levels necessary to obtain air velocities around 10^4 cm sec^{-1}. The straight tube containing the liquid was connected at one end to the pressurized tank and at the other end to a solenoid valve that could be opened rapidly ($\approx$0.05 sec) to initiate flow. Slugs of Newtonian (glycerine/water) or non-Newtonian pseudoplastic fluid (guaran gel) were used and were blown out of the tube by the turbulent stream of gas (10,11).

Mucus and Mucus–like Liquids

Human bronchial mucus (which may be difficult to gather in the fresh state), as well as sputum, has been used in the test models. A wide variety of other test liquids of varying viscosities and elasticities have been used. These have the advantage of being more readily available and having more uniform and simple properties than mucus or sputum. They include Newtonian liquids, such as glycerol in water and oils, and non-Newtonian liquids, such as sodium carboxymethylcellulose (SCMC), a viscous liquid, polymethoxide (Polyox), a viscoelastic liquid, and others, such as guaran gel, hog gastric mucin, or locust bean gum crosslinked with $Na_2/B_4/O_7$ (7).

Viscoelasticity

In early studies, the flow properties of non-Newtonian solutions were determined in a tube viscometer. These fluids were mainly of a pseudoplastic type, and their flow properties could be represented by logarithmic graphs of shear stress against shear rate.

The falling sphere method involves allowing steel spheres of different sizes to fall separately through the liquid in a cylindrical container of known diameter. The rate of fall is obtained by timing the passage of the sphere between fixed marks on the container. With a high diameter ratio between the steel sphere and liquid container, there is relatively little disturbance of the liquid during passage

---

* A Newtonian liquid is one in which the relationship between shear stress and strain is linear, whereas a non-Newtonian liquid exhibits nonlinear characteristics (i.e., viscosity decreasing with increasing shear rate).

of the sphere, and the effect of thixotropy is minimal. The Ladenburg wall correction factor can be applied (2).

The syringe method first applied to sputum in 1953 uses a conventional 20-ml glass syringe in which the nozzle is sealed and the end of the hollow plunger is removed and replaced by a brass plate of 2 cm diameter and 1 cm thickness through which are drilled 12 holes of 0.1 cm diameter. The syringe is mounted vertically, and different weights are placed on top of the plunger through which a hole is made for air release. The liquid sample is poured into the sealed barrel of the syringe, the plunger is depressed until liquid flows through the 12 holes in the plate, a known weight is placed on the plunger, and the rate of descent is measured. This method does not correlate closely with the previous method because of the much higher shear rates involved. This is an important point to bear in mind when comparing results.

Some workers use the magnetic rheometer technique, whereby a small steel ball is inserted in a drop of mucus and oscillated magnetically over a range of frequencies. The amplitude of vibration of the phase lag with respect to the driving force is used to determine the elasticity and the viscosity as a function of radian frequency. Other methods include the microdouble capillary method (4), and the Ferranti-Shirley cone and plate viscometer.

In general, it is important and should be emphasized that when comparing different rheological results the methods be similar. Otherwise, the results can be widely discrepant, particularly if different shear rates are used. These methods are appraised more fully in some of the other chapters in this book.

RESULTS: MEANS OF EXPRESSION

With two-phase gas–liquid flow, the results may be expressed as pressure gradient versus gas flow rate (Fig. 2). In the annular flow regimen, there is a very rapid buildup of pressure drop that occurs more readily in viscous solutions than in viscoelastic solutions (e.g., Polyox). This indicates the presence of a large energy-consuming interaction between the gas and liquid phases. The results may also be expressed as the Lockhart Martinelli correlation (8), which gives a fairly good estimate of two-phase pressure drop in Newtonian systems, although the predicted values are too high in the case of non-Newtonian systems.

Isoflow pressure viscosity curves have been constructed with liquid layers of different thicknesses (2). Alternatively, pressure flow curves may be plotted logarithmically. The effect of different depths of the mucus-lining layer can be normalized by plotting the pressure–flow relationships in a Moody diagram where friction factor versus Reynolds number* (7).

Analysis of the cough experiments (10,11) indicates that during the flow a

---

* Reynolds number (Re) is the non-dimensional ratio of gas density × linear velocity/viscosity. Under ideal conditions, laminar flow changes to turbulent flow at Re ≃ 2,000.

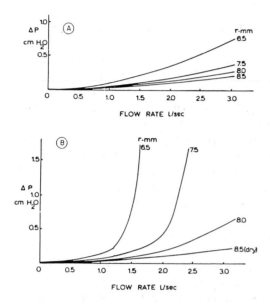

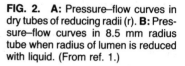

FIG. 2. **A:** Pressure–flow curves in dry tubes of reducing radii (r). **B:** Pressure–flow curves in 8.5 mm radius tube when radius of lumen is reduced with liquid. (From ref. 1.)

steady-state balance exists between the shear force exerted on the flowing liquid layer by the flowing gas and the shear force required to maintain the liquid layer in steady laminar flow along the tube wall. This steady-state shear force balance was used to obtain quantitative estimates for the serous layer velocities induced by cough in various generations of the tracheobronchial tree. These velocities appear to be significant down to about the 12th generation of Weibel for cough in a healthy person. The serous layer velocities were strongly dependent on the serous layer thickness and viscosity.

Values of cough-induced curves and normal ciliary serous layer or mucus layer mean velocity were plotted versus the Weibel generation. Cough-induced mean velocities were high for the first three generations, which were assumed to be collapsed to about 30% of their normal cross-sectional area during cough.

RESULTS FROM PREVIOUS STUDIES

In general, the studies cited, although performed in model tube systems, all confirm the likelihood of two-phase gas–liquid flow taking place at flow rates down to those seen during tidal breathing and in both central and more peripheral airways.

This two-phase interaction is not due to luminal narrowing or surface roughness alone but to energy transfer between the two phases. During coughing, for instance, this will have the advantage of tending to clear secretions cephalad, and it now seems clear that this is an integral and important part of the cough mechanism leading to expectoration of sputum.

The two-phase interaction is dependent on the thickness of the liquid layer and its viscoelastic properties.

The criteria for mucus transport in the airways by this mechanism were established in tube models positioned vertically (Fig. 3) in such a way that the liquid could form a uniform layer while traveling upward through the tube with a continuous upward airflow (6). The critical airflow rate was found to be Re 142 to 1,132 (for a 0.5 cm id model) and Re 708 to 2,830 (for a 1.0 cm id model), depending on the liquid tested. In both, the critical airflow rate was lower with viscoelastic liquids than with viscous oils. The critical liquid layer thickness ranged from 0.2 to 0.5 mm in the smaller tube and 0.8 to 1.4 mm in the larger tube at Re 2,800. These values decreased with increasing airflow rate. The critical thickness relative to the tube diameter ranged from 3 to 15% and was lower by 30 to 50% in the smaller tube. These results supported the hypothesis that two-phase gas–liquid flow may be relevant in patients with bronchial hypersecretion during normal breathing.

In a further study, the same authors used the same glass tubes positioned either vertically or horizontally to measure the transport speed of the mucus (5). In the vertical tube, this ranged from 1.1 to 3.1 cm/min at a given mucus feed and airflow rate, increasing with airflow but decreasing with higher mucus viscosity (Fig. 4). More elastic mucus caused lower flow resistance. The transport speed in the horizontal tube was 5 to 60% faster than that in the vertical tube. From

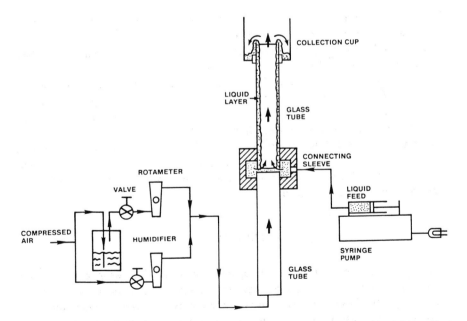

FIG. 3. Schematic diagram of experimental system for measuring two-phase flow with a continual liquid feed (5,6). (From ref. 3.)

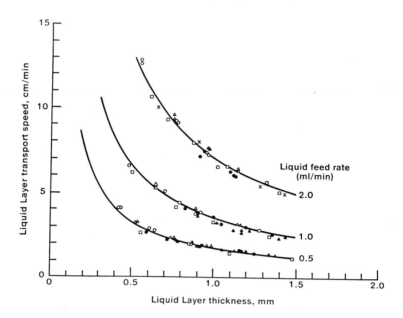

FIG. 4. Relationship between liquid layer transport speed and thickness in a two-phase vertical flow model. Solid lines are theoretical predictions and symbols are experimental data (6). (From ref. 5.)

these data, the transport speed could be functionally related to airway diameter mucus layer thickness and mucus production rate.

Studies with oscillatory flow show that flow resistance at low amplitude increased only to the extent of that expected from simple constriction of the tube cross-section area (7). At high amplitude, oscillatory flow resistance increased beyond that indicating the onset of two-phase gas–liquid flow. This is important, since it may lead either to improved mucus clearance or mucus impaction in the lungs, depending on the type of oscillatory flow.

Cough clearance by two-phase flow is a prime example of the usefulness of this function within the lungs (10). It depends on a high linear airflow velocity, which may be critically reduced in patients with airflow obstruction and which may, therefore, render cough inefficient (2).

CONCLUSIONS

Studies so far have led to the inescapable conclusion that two-phase gas–liquid flow can exist within the human tracheobronchial tree, particularly if there is mucus hypersecretion, whether from viral respiratory infection, chronic bronchitis, or other causes. Most studies, however, have been performed on straight rigid tubes, with one or two attempts with branching models, none of which have had the flexible compliance of the human airway.

It follows that studies using actual casts of the human airway may be valuable, as would studies of postmortem lungs, although the problems presented by these studies are significant. *In vivo* studies in humans have not yet been attempted, and it may be that the methods sensitive enough to pick up the increased resistance in this type of flow are not yet available. Nevertheless, these possibilities should be kept in mind. This work does focus attention on the physical aspects of mucus clearance from the lungs in general and on its undoubted importance in disease states.

ACKNOWLEDGMENT

The author thanks Miss Lorraine Campbell for typing the manuscript.

REFERENCES

1. Agnew, J. E., Little, F., Pavia, D., and Clarke, S. W. (1982): Mucus clearance from the airways in chronic bronchitis: Smokers and non-smokers. *Bull. Eur. Physiopathol. Respir.*, 18:473–484.
2. Clarke, S. W. (1973): The role of two-phase flow in bronchial clearance. *Bull. Physiopathol. Respir.*, 9:359–372.
3. Clarke, S. W., Jones, J. G., and Oliver, D. R. (1970): Resistance to two-phase gas–liquid flow in airways. *J. Appl. Physiol.*, 29:464–471.
4. Kim, C. S., Brown, L. K., Lewars, G., and Sackner, M. A. (1983): Deposition of aerosol particles and flow resistance in mathematical and experimental airway models. *J. Appl. Physiol.*, 55:154–163.
5. Kim, C. S., Greene, M. A., Sankaray, S., and Sackner, M. A. (1986): Mucus transport in the airways by two-phase gas–liquid flow mechanism: Continuous flow model. *J. Appl. Physiol.*, 60:901–907.
6. Kim, C. S., Rodriguez, C. S., Mungen, A. E., and Sackner, M. A. (1986): Criteria for mucus transport in the airways by two-phase gas–liquid flow mechanism. *J. Appl. Physiol.*, 60:908–917.
7. King, M., Chang, H. K., and Webber, M. E. (1982): Resistance of mucus-lined tubes to steady and oscillatory airflow. *J. Appl. Physiol.*, 52:1172–1176.
8. Lockhart, R. W., and Martinelli, R. C. (1949): Proposed correlation of data for isothermal two-phase two-component flow in pipes. *Chem. Eng. Prog.*, 45:39–48.
9. Oliver, D. R., and Young Hoon, A. (1968): Two-phase non-Newtonian flow. *Trans. Inst. Chem. Eng.*, 46:T106–T115.
10. Scherer, P. W. (1981): Mucus transport by cough. *Chest,* 80:830–833S.
11. Scherer, P. W., and Burtz, L. (1976): Fluid mechanical experiments relevant to coughing. *J. Biomech.*, 11:183–187.
12. Sturgess, J. M.; Palfrey, A. J., and Reid, L. (1970): The viscosity of bronchial secretions. *Clin. Sci.*, 38:145–156.
13. Weibel, E. R. (1963): *Morphometry of the Human Lung.* Springer, Berlin.

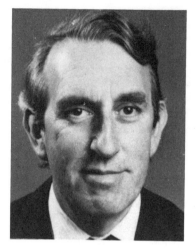

Stewart William Clarke was born in Eastwood, England, in 1936. He received the M.B. degree in 1959 and the M.D. degree in 1969 from the University of Birmingham (England). He is currently Head of the Department of Thoracic Medicine, Consultant Physician and Senior Lecturer, the Royal Free Hospital and School of Medicine, and Brompton Hospital and Cardiothoracic Institute (Hon.), London. Fields of interest include clinical thoracic medicine, lung clearance, and aerosols.

Methods in Bronchial Mucology,
edited by P. C. Braga and L. Allegra.
Raven Press, Ltd. © 1988.

2.4. Rheological Properties Other than Viscoelasticity and Adhesivity

E. Puchelle and J. M. Zahm

INSERM U314, Faculté de Medecine, 51095 Reims Cedex, France

Spinability
Pourability
Yield stress
Thixotropy

SPINABILITY

Spinability is the ability of bronchial mucus to be drawn into threads when stretched. This parameter can be measured with an automatic apparatus (Filancemetre Sefam) (10) derived from that developed by Burnett et al. (2) and Chretien et al. (3) for cervical mucus. The principle of measurement is described in Fig. 1.

A calibrated volume of the mucus to be studied is introduced into the bottom reservoir. A part of this sample is then sucked in by the prehension system. A low current is applied to the sample from a voltage supply. By raising the prehension system vertically at constant speed, the sample is stretched, and the electronic device measures the maximum length of the thread at the moment of thread rupture.

In pathological bronchial secretions collected in patients suffering from chronic

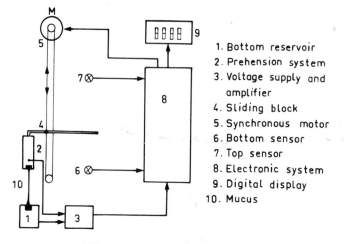

FIG. 1. Synoptic of the filancemeter.

1. Bottom reservoir
2. Prehension system
3. Voltage supply and amplifier
4. Sliding block
5. Synchronous motor
6. Bottom sensor
7. Top sensor
8. Electronic system
9. Digital display
10. Mucus

obstructive pulmonary disease (COPD), the mean coefficient of variation obtained for three measurements carried out on the same mucus sample is about 20%. This relatively high mean coefficient of variation is likely to be due to the heterogeneity of sputum. In fact, when using a solution (50% w/w in water) of porcine stomach mucin (Sigma Chemical) as a simulant of mucus, the coefficient of variation is only 8%.

In patients with COPD, large variations in spinability are observed from one patient to another. In 60 patients, the bronchial mucus spinability, measured at a stretching rate of 10 mm sec^{-1}, ranged between 15 and 150 mm.

Spinability is a rheological index, giving information about the internal cohesion forces of mucus. The concentration of mucus glycoproteins, the degree of intermolecular and intramolecular crosslinkings, and the hydration of mucus are factors that control mucus spinability. This parameter is not directly dependent on the degree of viscosity and elasticity. A definite spinability may be observed for mucus samples with quite different viscosities. Furthermore, a nonelastic solution may be spinable.

Spinability measurement can be useful in the routine screening of clinical samples and the initial evaluation of mucus-modifying agents.

POURABILITY

Keal and Reid (7) described a very simple clinical test that did not require any apparatus to estimate the physical properties of the sputum samples expectorated by patients. This simple rheological index represents the capacity of a fluid to adhere to the walls of a container and flow under gravity. They determined four grades according to the scale of pourability:

Grade I	Adhering closely to the container
Grade II	Moving slowly with gravity
Grade III	Moving rapidly with gravity
Grade IV	Moving instantaneously as soon as container is reversed

Keal and Reid (7) observed a significant and inverse correlation between the pourability and viscosity. According to these authors, the clinical assessment of pourability could have some predictive value of viscosity. In fact, pourability is an index that includes several rheological factors, such as viscosity, surface tension, and adhesiveness or stickiness of mucus. Depending on the method of collection and the quantity of sputum present in the container, the pourability grade will differ markedly. Therefore, this index must be interpreted with great care and should be determined on sputum samples protected from salivary contamination (9). We have observed that the pourability of sputum samples collected in patients with cystic fibrosis (CF) is low (grade I or II) in 73% of samples (8). These results are in agreement with the classic clinical concept of the stickiness of CF mucus samples.

YIELD STRESS

Yield stress is defined as the minimal shear stress necessary to apply to a substance for it to flow. If the shearing stress is less than this critical value τy called "yield stress" (or yield value), the sample will not flow but will behave as an elastic solid. It will deform and recover its initial position as soon as the stress is interrupted. If the shear stress is higher than τy, the sample will flow. Such a behavior, characteristic of plastic materials, is shown in Fig. 2, where shear stress τ is plotted against shear rate $\dot{\gamma}$.

Different techniques can be applied to the measurement of the yield value.

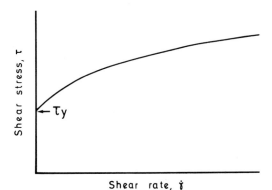

FIG. 2. Shear stress–shear rate rheogram for a fluid with yield stress. (τy) Yield stress.

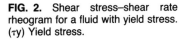

Flow Curve Extrapolation

Cone-plate viscometers (such as the Ferranti-Shirley) have been proposed not only for measuring viscosity but also for determining yield stress of mucus. Such viscometers can be programmed to give a linear increase in shear rate and to measure the resulting shear stress. From the rheograms obtained, static and dynamic yield values have been derived, showing that sputum exhibits yield values ranging between 10 and 70 pascal (Pa). Purulent secretions had higher values than mucoid samples (6). As noted by Davis (4), continuous shear rate experiments are not adapted to the correct estimation of yield stress. In fact, the sample is forced to flow, and the typical points in the rheograms obtained were probably due to inertial and slippage effects.

Stress Relaxation

Stress relaxation technique after cessation of steady-state flow (1) also has been used for determining the yield stress of sputum samples. The yield stress was measured with a concentric cylinder rheometer (Rotovisko, Haake) by torque relaxation, after manual application of a torque on the inner cylinder, which was then allowed to relax to an equilibrium position corresponding to yield value. Although this technique was limited by the low sensitivity of the torsion wire used for measuring stress and by mechanical friction of the apparatus, yield values obtained were lower than 2.3 Pa. A new rheometer (viscoelasticimetre, Sefam) has been designed for measuring viscoelastic and yield values properties (5). A constant shear rate is applied to the sample, and after obtaining steady-state stress, the shear rate is stopped and the shear stress relaxes to yield value. Using this technique, the mean yield value obtained for pathological bronchial mucus was 1.9 ± 1.2 Pa.

Creep Test

Another way to measure yield stress is to apply to the sample a shear stress that is increased step by step and to record the resulting deformation of the sample. Until the stress is less than the yield value, the strain versus time remains constant. If the stress is beyond the yield value, the strain increases continuously with time.

This method, used with controlled stress rheometers (Carri-Med, Haake), is probably the most accurate method for determining yield stress.

THIXOTROPY

Bronchial mucus possesses an internal structure that involves time-dependent properties, such as thixotropy. According to the rheology dictionary, thixotropy

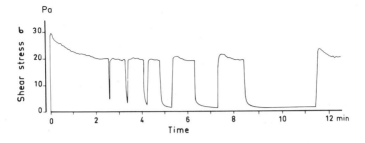

FIG. 3. Shear stress time response of 10% reconstituted mucus with increasing time periods.

can be defined as the reversible decrease of apparent viscosity with time when a constant shear rate is applied. In response to a rectangular shear rate step higher than 1 sec^{-1}, the shear stress behavior of respiratory mucus is characterized by a typical overshoot followed by a shear thinning of the sample. After attainment of a steady-state shear stress and allowing the sample to rest for a progressively increasing time, the restructuring of mucus occurs. One can observe that the overshoot does not occur if rest time is short. It progressively reappears after a rest interval of several minutes (Fig. 3).

Thixotropy is a reversible behavior depending on the concentration of the coupling that maintains the structure of mucus.

REFERENCES

1. Benis, A. M., Puchelle, E., and Sadoul, P. (1972): Adaptation of a concentric cylinder viscometer to the routine measurement of the viscoelastic properties of sputum. In: *Rheology of Biological Systems,* edited by M. Litt and H. L. Gabelnick, pp. 218–259. Charles C Thomas, Springfield, IL.
2. Burnett, J., Glover, F. A., and Scott Blair, G. W. (1967): Field measurements of the spinability of bovine cervical mucus. *Biorheology,* 4:41–45.
3. Chretien, F. C., Ozenda, M., and Volochine, B. (1977): Automatic device for measuring the spinability of cervical mucus in women. *Med. Biol. Eng. Comput.,* 15:673–678.
4. Davis, S. S. (1973): Techniques for the measurement of the rheological properties of sputum. In: *Rheology of Bronchial Secretions and Respiratory Functions,* edited by E. Puchelle, pp. 47–90. Masson et Cie, Paris.
5. Duvivier, C., Didelon, J., Arnould, J. P., et al. (1984): A new viscoelastometer for studying the rheological properties of bronchial mucus in clinical practice. *Biorheology (Suppl.),* 1:119–122.
6. Feather, E. A., and Russel, G. (1970): Sputum viscosity in cystic fibrosis of the pancreas and other pulmonary diseases. *Br. J. Dis. Chest,* 64:192–200.
7. Keal, E., and Reid, L. (1970): Méthodes d'étude des modifications de la secrétion bronchique et de sa viscosité. Poumon Coeur, 26:5258.
8. Puchelle, E., Jacquot, J., Beck, G., Zahm, J. M., and Galabert, C. (1985): Rheological and transport properties of airway secretions in cystic fibrosis. Relationships with the degree of infection and severity of this disease. *Eur. J. Clin. Invest.,* 15:389–394.
9. Puchelle, E., Tournier, J. M., Zahm, J. M., and Sadoul, P. (1984): Rheology of sputum collected by a simple technique limiting salivary contamination. *J. Lab. Clin. Med.,* 103:347–353.
10. Zahm, J. M., Puchelle, E., Duvivier, C., and Didelon, J. (1986): Spinability of respiratory mucus. Validation of a new apparatus: The filancemeter. *Bull. Eur. Physiopathol. Respir.,* 22:609–613.

Methods in Bronchial Mucology,
edited by P. C. Braga and L. Allegra.
Raven Press, Ltd. © 1988.

2.5.1. ADHESIVITY ASSESSMENT

2.5.1. Tack Test Technique

M. T. Lopez-Vidriero

Boehringer Ingelheim GMBH, Zentrale Abteilung Medizinische Dienste, Ingelheim am Rhein, Federal Republic of Germany

---

Tack
Methods for measuring tack
Measurement of tack of sputum using a probe test

Several biological substances, such as blood and secretions, are known to have adhesive properties and have been used in the past as glues to join together materials of different nature. Airway mucus adheres to surfaces, and this property has been studied in the past as pourability (4), that is, the stronger the adherence, the longer it takes for the secretion to slide down the wall of the container. This simple test was used as an index of viscosity, and it correlates with apparent viscosity but only when the secretion is not infected. From this observation one can conclude that the nature of the chemical and physical properties of the adhesive will influence its adherence to a surface. In the clinical situation, patients complain of difficulty in shifting the phlegm because the mucus sticks to their throat. This symptom most likely reflects the adherence of abnormal mucus to diseased epithelium.

Zygology is the science of joining things, and adhesion is part of this science. An adhesive is a substance that is capable of holding materials together by surface attachment. Adhesion has been defined as the state in which two surfaces are held together by interfacial forces, which may be valence forces or interlocking action or both (6). The process of adhesion is complex, and it is influenced by many variables, such as physical and chemical properties of both the adhesive and the surface. Depending on the mechanism involved, different types of adhesion

141

have been described: mechanical or entanglement, electrostatic, diffusion, and adsorption. In mechanical adhesion, the morphology of the surface, its roughness, plays an important role in determining the strength of the joint. In this type of adhesion, the adhesive must penetrate into the irregularities of the surface, thus acting as a mechanical interlocking system. The morphology of the epithelium, particularly the ciliated epithelium, offers ideal conditions for mechanical adhesion, but the nature of the surface—glycocalix—can also influence adhesion to the cell membrane by other mechanisms, such as electrostasis or adsorption. In diseased airways where the epithelium has been shedded, such as in asthma and viral infections, the roughness of the surface is also suitable for mechanical adhesion.

Electrostatic adhesion is based on the concept of an electrical double layer, where the adhesive is compared to a condenser and the double electric layer produced at the interface with the plates of a condenser.

Adhesion by diffusion can take place only when the adhesive materials—polymers—show autohesion. This is the type of adhesion observed with contact adhesives, when the glue is applied to both surfaces and the union of the adhesive is by a diffusion process. In this type of adhesion, the nature of the adhesive, which is always a polymer, is the principal factor and depends on the chain structure and flexibility of the molecules as well as their ability to exhibit microbrownian motion. It is likely that in small airways, where the thickness of the mucus layer is increased, adhesion by diffusion of glycoprotein molecules can take place and thus contribute to airflow limitation.

Adsorption adhesion refers to the bonding of dissimilar materials when the molecules of the adhesive are brought into close molecular contact with those of the surface, and intermolecular interforces maintain the adhesive and substrate together. The van der Waals forces are mainly responsible for this type of adhesion, and they include the London forces, the Keesom dipole–dipole interaction, and the Debye dipole–molecule interaction. Adhesion by adsorption can, therefore, take place between the cationic/anionic part of the epithelial glycoprotein and those of the cell membranes and glycocalyx.

Increasing interest has been focused on the thermodynamic theory of bond formation, which is beyond the scope of this chapter. However, one topic should be mentioned that may explain some of the technical difficulties faced when measuring adhesiveness. The wetting of the surface by the adhesive is the first step involved in bond formation, and it depends on the free energies of the surface (adherend) and the liquid (adhesive) as well as the interfacial free energy. Therefore, the surface tension of the airway mucus will influence the degree of wettability and, hence, its adherence to the airway wall. Another important factor involved in adhesion of polymers is the flow (viscosity) and deformation (elasticity) of the adhesive (7).

The surface tension of the material as well as its viscoelastic properties will determine the degree of contact and spreading and, hence, the strength of the bond and should be taken into account when measuring adhesiveness.

TACK

Adhesive materials of different nature can exhibit tack. Tack has been defined as the property or characteristic of different adhesive materials to bind tenaciously and rapidly under conditions of light contact pressure and short contact time (1,3). Contact pressure and time of contact are the main features and are of major importance for standardization of the techniques for measuring tack.

Tack, or tackiness, is not a physical property, such as viscosity, elasticity, or surface tension. It is the result of a particular combination of these properties. Rubber, paints, printing inks, varnishes, and adhesive tapes exhibit tack, although they differ in physical and chemical properties. The magnitude of tackiness of a substance depends on several factors, some related to the substance itself—surface adhesive forces and viscoelastic properties—and others related to the surface— geometry or roughness—as well as to external factors, such as magnitude of the pressure and the time of contact.

In diseases characterized by acute or chronic mucus hypersecretion, all these factors can be present, resulting in adherence of mucus to the bronchial wall, particularly during cough or forced expiration. Light pressure on the mucus can occur during cough when the intrathoracic pressure narrows the airway lumen. During forced expiration, the high airflow can increase the normal force of the mucus and thus apply light pressure. During both cough and forced expiration, the time of contact is short, which is one of the criteria for defining tack.

METHODS FOR MEASURING TACK

The first known attempts to measure tack were made as early as the midnineteenth century by Stefan (1847) and by Reynolds (1886) (2). These authors measured tack as the force required to separate two flat surfaces, at a given rate, when immersed in a liquid. Tack can be measured by hand, but this method gives only qualitative data. Quantitative measurement of tack can be carried out by three main test procedures: peel tests, rolling ball or cylinder tests, and the probe test.

Peel Tests

Peel tests are based on the principle of spreading the material on a flexible substrate under controlled conditions of pressure and time of contact. The force required to peel apart the bonded complex is a measure of tack (2). Another peel method uses a similar principle, but the flexible substrate with the adhesive is placed on a nonflexible surface, which is usually glass or stainless steel. Tack is measured as the force required for debonding the flexible substrate or as the time taken to achieve separation.

The loop test is not widely used, since the interpretation of results is difficult. A loop is made with a coated tape and a force is applied at both ends of the tape.

In the rotating drum test, the drum is covered with adhesive tape, and a rigid rotatable wheel is placed in contact with the adhesive. The drum is rotated at a constant speed, and the force required to keep the wheel stationary is the measure of tack.

Rolling Ball or Cylinder Tests

The rolling ball or cylinder tests are easy to set up, but the mathematical equations are difficult, since the time of contact is considered not to be constant.

The principle of this test is that the adhesive is spread on a flat plane that is inclined to a given degree. The adhesive is laid on only the lower portion of the surface so that when the sphere or cylinder is released from the top of the plane, it can roll down freely before reaching the adhesive. Tack is measured as the distance that the ball or cylinder can travel on the adhesive before stopping. The main disadvantage of this method is that the distance is not measured accurately, and many replicates are required. In addition, the test is based on the assumption that the ball rolls on the surface and that the velocity is linear. It has been shown, however, that the ball tends to slide and that the velocity is not constant. This method is used mainly for quality control.

Probe Test

The probe test was first developed by Stefan (1874). He used two parallel disks of known radius, which were immersed in a liquid of a given viscosity. The force required to move the plates a given distance is a function of time, expressed as:

$$Ft = 3/4\pi a^4 \eta \left[\frac{1}{h2^2} - \frac{1}{h1^2} \right]$$

in which t is time; a is radius of the plates; η is viscosity of the liquid; h is position before (h1) and after (h2) separation.

This formula can be applied only when studying Newtonian liquids immersed in a liquid. When the plates are not immersed in liquid the surface tension of the liquid will influence the force required to separate the plates. The formula changes accordingly:

$$\frac{4\eta}{h^3} \frac{dh}{dt} = \frac{Fh^3 l^2}{v^3} - \frac{2\gamma h l^2}{v^2}$$

where v is liquid volume; γ is liquid surface tension; l is $2a$.

This formula can be applied to Newtonian liquids, but with non-Newtonian liquids, such as mucus, a more complex formula should be used.

The basic principle of the probe test is that a surface is brought into contact with an adhesive material, and it is allowed to be in contact for a fixed time and under fixed-load conditions. The probe is then pulled off at a defined rate, and the force is recorded. Other instruments express tack as the work per distance using integrating devices connected to the instrument.

A tensile machine, such as the one shown in Fig. 1, can be used for measuring tack of airway mucus/sputum. Several factors should be taken into account when measuring tack, since they can influence the results. The most important factors are probe composition, adhesive film thickness, applied probe force, dwell time, cross-head speed, and temperature.

Probe Composition

The characteristics of the probe material—metal, glass, airway epithelium—as well as the shape—hemispherical or flat—and dimensions should be known and

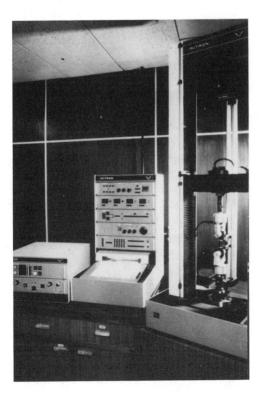

FIG. 1. Tensile machine for measuring rack.

standardized. In the method described here, the probe used was metal of low surface roughness with a diameter of 1 cm.

Adhesive Film Thickness

The adhesive film should be thin and uniform. This is relatively easy with homogeneous liquids of low viscosity, but it is difficult to standardize with such materials as mucus. Since all the other factors can be controlled with accuracy, it is possible to obtain reproducible thickness by measuring accurately the volume of the material. The volume required depends on the size of the probe; in this method 1 ml of material was used.

Applied Force Probe

The applied force of the probe will depend on its weight and varies with the type of tensile machine used, which is dictated by the nature of the material to be tested. The tensile machine used in this study was fitted with a probe weighing 119.85 g, which is equivalent to a force of 1.175 Newton (N). Since the weight of the probe will influence the thickness of the film, it is important to establish a suitable weight to achieve a thin film.

Dwell Time

Dwell time, that is, the time that the probe is in contact with the material, is one of the most important factors influencing the measurement of tack. The effect of dwell time has been studied in several adhesives. It has been shown that the relationship between dwell time and tack is linear, and this applies to many different types of adhesives over a wide range of dwell times—0.4 sec to 238 hr (1,3).

Sputum shows similar behavior; an increase in dwell time from less than 1 sec to 180 sec results in an increase in tack (Fig. 2). In this experiment, the relationship was linear only between <1 sec and 60 sec, and then the increase reached a plateau. The dwell time selected was 60 sec, although this was later found to be too long (5). Shorter times, less than 1 sec, are recommended.

Cross-Head Speed

The cross-head speed, that is the rate at which the probe is withdrawn from the adhesive, has a marked influence on tack (1,3). Tack increases with increasing cross-head speed, and the relationship for most adhesives is curvilinear.

The influence of cross-head speed on tack of sputa is shown in Fig. 3. The

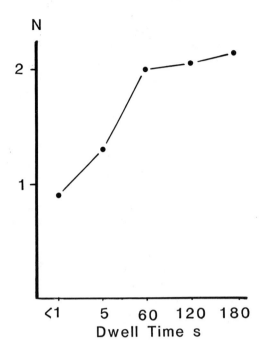

FIG. 2. Effect of dwell time on tack of sputum.

FIG. 3. Effect of cross-head speed on tack of sputa.

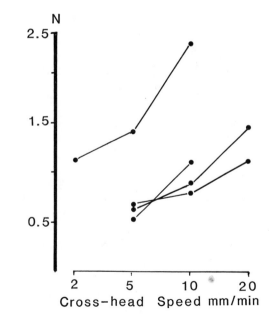

speeds tested were 2, 5, 10, and 20 mm/min. In all samples tested, there was an increase in tack that was more marked at higher speeds—10 and 20 mm/min. No higher speeds were studied, but because of the nature of the material, it is necessary to use even higher speeds, such as those used for other adhesives, up to 80 mm/min (3).

Temperature

Tack is influenced by temperature, and this has been studied in great detail with natural rubber (1,2). The changes in tack with decreasing temperature from +40°C to −20°C show a bell-shaped curve; i.e., there is a gradual increase in tack with decreasing temperature until a peak is reached and then tack sharply decreases. Each material exhibits a particular type of bell-shaped curve regarding the temperature at which the peak is observed and the width of the curve. It is of interest to note that when tack is measured at increasing temperature, it decreases, and a temperature is reached at which cohesive failure rather than tack is measured.

The behavior of tack with temperature can be explained by changes in stiffness of the material. Changes in viscoelastic properties of materials, particularly polymers, are well documented.

No data are available on the relationship between tack and temperature in sputum. Ambient temperature was used for the experiments, and more work is required in this area.

MEASUREMENT OF TACK OF SPUTUM USING A PROBE TEST

A tensile machine (Fig. 1) was used for measuring tack of sputa. The probe, a semihemispheric plunger, was modified by attaching a flat metal surface 1 cm in diameter. The method was standardized as follows:

Temperature	20°C
Probe weight	119.85 g (1.175 N)
Dwell time	60 sec
Cross-head speed	10 mm/min

Tack was measured on sputum, dried sputum, gel phase, and sol phase. Dried sputum was fresh sputum that had been dried with filter paper to remove the watery capsule. Gel and sol phases were obtained by high-speed ultracentrifugation (160,000 g × 30 min at 4°C).

The results are diagrammatically represented in Fig. 4. It is of interest that by removing liquid from the sputum, tack decreases, and this is even more apparent in the gel phase. Sol phase of sputum does not exhibit tack. These results are preliminary and are only an attempt to measure tack of sputum. It is likely that the experimental conditions, particularly dwell time and cross-head speed, were

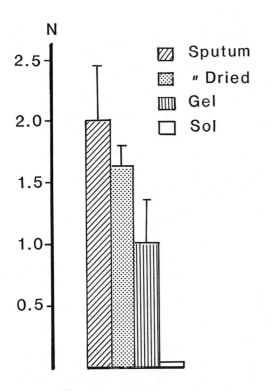

FIG. 4. Tack of sputum, dried sputum, gel phase, and sol phase.

not suitable for this type of polymer, and shorter dwell time and higher cross-head speeds should be investigated.

The probe test is based on separating two surfaces with the test material between them. Therefore, it is possible that deformation and flow could be measured as well as or instead of tack. This is shown in Fig. 5, which represents the flow chart of force (N)/time (mm/min). When the probe is lower, the material is compressed and deformation is observed; when the probe is stopped and during the dwell time, the material recovers; when the probe is withdrawn—tensile force—the material flows. It is important that the separation between the probe and the material be clean and that no threads or strings form. If this happens, what is measured is the tensile property of the material (cohesive failure) and not tack.

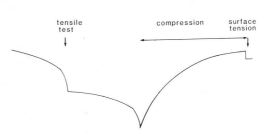

FIG. 5. Recording of tack test showing deformation, recovery, and flow of sputum under test conditions.

REFERENCES

1. Bates, R., and Counsell, P. J. C. (1976): The nature of tack. In: *Industrial Adhesives and Sealants*, edited by B. S. Jackson, pp. 73–90. Hutchinson Benham, London.
2. Busse, W. F., Lambert, J. M., and Verdery, R. B. (1946): Tackiness of GR-S and athor elastomers. *J. Appl. Physiol.*, 17:376–385.
3. Counsell, P. J. C., and Whitehouse, R. S. (1977): Tack and morphology of pressure-sensitive adhesives. In: *Developments in Adhesives*, edited by W. C. Wake, pp. 99–126. Applied Science Publishers, London.
4. Keal, E. (1970): Méthodes d'étude de las secretion bronchique et de la viscosite. *Poumon Coeur*, 26:52–58.
5. Lopez-Vidriero, M. T., Allegra, L., Sackner, M. A., and Puchelle, E. (1986): The physical properties of mucus and their clinical relevance. *Bull. Eur. Physiopathol. Respir.*, 22:207–212.
6. Patrick, R. L. (ed.). (1967): *Adhesion and Adhesives, Vol. 1*. Edward Arnold, London.
7. Vohralik, V., and Wake, W. C. (1976): Theories of adhesion and joint strength. In: *Industrial Adhesives and Sealants*, edited by B. S. Jackson, pp. 30–48, Hutchinson Benham, London.

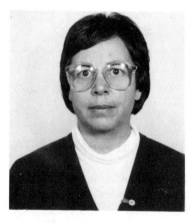

Maria Teresa Lopez-Vidriero was born in Madrid, Spain, in 1940. She received the M.D. degree in 1973 from the University of Madrid (Spain) and the Ph.D. degree in 1976 from London University (England). Fields of interest include mucus biochemistry and mucoactive drugs.

Methods in Bronchial Mucology,
edited by P. C. Braga and L. Allegra.
Raven Press, Ltd. © 1988.

2.5.2. Mucus Adhesiveness

E. Puchelle and J. M. Zahm

*INSERM U314, Faculté de Medecine,
51095 Reims, France*

Adhesiveness is a phenomenon that characterizes the attraction between an adherent surface (the mucosa) and an adhesive system (the mucus). This parameter plays a role in the cilia–mucus, cough–mucus, and bacteria–mucus interaction mechanisms. The adhesive properties of bronchial mucus can be analyzed by measuring the strength that must be applied in order to achieve separation between the adhesive fluid and the adherend surface.

The platinum ring method allows the measurement of these adhesive properties. The platinum ring is put into close contact with a sample of mucus or with a mucus-coated mucosa. This ring is then moved at a constant rate. A strain gauge, connected to the ring, measures the force required for effecting separation between the ring and the mucus. For a reliable analysis of the adhesive properties of mucus, it is necessary to obtain a true separation, with no thread formation between the ring and the mucus. We obtained such optimal conditions using a 10 mm diameter and 0.7 mm thickness platinum ring vertically raised at a rate of $10 \text{ mm} \cdot \sec^{-1}$. In patients with chronic bronchitis, the mucus adhesiveness varied between 57 and $137 \text{ m}N \cdot \text{m}^{-1}$, with an intraindividual and interindividual variation of 7% and 25%, respectively. Purulent secretions with low water content collected in patients with chronic bronchitis or cystic fibrosis exhibit the highest values of adhesiveness. Figure 1 shows the *in vitro* effect of a surface tension-lowering agent, sodium dodecyl sulfate (SDS), on bronchial secretions.

At final concentration of 2% SDS gives a significant 24% decrease of adhesive properties by reference to control values.

The study of the adhesive properties of mucus will allow the determination of the optimal values for mucus transport by ciliary and cough mechanisms.

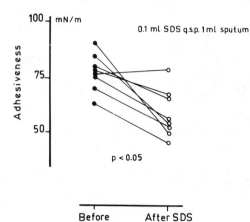

FIG. 1. Effect of sodium dodecyl sulfate (SDS) on the adhesive properties of bronchial secretions.

3. Chemical Methods of Analysis

Methods in Bronchial Mucology,
edited by P. C. Braga and L. Allegra.
Raven Press, Ltd. © 1988.

3.1. MACROMOLECULE AND ION IDENTIFICATION

3.1.1 Glycoproteins

M. Lusuardi and C. F. Donner

Centro Medico di Riabilitazione, Divisione di Fisiopatologia Respiratoria,
Veruno, Italy

Degradative methods
Marker determination
Results
Discussion
Appendixes

Human respiratory mucus composition includes about 1% (by weight) salts and other dialyzable constituents, 1% lipids, 0.5 to 1% free proteins, 0.5 to 1% carbohydrate-rich glycoproteins, and 95% or more water (4,8).

Rheological properties of mucus are primarily attributed to glycoprotein components (20). Biochemical characterization of glycoproteins is thus necessary to better understand the functions of respiratory mucus in health and disease and the possible role of drug treatment. Human respiratory mucus glycoproteins (MG) are macromolecules averaging 10^6 daltons (variation range from 2×10^5 to 2×10^7 daltons) of molecular weight and consisting of 70 to 80% carbohydrates, 20 to 30% proteins, and 1 to 2% sulfates (20). Each molecule is composed of a threonine-, serine-, and proline-rich protein core with many *O*-glycosidic linked, branched oligosaccharide chains. The molecular structure is similar to a bottle brush in which oligosaccharide chains radiate from a straight peptide backbone, with the exception of limited oligosaccharide-free naked protein zones (6). The *O*-glycosidic bond is usually between serine or threonine amino acidic residues and *N*-acetylhexosamine (*N*-acetylgalactosamine and, less frequently, *N*-acetylglucosamine) (4,19). Oligosaccharidic sidechains vary in length from 1 to 20 sugars (4,19); monosaccharide constituents in order of decreasing quantity are, respectively, *N*-acetylglucosamine, galactose, *N*-acetylneuraminic acid, fucose, and *N*-acetylgalactosamine (20).

155

Two different approaches can be followed in the biochemistry of mucus, i.e., an *in vivo* and an *in vitro* approach, differing in the conditions of producing mucus. In addition, there are two different ways of analyzing mucus, i.e., dosage of markers and isolation and characterization of different constituents, glycoproteins in our case (24). We discuss in detail the most widely used methods in the study of human respiratory MG and briefly cite more complex and *in vitro* biochemical methods.

DEGRADATIVE METHODS

Different methods of analysis are suitable for use in the biochemical definition of MG, both in normal and in pathological conditions, but first it is necessary to solubilize mucus. Treatment of sputa before biochemical studies is necessary for two obvious reasons: (a) mucus inhomogeneity and viscoelasticity do not allow appropriate treatment of samples for dosage procedures, and (b) the different macromolecular components of sputum are complexed with each other, with covalent or noncovalent bonds being broken for a precise qualitative and quantitative identification of the single fractions. Creeth reviewed various methods (8), the most common of which are summarized here in order of decreasing degree of degradation:

1. Proteolysis uses, e.g., trypsin, papain, or pronase (most effective; see Appendix I, Flow Chart 1 for procedure).
2. Thiol reduction is the most common chemical method of solubilizing mucus. It is based on the reducing property of thiol-containing molecules, such as cysteine, *N*-acetylcysteine, mercaptoethanol, and dithiothreitol (0.01–0.1 M in 0.1 M Tris–HCl buffer, pH 8.0, for 1 hr at room temperature) (9,31).
3. Ultrasonic disruption is a simple and quick physical method to solubilize mucus, probably mediated by free hydroxyl radicals produced by cavitation (8).
4. Dispersion with urea or guanidinium salts. A 6 to 8 M urea or 6 M guanidine hydrochloride solution is usually employed to disperse native mucus or the gel component of sputum obtained with ultracentrifugation procedures (30).
5. Combinations of the previous procedures, e.g., reduction with 5 mM dithiothreitol in the presence of deionized 8 M urea, eventually followed by carboxymethylation under nitrogen with 15 mM iodoacetamide at pH 9.0 for 30 min (5).

Described pretreatment methods are all degradative, and, apart from urea extraction, they should thus be used preferentially if we adopt the biochemical approach of marker or mono/oligosaccharide dosage. For isolation of MG molecules, a sol–gel separation usually is performed first, followed by a dispersion of the sol–gel components in salt or urea solutions for further steps of analysis (8). Boat et al. consider unsuitable a preliminary centrifugation step in the case of nonpurulent secretions (5).

MARKER DETERMINATION

Marker substances are useful to estimate sputum glycoproteins. This relatively simple approach has been permitted by a complex and complete molecular definition of MG and serum glycoproteins (SG) obtained with isolation procedures. SG are present in pathological secretions as a result of plasma transudation related to phlogosis.

Fucose and sulfate are markers of MG, in which they are well represented, whereas in SG there are low levels of fucose, and sulfate is absent (24,29). On the contrary, mannose can be considered a marker of SG (24,29). Sialic acid is almost equally represented in both MG and SG, and thus it is not a specific marker. However, its dosage can be useful because the sialic acid/fucose ratio is a reliable index for different types of sputum (23). Detecting methods for these markers can be performed simply with a spectrophotometer and commonly available chemical reagents. Fucose can be dosed using the method of Gibbons (15) (Appendix I, Flow Chart 2) or Dische and Shettles (12); sulfate with the method of Antonopoulos (2) or Terho and Hartiala (36) (Appendix I, Flow Chart 3); mannose according to the procedure reported by Dische (11) (Appendix I, Flow Chart 4) or with the more specific enzymatic assay of Das et al. (10). Apart from specific markers, it is possible also to evaluate the quantity of other important saccharidic constituents: hexosamines with the method of Boas (3) or Cessi and Piliego (7), neutral exoses with Roe's anthrone method (33), sialic acid with the method of Warren (37) (Appendix I, Flow Chart 5) or Aminoff (1).

Results can be expressed in relation to total sputum volume or, better, to dry weight measured after lyophilization. If mannose is not reliably detectable, normalization of data as a ratio to albumin can be useful in evaluating the variation of different components of sputum in relation to phlogistic transudation of bronchial mucosa (28). Actually, albumin is a good standardization factor for other proteins derived from serum and of comparable molecular size (35). Albumin can be dosed with radial immunodiffusion plates according to Mancini et al. (26).

Estimation of Sputum Glycoproteins with Isolation and Characterization of Single Macromolecular Components

In this kind of study, more complex equipment and time-consuming biochemical procedures are necessary (30,31). As stated, a preliminary ultracentrifugation step separates sputum into a sol and a gel phase (45,000 g for 1.5 hr at 4°C). Proteins and glycoproteins extraneous to gel formation can thus be eliminated. The sol phase is dialyzed to zero ionic strength, lyophilized, and fractionated by molecular-exclusion chromatography (Fig. 1) on Sepharose (a polysaccharide derivative produced by Pharmacia) 4B columns using 0.15 M NaCl. Fractions are collected at 20 ml/hr, and their absorbance is measured at 280 nm and at 620 nm after reaction

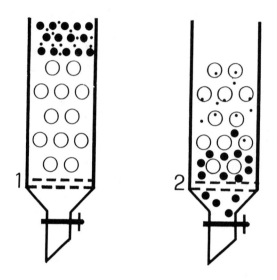

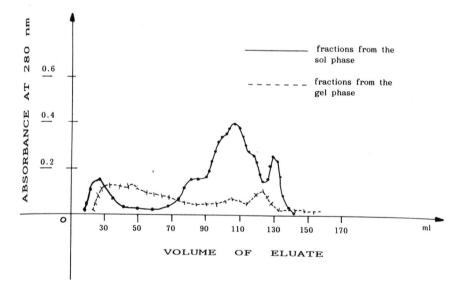

FIG. 1. Principle of molecular-exclusion (or gel-filtration or molecular-sieve) chromatography. Smaller molecules (·) are retarded because they penetrate into the pores of Sephadex beads (○), whereas larger molecules (●) move faster down the column, being excluded from the pores.

with anthrone (Figs. 2 and 3). In the former case, fractions are identified according to their protein content; light absorbance at 280 nm is in fact due to tryptophan and tyrosine residues (22). In the latter case, anthrone reaction puts in evidence the exose sugars, thus allowing an identification of MG related to the saccharidic component.

The gel phase is treated with twice its volume of 0.3 mM sodium azide for 4

——————— fractions from the sol phase

– – – – – – – fractions from the gel phase

FIG. 2. Example of results from column chromatography of sol (solid line) and gel (broken line) phases obtained from sputum samples with ultracentrifugation. Absorbance profile at 280 nm of consecutive eluate fractions. (Modified from ref. 30.)

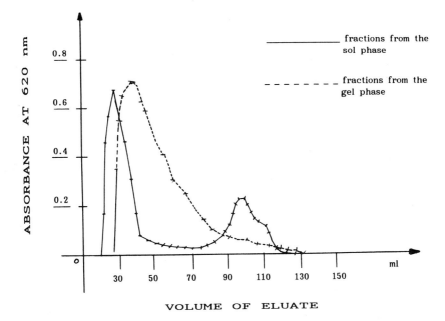

FIG. 3. Example of results from column chromatography of sol (solid line) and gel (broken line) phases obtained from sputum samples with ultracentrifugation. Absorbance profile at 620 nm of consecutive eluate fractions after anthrone reaction. (Modified from ref. 30.)

hr at 4°C to remove soluble proteins. Ultracentrifugation washing with sodium azide is repeated twice. Two or three washes are usually sufficient. A treatment follows with 6 M urea and 0.1 M NaCl (final concentrations), adding the solid reagents and gently stirring at room temperature until complete dispersion (time required is from 30 min to 3 days or longer). A 30-min centrifugation at 2,000 *g* follows in order to remove insoluble components. Supernatants are retrieved and slowly mixed with ethanol at 4°C to a final concentration of 40% (v/v). Samples then undergo another centrifugation step (2,000 *g* for 20 min), followed by an incubation period at 4°C for 4 hr. The precedure is repeated after adding ethanol to the supernatant to a 55% final concentration. The precipitate obtained, after discarding the supernatant, is composed almost completely of bronchial glycoproteins. Minor glycoprotein fractions can be separated at 60% and 90% (v/v) ethanol. Precipitates are then dissolved in water, dialyzed, and lyophilized. At this point, a chromatographic procedure using a diethylaminoethyl (DEAE) derivative of Sephadex is applied, thus combining the principles of ion-exchange and molecular-exclusion chromatography (22).

Glycoproteins can thus be fractionated on the basis of both their molecular size and their electric charge. One hundred milligram aliquots of bronchial glycoproteins are resuspended in 8 ml of 6 M urea and applied to a DEAE-Sephadex A-25 column (31.5 × 1.5 cm) previously washed with deionized 6 M urea. Column elution is first done with 6 M urea (70 ml), then with a linear gradient of NaCl obtained by passing 1 M NaCl in 6 M urea (250 ml) into a mixing chamber containing 6 M urea (250 ml). Fractions are collected at an elution rate of 20 ml/hr. Absorbance of each fraction is read at 280 nm and 620 nm after anthrone reaction (Figs. 2 and 3), and then chemical analyses for sugar and protein components are performed.

Previously described spectrophotometric methods can be used to determine carbohydrates, since they are the simplest and are quite precise (enzymatic procedures are preferred for specificity). Other more complex and expensive methods have been used by different authors, such as gel-filtration chromatography, ion-exchange chromatography of alkaline borohydride-cleaved sugars (13,30), gas–liquid chromatography of alditol acetate or trimethyl-silyl-ether derivatives (18,30), and high-performance liquid chromatography (17).

Total protein component can be evaluated by Lowry's procedure (25). Amino acid profile determination requires a complete hydrolysis of the sample, e.g., with a 24-hr incubation at 110°C of the mucus resuspended in 5.6 M HCl in a tube sealed under vacuum (18). Samples are dosed with an amino acid autoanalyzer. Such instruments are based on the principle of ion-exchange chromatography; cation-exchange resin-filled columns are usually employed to fractionate amino acids. The ninhydrin reaction is applied to quantitate amino acids in each elution fraction (22).

A similar procedure to those of Roberts (30,31) has been applied to the study of respiratory tract secretions from healthy subjects by Williams et al. (38). Mucus samples are dissolved in 8 M urea (1:4 v/v) and concentrated to 2 ml with ultrafiltration membranes (Amicon XM50) selecting molecules of mol wt > 50,000 daltons. Molecular-sieve chromatography is then performed on Sepharose CL2B columns (ϕ 2.6 cm × 70 cm), using 6 M urea and 0.01% (w/v) sodium azide in 10 mM sodium phosphate buffer (pH 7.2) as elution solution. Forty-five 9 ml eluate fractions are collected from the column, and their absorbance is spectrophotometrically read at 280 nm. A dialysis step follows against 0.1 M sodium acetate/acetic acid buffer (pH 5.8) containing magnesium chloride (25 mM) and sodium azide (0.01% w/v). One milliliter of alcian blue 0.1% in the buffer is mixed to 3 ml of the dialyzed fractions, and the solution is kept at room temperature for at least 2 hr to allow precipitation of glycoprotein/dye complexes, whose separation is completed with a centrifugation step. Precipitates are washed and redissolved according to Hall et al. (16), and absorbance of each fraction is spectrophotometrically read at 620 nm. The principle of this method is that alcian blue, a cationic dye, is able to interact with acidic residues of MG, i.e., sulfate and sialic acid, forming insoluble complexes (38). This method is limited to normal secretions because alcian blue also interacts with glycosaminoglycans and nucleic acids, which are important components of pathological purulent sputum. Some authors have used analytical density-gradient ultracentrifugation with CsBr as the gradient-forming salt to separate and characterize MG. For detailed procedure, see references 8 and 9.

A different approach to the biochemistry of MG is represented by study of the *in vitro* incorporation of specific radiolabeled precursors. In fact, organ cultures of human trachea produce MG almost identical to those isolated in sputa (14). Fragments of bronchial mucosa kept in adequate culture media and incubation conditions (27) are able to incorporate ^{14}C- or ^{3}H-radiolabeled sugars, amino sugars, threonine, or ^{35}S sulfate (19,20,27). MG fractions can then be isolated and purified as described and evaluated according to their composition of radiolabeled constituents. Cultures of airway tissues can be maintained for long periods (weeks to months) (27).

RESULTS

Proteolysis allows digestion of the free protein components of sputum and also of the naked segment of MG, which is the naked part of the protein core not protected from the enzymatic action by oligosaccharide chains. This method can be useful in the study of the oligosaccharide component, which is not degraded, but it cannot be extended to the investigation of the entire glycoprotein macromolecule or of the protein core (8).

Thiol reduction splits disulfide bonds so acting mainly on the protein component. This is a less degradative procedure in glycoproteins than is proteolysis, but it is more degradative than isolation procedures (8). This method should be reserved to the study of carbohydrate constituents and MG markers.

Ultrasonic disruption has degradative effects on both oligosaccharide and protein components (8), but at specific operative conditions, certain plasma (glyco)proteins are not antigenically altered and can thus be immunologically dosed (see Chapter 3.1.2.). If a sonifier is available, sonication is probably the best method of mucus pretreatment for dosing MG markers, but it is not suitable for MG isolation.

Dispersion with urea or guanidinium salts leads to a complete denaturation of the protein component of the secretions (8) acting on hydrogen bonds (32). When it is compared with the previous methods, it has the advantage that the primary structure of MG macromolecules is not altered, whereas molecular conformation probably is (8).

Combinations of the reported procedures often are adopted usefully for complete solubilization of nonpurulent tracheobronchial secretions, thus avoiding a centrifugal separation into a sol and a gel phase (5). According to Boat et al., ultracentrifugation preliminary procedures are ineffective as fractionation step for at least two reasons: (a) many macromolecules are found in both sol and gel phases, and (b) MG can be physically damaged or chemically altered because of release of sialyl residues (5).

DISCUSSION

Qualitative and quantitative evaluation of biochemical markers does not give results that can be considered pathognomonic to a particular disease, although some characteristics are evident. In cystic fibrosis, fucose concentration is lower and the NANA/fucose ratio is higher than in chronic bronchitis or asthma, suggesting an increase in the serum glycoprotein component (23). In purulent sputum from chronic bronchitis, sialyl and sulfate groups are increased, but fucose is not (23). Patients affected by extrinsic asthma without chronic bronchitis show an increase in serum components with low intragroup variations, whereas in intrinsic asthma with or without chronic bronchitis, there are many similarities with chronic bronchitis and high intragroup variations (23). According to Lopez-Vidriero and Reid (23), "sputum chemistry does not diagnose disease but tells the relative importance of the various processes," i.e., gland hypertrophy with mucus glycoprotein markers and inflammatory process with serum glycoprotein markers.

References 9, 13, 18, 21, 30, 31, 34, 38, and 39 give detailed results of methods of MG separation into many fractions. We here summarize the main results, i.e., the isolation of a major glycoprotein component in the gel phase with a carbohydrate content ranging from 60 to 70% (w/w), composed of fucose, galactose, galactosamine, glucosamine, and sialic acid, and with an amino acid pattern of the protein core accounting for 40 to 50% of total amino acid residues by hydroxyamino acids (serine, threonine) and proline (30,32). A further fractionation of this glycoprotein yields fractions rich in sulfate and sialic acid, but it is not possible to separate single fuco, sialo, and sulfoglycoproteins, as it was previously thought of (4,30,32).

Different MG show a continuous variation according to their sulfate and sialic acid content (32). Sulfate content is greater in larger oligosaccharides, and sialic acid content is highest in the small oligosaccharides (9). Blood group activity has been found in oligosaccharidic chains of the neutral MG units (4,32). According to ion-exchange chromatography and isoelectric focusing, MG show a strong net acid charge, which is a uniform characteristic independent of molecular size (19).

Different approaches to MG biochemistry have been discussed according to their increasing complexity. Physicians interested in such a field of mucology can choose the level of research according to the availability of equipment and to the parameters they want to consider. Marker dosage is the most simple and the cheapest solution and gives good results in both clinical and applied pharmacological studies. MG fraction separation is far more complex and expensive, but it is the preferred method for fine biochemical and basic pharmacological studies. The use of radiolabeled compounds is complex, too, but it allows the performance of dynamic studies on MG synthesis under different conditions.

REFERENCES

1. Aminoff, D. (1961): Methods for the quantitative estimation of *N*-acetylneuraminic acid and their application to hydrolysates of sialomucoids. *Biochem. J.*, 81:384–392.
2. Antonopoulos, C. A. (1962): A modification for the determination of sulfate in mucopolysaccarides by the benzidine method. *Acta Chem. Scand.*, 16:1521–1522.
3. Boas, N. F. (1953): Method for the determination of hexosamines in tissues. *J. Biol. Chem.*, 204:553–563.

4. Boat, T. F., and Cheng, P. W. (1980): Biochemistry of airway mucus secretions. *Fed. Proc.*, 39:3067–3074.
5. Boat, T. F., Cheng, P.W., Iyer, R. N., Carlson, D. M., and Polony, I. (1976): Human respiratory tract secretions. (Mucous glycoproteins of nonpurulent tracheobronchial secretions, and sputum of patients with bronchitis and cystic fibrosis.) *Arch. Biochem. Biophys.*, 177:95–104.
6. Carlstedt, I. (1982): "Normal" respiratory mucin. *Eur. J. Respir. Dis.*, 63:493–495.
7. Cessi, C., and Piliego, F. (1960): The determination of amino sugars in the presence of amino acids and glucose. *Biochem. J.*, 77:508–510.
8. Creeth, J. M. (1978): Constituents of mucus and their separation. *Br. Med. Bull.*, 34:17–24.
9. Creeth, J. M., Bhaskar, K. R., Horton, J. R., Das, I., Lopez-Vidriero, M. T., and Reid, L. (1977): The separation and characterization of bronchial glycoproteins by density-gradient methods. *Biochem. J.*, 167:557–569.
10. Das, L., Lopez-Vidriero, M. T., and Reid, L. (1974): A simple sensitive enzymatic assay method for determination of mannose in glycoproteins. *Abstr. Commun. 9th Meet. Fed. Eur. Biochem. Soc.*, p. 438.
11. Dische, Z. (1955): New color reactions for determination of sugars in polysaccharides. In: *Methods of Biochemical Analysis*, edited by D. Glyck, Vol. II, pp. 313–358. Interscience Publishers, New York.
12. Dische, Z., and Shettles, L. B. (1951): A new spectrophotometric test for the detection of methylpentose. *J. Biol. Chem.*, 192:579–582.
13. Feldhoff, P. A., Bhavanandan, V. P., and Davidson, E. A. (1979): Purification, properties, and analysis of human asthmatic bronchial mucin. *Biochemistry*, 18:2430–2436.
14. Gallagher, J. T., and Kent, I. W. (1975): Structure and metabolism of glycoproteins and glycosaminoglycans secreted by organ cultures of rabbit trachea. *Biochem. J.*, 148:187–196.
15. Gibbons, M. N. (1955): The determination of methylpentoses. *Analyst*, 80:268–276.
16. Hall, R. L., Miller, R. J., Peatfield, A. C., Richardson, P. S., Williams, I., and Lampert, I. (1980): A colorimetric assay for mucous glycoproteins using alcian blue. *Biochem. Soc. Trans.*, 8:72.
17. Honda, S. (1984): High-performance liquid chromatography of mono- and oligosaccharides. *Anal. Biochem.*, 140:1–47.
18. Houdret, N., Le Treut, A., Lhermitte, M., Lamblin, G., Degand, P., and Rouseel, P. (1981): Comparative action on reducing agents on fibrillar human bronchial mucus under dissociating and non-dissociating conditions. *Biochim. Biophys. Acta*, 668:413–419.
19. Kaliner, M., Marom, Z., Patow, C., and Shelhamer, J. (1984): Human respiratory mucus. *J. Allergy Clin. Immunol.*, 73:318–323.
20. Kaliner, M., Shelhamer, J. H., Borson, B., Nadel, J., Patow, C., and Marom, Z. (1986): Human respiratory mucus. *Am. Rev. Respir. Dis.*, 134:612–621.
21. Lamblin, G., Lhermitte, M., Degand, P., Roussel, P., and Slayter, H. S. (1979): Chemical and physical properties of human bronchial mucus glycoproteins. *Biochimie*, 61:23–43.
22. Lehninger, A. L. (1977): *Biochemistry*. Worth Publishers, New York.
23. Lopez-Vidriero, M. T., and Reid, L. (1978): Chemical markers of mucous and serum glycoproteins and their relation to viscosity in mucoid and purulent sputum from various hypersecretory diseases. *Am. Rev. Respir. Dis.*, 117:465–477.
24. Lopez-Vidriero, M. T., and Reid, L. (1978): Bronchial mucus in health and disease. *Br. Med. Bull.*, 34:63–74.
25. Lowry, O. H., Rosebrough, N. J., Farr, A. L., and Randall, R. J. (1951): Protein measurement with the Folin phenol reagent. *J. Biol. Chem.*, 193:265–275.
26. Mancini, G., Carbonara, A., and Heremans, J. F. (1965): Immunochemical quantitation of antigens by single radial immunodiffusion. *Immunochemistry*, 2:235–254.
27. Marom, Z., Shelhamer, J., Alling, D., and Kaliner, M. (1984): The effects of corticosteroids on mucous glycoprotein secretion from human airways "in vitro." *Am. Rev. Respir. Dis.*, 129:62–65.
28. Moretti, M., Giannico, G., Marchioni, C. F., and Bisetti, A. (1984): Effects of methylprednisolone on sputum biochemical components in asthmatic bronchitis. *Eur. J. Respir. Dis.*, 65:365–370.
29. Reid, L., and Clamp, J. R. (1978): The biochemical and histochemical nomenclature of mucus. *Br. Med. Bull.*, 34:5–8.
30. Roberts, G. P. (1974): Isolation and characterisation of glycoproteins from sputum. *Eur. J. Biochem.*, 50:265–280.

31. Roberts, G. P. (1976): The role of disulfide bonds in maintaining the gel structure of bronchial mucus. *Arch. Biochem. Biophys.*, 173:528–537.
32. Roberts, G. P. (1978): Chemical aspects of respiratory mucus. *Br. Med. Bull.*, 34:39–41.
33. Roe, J. H. (1955): The determination of sugar in blood and spinal fluid with anthrone reagent. *J. Biol. Chem.*, 212:335–343.
34. Rose, M. C., Lynn, W. S., and Kaufman, B. (1979): Resolution of the major components of human lung mucosal gel and their capabilities for reaggregation and gel formation. *Biochemistry*, 18:4030–4037.
35. Stockley, R. A. (1984): Measurement of soluble proteins in lung secretions. *Thorax*, 39:241–247.
36. Terho, T. T., and Hartiala, K. (1971): Method for determination of the sulfate content of glycosaminoglycans. *Anal. Biochem.*, 41:471–476.
37. Warren, L. (1959): The thiobarbituric acid assay of sialic acids. *J. Biol. Chem.*, 234:1971–1975.
38. Williams, I. P., Hall, R. L., Miller, R. J., and Richardson, P. S. (1982): Analyses of human tracheobronchial mucus from healthy subjects. *Eur. J. Respir. Dis.*, 63:510–515.
39. Woodward, H., Horsey, B., Bhavanandan, V. P., and Davidson, E. A. (1982): Isolation, purification, and properties of respiratory mucus glycoproteins. *Biochemistry*, 21:694–701.

APPENDIX I. TECHNICAL DETAILS

Flow Chart 1

Pronase digestion of sputum (31)

1. Suspend mucus sample at a concentration of about 5 mg/ml in 0.5 M Tris–HCl buffer, pH 8.0, containing 2 mM calcium acetate.

2. Add pronase (0.5 mg/ml final concentration) and a drop of toluene to prevent microbial growth.

3. Incubate the solution at 37°C for 24 hr.

4. At 22 hr, add a further quantity of pronase to a final concentration of 0.7 mg/ml.

Flow Chart 2

Dosage of fucose according to Gibbons (15)

1. Prepare standard solution with L(-)fucose.

2. Put in duplicate test tubes (labeled A and B) 0.5 ml of standard solution and of mucus sample diluted 1:100.

3. Add sulfuric acid (2.2 ml of a 6 + 1 solution) in ice-cold bath, incubate in boiling water for 10 min, and then cool in tap water.

4. Add 50 μl of tioglicolic acid (3.3% v/v) in tubes labeled A.

5. Shake and keep in dark for 3 hr.

6. Read samples spectrophotometrically at 400 and 430 nm wavelengths.

7. Results are obtained according to this formula:

$$(A400 - A430) - (B400 - B430) = \text{reading}$$

8. Calculate the quantity of fucose giving values on a standard curve obtained with L(-)fucose.

Flow Chart 3

Determination of the sulfate content of MG according to Terho and Hartiala (36). Two different methods can be used.

Procedure with Sodium Rhodizonate

1. Prepare a $BaCl_2$ buffer solution composed of 2 M acetic acid, 5 mM $BaCl_2$, and 0.02 M $NaHCO_3$, 10%, 2%, and 8% (v/v), respectively, in absolute ethanol (solution A).

2. Prepare a solution of sodium rhodizonate 25% (w/v) in water, add 100 mg L-ascorbic acid, and shake until complete dissolution is achieved. Add ethanol up to a volume of 100 ml. The solution, which is light brown, should be used after 30 min and is stable for 2 days (solution B).

3. Prepare sulfate standard solutions in the concentration range 4 to 24 μg/ml of water with Na_2SO_4 or sulfuric acid.

4. Add 0.5 ml each of samples, standards, and water (blank) in test tubes containing 2.0 ml ethanol.

5. Centrifuge test tubes until contents are clear.

6. Pipette 1.0 ml of solution A and 1.5 ml of solution B into each test tube and shake well.

7. Let the tubes stand 10 min in the dark at room temperature.

8. The intensity of the developed color is spectrophotometrically read at 520 nm; color is stable for 30 min.

Note. Do not clean glassware with sulfuric acid but with nitric acid. Rinse repeatedly in distilled water.

Procedure with Benzidine

1. The following solutions are prepared:
   A. 0.5% benzidine in 94% ethanol
   B. 1:1 (v/v) acetone/94% ethanol
   C. 0.5% thymol in 2 M NaOH
   D. 0.1 M $NaNO_2$
   E. Standard solutions are described in previous procedure

2. Pipette 1.0 ml each of samples, standards, and water into 10 ml centrifuge tubes with sharp pointed bottoms.

3. Add glacial acetic acid (1.0 ml), solution B (3.0 ml), and solution A (1.0 ml), shake tubes well, and leave them standing overnight at 4°C.

4. Centrifuge test tubes (3,000 g × 20 min) to remove benzidine sulfate precipitates and discard supernatants.

5. Wash away the excess benzidine from the precipitates, resuspending them with 9.0 ml of solution B and repeating the centrifugation step.

6. Dissolve precipitates in 1.5 ml 1.0 M HCl, shake test tubes, and leave them standing at room temperature for 30 min.

7. Add water (1.0 ml) and solution D (0.5 ml).

8. After 5 min add solution C (2.5 ml); a red color develops whose intensity is spectrophotometrically measured at 505 nm.

Note. Do not clean glassware with sulfuric acid but with nitric acid. Rinse repeatedly in distilled water.

Flow Chart 4

Dosage of mannose according to Dische (11)

1. Prepare standard solution with mannose (50 μg/ml).

2. Place in test tubes 0.9 ml of standard solution or of mucus sample and prepare a blank of water.

3. Add 0.1 ml of a 3% solution of cysteine hydrochloride.

4. Add 5 ml of sulfuric acid 75% (w/w).

5. Shake and heat at 100°C for 10 min.

6. Cool to room temperature.

7. Leave samples for 48 hr at room temperature. A faint yellow color may appear, which is not specific and does not affect the final reading.

8. Read samples spectrophotometrically at a wavelength of 340 to 355 nm.

9. Calculate the value of mannose quantity, reporting reading values on a standard curve obtained with a solution of mannose.

Notes

1. Best results are obtained when the mucus samples contain 10 to 100 μg/ml of mannose.

2. For the detection of mannose in the presence of other exoses, the optical density is determined at four different wavelengths, 400, 370, 375, and 350 nm. The ratio OD370 − OD400/OD350 − OD375 is <1 for mannose, 1 for galactose, and 2 for glucose. When twice as much (or more) glucose than mannose is present in solution, detection of mannose using this method becomes impossible.

Flow Chart 5

Dosage of *N*-acetylneuraminic (NANA) acid with the thiobarbituric acid assay according to Warren (37)

1. Prepare the following aqueous solutions with warming:
   A. Sodium periodate (meta) 0.2 M in 9 M phosphoric acid
   B. Sodium arsenite 10% in a solution of 0.5 M sodium sulfate − 0.1 N H_2SO_4
   C. Thiobarbituric acid 0.6% in 0.5 M sodium sulfate
   All solutions can be stored at room temperature and are stable for a month at least.
2. Prepare a standard solution with *N*-acetylneuraminic acid.
3. Put in test tubes 0.2 ml of water (blank), standard solution, and mucus sample (eventually diluted).
4. Add 0.1 ml of solution A.
5. Shake and allow samples to stand at room temperature for 20 min.
6. Add 1 ml of solution B and shake the tubes until the yellowish brown color disappears.
7. Add 3 ml of solution C, shake, and cap the tubes with a glass bead.
8. Heat in a vigorously boiling water bath for 15 min.
9. Remove the tubes and place in cold water for 5 min. The red color fades, and the solution often becomes cloudy, but this does not affect the final reading.
10. Transfer 1 ml of this solution to a tube containing 1 ml of cycloexanone.
11. Shake twice and centrifuge for 3 min at 4,000 rpm.
12. Spectrophotometrically read the absorbance of the organic phase at 549 nm against the blank.
13. The amount of NANA can be determined by this formula:

$$\mu M \text{ of NANA} = V \times OD549/57$$

where V is the final volume of the test solution.

Notes.

1. The following equation corrects for the absorbance at 549 nm, which does not derive from NANA:

$$\mu M \text{ of NANA} = 0.09 \times OD549 - 0.033 \times OD532$$

2. In the presence of large amounts of 2-deoxyribose, there is a second method of correction:

$$\mu M \text{ of NANA} = 0.138 \, OD562 - 0.009 \, OD532.$$

APPENDIX II. CHEMICAL, EQUIPMENT, AND INSTRUMENT MANUFACTURERS

Chemicals

Sigma Chemical Company, P.O. Box 14508, St. Louis, MO 63178, USA
BDH (British Drug Houses) Ltd, Poole, Dorset, UK

Pharmacia Fine Chemicals, Box 175 S-75104, Uppsala, Sweden
Serva Feinbiochemica, 6900 Heidelberg-I, Carl-Benz-Str 7, P.O. Box 105260,
  West Germany

Equipment for Chromatographic Procedures

Amicon Corporation, 17 Cherry Hill Drive, Danvers, MA 01923, USA
Alltech, 2051 Waukegan Rd, Deerfield, IL 60015, USA
Pharmacia Fine Chemicals, Box 175 S-75104, Uppsala, Sweden
NEN Chemical GmBH, D 6072 Dreieichenhain, Daimlerstrasse 23, Postfach 1240,
  West Germany

Instruments

Beckman, Rue des Pierres-du-Niton 17, CH-1207, Geneva, Switzerland; Fullerton,
  CA, USA (centrifuges, ultracentrifuges, spectrophotometers, amino acid analyz-
  ers)
Branson Sonic Power Company, Danbury, CT, USA
LKB-Produkter AB, Box 305, S-161 26, Bromma, Sweden (spectrophotometers,
  HPLC systems, amino acid analyzers)

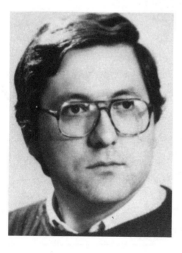

Mirco Lusuardi was born in Novellara (RE), Italy, in 1957. He received the M.D. degree in 1983 from the University of Modena, Italy. He is Hospital Assistant of the Division of Pulmonary Disease of the Clinica del Lavoro Foundation, Medical Center of Rehabilitation in Veruno (No), Italy. His interests are cytology and biochemistry of lung fluids.

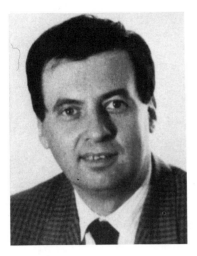

Claudio Ferdinando Donner was born in Varese, Italy, in 1948. He received the degree of Medical Doctor in 1972 from the University of Pavia, Italy. He is Chief of the Division of Pulmonary Disease of the Clinica del Lavoro Foundation, Medical Center of Rehabilitation in Veruno (NO), Italy. His research interests include pulmonary rehabilitation and home management of chronic respiratory failure, lung cytology, and biochemistry.

Methods in Bronchial Mucology,
edited by P. C. Braga and L. Allegra.
Raven Press, Ltd. © 1988.

3.1.2. Proteins, Deoxyribonucleic Acid, and Ion Identification

M. Moretti

*Istituto di Tisiologia e Malattie, Dell'Apparato Respiratorio, Università di Modena,
Modena, Italy*

Since the early 1950s, some authors have focused their interest on the protein components of bronchial secretion. The progress in this research was related strictly to the improvement of the electrophoretic techniques combined with the production of specific antisera against human proteins. Initially, the sputum protein components were studied by electrophoresis on paper or cellulose acetate (40), but the various proteins were detected mainly by using immunoelectrophoresis and two-dimensional electrophoresis (6,17,41). The concentration of sputum proteins in bronchial secretion was assessed by single radial immunodiffusion (SRID) and electroimmunodiffusion (EID). These two methods are still widely employed in sputum research, and new immunological assays, such as immunonefelometry (IN) and enzyme-linked immunosorbent assay (ELISA), are coming into use (14, 15,42).

Concentrations of soluble proteins range from 0.1 to 0.5 g/100 ml, due particularly to different stages of bronchial inflammation (20). The term "protein" as used in this chapter means both the proteins themselves and the plasma-type glycoproteins, such as immunoglobulins, α_1-acid glycoprotein, and others. Some of the proteins found in sputum are transudated from serum, although a large percentage is produced locally either by bronchial tract cells or by systemic cells located in the respiratory tract (Table 1). The protein profile of sputum is similar to that of bronchial secretion

TABLE 1. *Proteins detected in sputum and their origin*

Proteins	Origin	Reference
Albumin Proalbumin Ceruloplasmin Haptoglobin Transferrin α_1-Acid glycoprotein α_1-Antichimotrypsin Hemopexin Fibrinogen Antithrombin III	*Passive diffusion from plasma*	17, 41, 42
	Bronchial production and passive diffusion	
IgA, IgG, IgM, IgE	Plasmacells	17, 42
C_3	Macrophages	42
α_2-Macroglobulin	Fibroblasts	
	Bronchial mucosa(?)	42
Lysozyme	Macrophages	
	Leukocytes	Chapters 3.3, Section 3.5
	Serous cells (submucosal glands)	
α_1-Antitrypsin	Macrophages	43
	Bronchial production	
Free secretory piece	Mucus cells (submucosal glands)	Chapter 3.3
S-IgA	Plasma cells and mu- cus cells	Chapter 3.3
Lactoferrin	Serous cells (submucosal glands)	Section 3.5
Low molecular weight inhibitor of elastase		34
Bronchial amylase		17

obtained during bronchoscopy. The latter has a lower protein concentration than the sputum sample because of the dilution effect of the anesthetic fluid (45).

This chapter describes the methods of sputum pretreatment and the techniques used for detecting the various proteins in the sputum sample. A list of manufacturers of chemicals, immunochemicals, and instruments used in these techniques can be found in Appendix I.

MATERIALS AND METHODS

Sputum Pretreatment

Sputum consists of a gel component dispersed in a continuous sol phase. Sputum physical inhomogeneity and viscoelasticity hamper pipetting and limit the electrophoretic resolution. A variable percentage of sputum proteins is bound to the mucus glycoproteins or entrapped in a fibrillar network. The purpose of mucus pretreatment is to homogenize sputum by reducing its viscosity and to solubilize all proteins without altering their native structure and the antigenic determinants. Chemical procedures to liquefy bronchial secretions have been used for several years, but recently the degradative effects of some preparative methods have been recognized.

Proteolytic Enzymes and Thiol Compounds

Proteolytic enzymes (chymotrypsin, trypsin, pronase, papain) and reducing agents (*N*-acetylcysteine, dithiothreitol, mercaptoethanol) solubilize mucus (19), but they also modify the structure of the sputum soluble proteins (17). Their liquefying activity is limited to preparative procedures for cytological analyses in bronchial secretions (28).

Electrolytes and Buffers

Several salts, such as sodium chloride and calcium chloride, have a good solubilizing effect on sputum (19). The electrolyte liquefying activity is due to the ionic strength of the solution rather than to the molar concentration (19); the ions work by reducing the electrostatic interactions between sputum proteins and mucus glycoproteins (14).

Harbitz et al. (14) evaluated the liquefying activity of various buffers at different pH values. The results of these experiments indicated that a sputum sample may be solubilized in phosphate buffer 0.07 M, pH 6.0, when NaCl 0.05 M is added. The sputum, diluted 1:6 with the buffer, was stirred gently at 4°C for 12 hr. The sample was then centrifuged at 17,000 *g* for 30 min, and the proteins in the supernatant were measured. The authors (14) reported that this procedure solubilized approximately 75% of the total amount of protein and carbohydrate in the sputum.

Some salts and buffers are compatible with the activity of degradative enzymes present in the sputum. Prolonged times of extraction expose the proteins to the risk of enzymatic degradation.

Miscellaneous Agents

Disodium versenate at concentrations greater than 0.25 M can liquefy sputum mainly because of its calcium-binding effect (19).

Urea in 4 M solution effectively solubilizes sputum, but at this concentration, it denatures the protein components (18,19).

Ion Exchange Cellulose

Mucus pretreatment consists of a protein extraction by means of an ion exchange cellulose. The sputum is mixed with a strong ionic exchanger (Ecteola-cellulose) in a phosphate–saline buffer. The acid mucins are fixed to the cellulose, and the proteins are extracted by the buffer. Sputum pretreatment is performed by adding 1 ml of sputum to 1 g of Ecteola-cellulose (wet substance) and 2 ml solution of phosphate buffer 0.001 M, pH 7.5 and NaCl 0.15 M. The mixture is subject to mild agitation for 4 hr at 4°C and centrifuged at 6,500 g for 15 min. The supernatant is collected for chemical analyses (17).

Sonication

Several authors (15,21,29,40) liquefied sputum by ultrasonic methods. The solubilizing activity of ultrasound seems to be due to hydroxyl radicals produced by a cavitation effect (9). Sonication breaks down the mucus fibrillar network into small flexible filaments, as shown by electron microscopy (39). Different procedures may be used to liquefy mucus. My method is to sonicate 2 to 3 ml of sputum sample in a 3 cm diameter test tube immersed in an ice bath. The tip of the sonicator is dipped just below the sample surface, which is submitted to six 20-sec bursts of ultrasound separated by equivalent periods of pause. The sonication is performed at 10 W and 20,000 Hz frequency. Very viscous samples may be sonicated even for 3 min, since this time of exposure does not destroy albumin, immunoglobulins, lysozyme, and lactoferrin (33). Girard et al. (13) showed that 19,500 Hz frequency and 2.5 min of sonication are the optimal conditions to homogenize sputum, when enzymatic activities are measured.

Centrifugation

High-speed centrifugations, such as 118,000 g for 4 hr (40), 160,000 g for 3 hr (21), 100,000 g for 1.5 hr (42), and 54,000 g for 1.5 hr (45), separate sputum into a clear liquid supernatant (sol phase) and a dense, viscous phase (gel phase). The sol phase contains the free proteins and, in some cases, a small amount of soluble glycoproteins, DNA, and lipids. The gel phase contains mainly the less soluble gel glycoproteins, together with a variable percentage of proteins and lipids bound to the mucus fibers (2). The sol/gel volume ratio varies significantly among sputa in relation to the speed and the time of centrifugation (21). The sol phase of ultracentrifuged samples does not always represent the concentration of proteins in the whole sputum. A variable proportion of albumin and immunoglobulins was found in the gel phase (2).

The isopyknic density-gradient centrifugation in cesium (9) separates sputum components on the basis of their buoyant densities: lipids, proteins, serum-type glycoproteins, mucus glycoproteins, and DNA, in order of increasing density. Density gradient ultracentrifugation is the method of choice to study native glycoproteins.

Various Techniques

Some authors (15) combine techniques, e.g., sputum is homogenized by ultrasound and then solubilized by agitation in a hypertonic buffer.

Estimation of Sputum Proteins

Immunological methods are used widely for quantitative analysis of sputum proteins. Such methods include SRID, EID, immunofluorimetric assay (IF), IN, and ELISA. The procedures for DNA and total protein assays are described also.

Single Radial Immunodiffusion

SRID is a quantitative technique that uses a layer of agarose in which a specific antiserum is uniformly incorporated. The antigen solution is placed in a hole within the antiserum containing gel. As the diffusion occurs, a circular immunoprecipitate area takes place, the diameter of which is related to the antigen concentration (8) (Appendix II).

Electroimmunodiffusion

EID, also called rocket immunoelectrophoresis or electroimmunoassay, is a quantitative method for the determination of antigens by a specific antigen–antibody reaction. The antigen solutions are placed in wells punched in an antiserum containing gel. During the electrophoretic migration through the gel, the antigen develops a long, rocketlike immunoprecipitate. The height of the precipitation peak is used to estimate the antigen concentration (12) (Appendix III).

Immunonefelometry

Appropriate concentrations of antigens and specific antibody form insoluble complexes that scatter the incident light in all directions. Nefelometers measure the scattered light by a detector generally situated at a 90 degree angle from the incident light. An electronic system transforms the variation of scattered light into protein concentration by using a calibration curve (38). The laser nefelometer differs because it detects the scattered light of a laser beam. IN has a good sensitivity, since it assesses protein concentrations greater than 20 mg/liter. Specific antisera for the most common plasma proteins are available for IN assay.

Fluorimetric Immunoassay

Some substances (fluorescent substances) may absorb light, rising to a high energy level that is dispersed in the form of heat and light. The fluorescent emission is proportional to the concentration of the substance and to the activating energy. Quantitative FI for human proteins uses the classic antigen–antibody reaction. The antigen is added to a solution of specific antibodies coupled to small hydrophilic immunobeds (immunoadsorbents). The antigen bonds to the immunoadsorbents, and a fluorescently labeled monospecific antiserum, added to the mixture, combines with the antigen–immunoadsorbent complex. The unreacted material is separated from the stable fluorescent antibody–antigen–immunoadsorbent complexes, which are assayed by a fluorimetric procedure (11). FI is a sensitive but time-consuming method and not easily automated. Only few FI kits are available for the estimation of proteins.

Enzyme-Linked Immunosorbent Assay

ELISA is an immunoassay that uses an enzyme-labeled reactant (an antigen or an antibody) to detect an unknown substance. At the end of the assay, the enzyme-labeled reactant bound to the unknown substance is measured by reaction with the specific enzyme substrate (24,44).

Various modifications of the ELISA have been used to assay both antigens and antibodies. The double antibody sandwich technique may be used to measure various proteins at low concentration in lung fluids, such as immunoglobulins. In this method a solid phase is coated with a specific antibody against the immunoglobulin being sought. The test solution, an enzyme-labeled specific antibody against the unknown immunoglobulin, and the enzyme substrate are added in succession.

The sensitized solid phase immobilizes the unknown immunoglobulin, which, in turn, is linked to the enzyme-labeled antibody. The color produced by the enzyme reaction is proportional to the concentration of the unknown immunoglobulin concentration.

ELISA is recommended for its ability to detect large size proteins in bronchial secretions. Immunoenzyme assay is considered less precise and sensitive than radioimmunoassay. However, the use of radioimmunoassay is limited by severe restrictions in the use of radioisotopes in the laboratory.

Estimation of Total Proteins

The Lowry method (copper-folin reaction) is widely accepted for the estimation of low quantities of proteins (25) because of its sensitivity and speed (Appendix IV). Some substances may interfere with the copper-folin reaction, reducing the its specificity (11).

Estimation of Deoxyribonucleic Acid

Dishie's diphenylamine method of DNA estimation at 100°C was modified by Croft and Lubran (10). Their method increases the sensitivity of the technique and offers a mathematical method for correcting the interference of sialic acid in the DNA estimation. The DNA measurement is an objective method to quantify sputum inflammation (20,32) (Appendix V).

Expression of Sputum Protein Concentration

The protein concentration is usually expressed as mg/ml of sputum or mg/g wet weight sputum. Some authors (37,46) showed a variability in sputum protein concentration within and between chronic bronchitis patients. The dilution of sputum proteins by saliva may account partially for the interpatient and intrapatient variability, but other factors must be considered, such as errors of estimation of bronchial proteins, the circadian rhythm of bronchial secretions, and different degrees of bronchial inflammation.

To overcome the dilutional factor by saliva, the results can be expressed as mg/g of total protein, or, preferably, either as mg/g of dry macromolecular weight (DMW) or by dividing each protein concentration, calculated in mg/ml of sputum, for the corresponding value of albumin.

The sputum/serum protein concentration ratio has been used to point out the local production or serum exudation of the proteins measured; this correction does not solve the problem of dilution.

Wiggins and Stockley (46) tried to overcome the interpatient and intrapatient variability by dividing the sputum/serum ratio of each protein by the sputum/serum albumin ratio. They concluded that "the standardization for albumin fails to overcome the problem . . . because the variability is not merely the result of a variable but simple dilutional effect caused by saliva" (46).

RESULTS

There are no sputum marker proteins that differentiate the major hypersecretive lung diseases (6,20). The degree of bronchial inflammation is the main responsible factor that influences the sputum protein concentration (42). In mucoid sputum, DMW, DNA, and small size plasma proteins are present in low concentrations, and the large serum proteins are detected primarily in the infected secretions. The purulent sputum has high values of albumin and serum acute phase proteins, such as α_1-acid glycoprotein, haptoglobin, and α_1-antitrypsin. Albumin particularly may be used as a marker of bronchial inflammation just because its small molecular size and high serum concentration favor its exudation.

Table 2 shows the average concentration of the most representative sputum proteins measured in four chest diseases, from various clinical investigations (5, 6,15,23). Albumin and serum acute phase proteins are significantly higher in patients

TABLE 2. *Sputum protein concentration in patients with chronic bronchitis, bronchiectasis, cystic fibrosis, and asthma*

	Chronic bronchitis[a]	Asthma[a]	Cystic fibrosis[a,b]	Bronchiectasis[c]
Albumin	24.0 (8.9)[d]	138.0 (100.0)	71.0 (40.0)[b]	87.5
Lactoferrin	27.0 (14.5)	27.0 (14.5)	94.0 (55.0)[b]	
Lysozyme	43.0 (27.6)	46.0 (25.7)	75.0 (21.0)[b]	
α_1-Acid glycoprotein	1.4 (1.1)	3.5 (3.4)	1.5 (1.5)[a]	2.5
Haptoglobin	2.2 (1.7)	6.5 (6.3)	2.0 (2.9)[a]	4.7
Transferrin	2.4 (1.2)	6.9 (3.9)	2.3 (1.5)[a]	6.5
α_1-Antitrypsin	2.4 (1.6)	11.0 (6.1)	20.0 (24.0)[b]	13.5
α_1-Antichymotrypsin	1.2 (0.7)	4.5 (1.8)	1.6 (1.4)[a]	2.5
IgA	76.0 (41.9)	14.0 (7.8)	64.0 (46.0)[b]	42.7
IgG	17.0 (9.7)	34.0 (26.3)	56.0 (41.0)[b]	35.5
IgM			13.0 (10.0)[b]	
C_3	1.1 (0.7)	2.3 (1.4)	1.0 (0.8)[a]	2.3
Dry molecular weight (DMW)[e]				
Mucoid sputum[f]	15.0 (4.9)	17.9 (11.9)	13.4 (5.9)	
Purulent sputum[f]	51.2 (16.2)		62.6 (7.2)	39.9 (10.5)

[a] Sputum sol phase, from ref. 6.
[b] Whole sputum, from ref. 15.
[c] Sputum sol phase, from ref. 5.
[d] Average protein concentrations are expressed in mg/dl ($\pm$SD).
[e] Average DMW is expressed in mg/ml ($\pm$SD).
[f] Whole sputum, from ref. 23.

with asthma, bronchiectasis, and cystic fibrosis. The asthmatic group was studied during an acute attack, and cystic fibrosis and bronchiectatic groups always included patients with chronically infected sputa. On the contrary, chronic bronchitics, who were investigated during a stable clinical period, had low sputum concentration of serum plasma proteins. The data in Table 2 clearly evidence the effect of inflammation on bronchial secretion, indicating that comparison among groups of patients must always take into account the percentage of infected sputa present in each group.

The study of sputum proteins gives prognostic information on bronchial diseases. In chronic bronchitics, the decrease in the sputum IgA/albumin ratio has been related to the progress of the disease (36). In fact, the increasing damage to bronchial mucosa is associated with a reduced IgA local secretion and increased plasma protein diffusion. In cystic fibrosis, Jacquot et al. (15) noticed a correlation between plasma proteins and the severity of the disease.

The clinical relevance of detecting sputum deficits in S-IgA and other local defense proteins is discussed in Chapters 3.3 and 3.4.

COMMENTS

Analysis of sputum proteins allows characterization of the bronchial secretion in terms of exudative component and deficit of local defense mechanisms. These data help the physician to choose adequate treatment and to evaluate the therapeutic results (29,31). Hence, easy and reliable techniques are required for sputum pretreatment and protein analysis.

The author compared the liquefying effect of four different mucus pretreatments on the same sputa collected from chronic bronchitics (30; Moretti, unpublished data). Four samples from each sputum were homogenized by, respectively, phosphate buffer pretreatment, sonication, sonication followed by solubilization in phosphate buffer, and ultracentrifugation at 59,000 g for 90 min. The concentrations of albumin, immunoglobulins, lysozyme, and lactoferrin were evaluated in the sputum samples after each treatment. The protein concentrations were similar in sputa sonicated or sonicated and then solubilized in phosphate buffer. In sputa either liquefied in phosphate buffer or ultracentrifuged, I found lower protein concentrations than in the sonicated samples.

SRID is the method of choice to measure sputum proteins. It is a brief technique that does not require sophisticated and expensive instruments. The SRID plates, for normal and low range concentrations (>10 mg/liter), are produced by several chemical industries. The evaluation of SRID precipitates by the endpoint method is recommended, even if the results are available after 48 to 72 hr. Errors of estimation may occur with SRID when S-IgA and α_1-antitrypsin are assessed (for further details, see Chapters 3.3 and 3.4). The underestimation of S-IgA may be overcome partially by using either a correction factor or 80% of S-IgA as the reference standard.

The IN is a good alternative to SRID because it slightly understimates S-IgA using 7S IgA as standard and speeds up the procedure of analysis in automated instruments. On the other hand, the required predilution of the sample for some IN assays decreases the sensitivity of the technique.

The EID has similar characteristics to SRID, but a limited number of samples are processed per electrophoretic chamber.

Less than 50 ng/ml of protein may be measured easily by ELISA, which is the method of choice to detect immunoglobulins or other proteins in highly diluted lung fluids, such as bronchoalveolar lavage fluid. There are no ELISA kits available on the market to assay the most common plasma proteins. Hence, setting up the ELISA technique for each sputum protein is time consuming.

ION IDENTIFICATION

pH

In normal subjects, the pH of airway mucus has been measured on sputum produced after inhalation of prostaglandin $F_{2\alpha}$ (22) or directly in the bronchial airway (4). Boden et al. (4) found an endobronchial pH of 6.58 in normal airways. This value did not vary significantly with the level of the bronchial tree, but it became acidic in the presence of pneumonia. The pH measurements were obtained by fibrobronchoscopy and represent more the epithelial surface pH than the true value of mucus plugs (4). In pathological studies, several authors (3,40) have noticed that there is a wide range of sputum pH between 6.0 and 8.5, although significant differences among the bronchial hypersecretive diseases have not been found. These results may be liable to criticism. The pH was measured at different times in the sputum collection and, in some cases, on the sol phase of ultracentrifuged sputum. It is well known that the sputum pH becomes increasingly alkaline in open air because of the loss of carbon dioxide. Hence, it is obvious that sputum pH measurement requires some precautions. The assay has to be performed on an homogenized, freshly produced sputum, which has been neither diluted nor centrifuged. A pH electrode connected to a pH meter is used.

Electrolytes

The electrolyte composition and osmolarity of bronchial secretions were studied both in laryngectomized patients considered as ''normal'' controls and in various hypersecretive bronchial diseases (3,35,40). The sputum ion content was found to be related to the degree of infection in the sample. Calcium, phosphorus, and potassium concentrations were higher in purulent than in mucoid sputum (35). Infected secretions had lower contents of sodium and chloride, and that was probably due to a back diffusion to keep an osmotic balance (35). Several authors (35,40) failed to differentiate bronchial diseases in terms of sputum ionic content. Neverthe-less, it has been suggested that, in cystic fibrosis, hydroelectrolytic disorders of bronchial mucosa could explain both the fundamental alterations of the disease and the colonization of lung secretions by only a few bacterial species (16).

Measurement of sputum electrolytes must be carried out on the whole sputum specimen that has been homogenized. Potassium and sodium are bound mainly to soluble macromolecules that are separated easily from the sputum gel phase by centrifugation (3), whereas calcium and chloride are partially tied to the macro-molecules of the gel phase (3). Sodium and potassium usually are estimated in sputum by flame photometry using lithium as an internal standard. Various methods, such as photometry, fluorimetry, and atomic absorption, were proposed to measure ions in biological fluids. The photometric technique was used frequently for measur-ing phosphate (1), chloride (47), calcium (7), and magnesium (27) in sputum. Photometric analysis is preferred because the technique is carried out without sophisticated, expensive equipment.

REFERENCES

1. Bartlett, G. R. (1959): Colorimetric assay methods for free and phosphorylated glyceric acid. *J. Biol. Chem.*, 234:466–475.
2. Bhaskar, K. R., and Reid, L. (1980): Application of density gradient methods to study the composi-tion of sol and gel phases of CF sputa and the isolation and characterization of epithelial glycoproteins from the two phases. In: *Perspectives in Cystic Fibrosis. Proceedings of the 8th International Cystic Fibrosis Congress,* Toronto. May 26–30, edited by J. M. Sturgess, pp. 113–121.
3. Boat, T. F., and Matthews, L. V. (1973): Chemical composition of human tracheobronchial secretions. In: *Sputum, Fundamentals and Clinical Pathology,* edited by M. J. Dulfano, pp. 243–273. Charles C Thomas, Springfield, IL.
4. Boden, C. R., Lampton, L. M., Miller, P., Tarka, E. F., and Everett, E. D. (1983): Endobronchial pH: Relevance to aminoglycoside activity in gram-negative bacillary pneumonia. *Am. Rev. Respir. Dis.,* 127:39–41.
5. Brogan, T. D., Davies, B. H., Ryley, H. C., Ross, P. I., and Neale, L. (1980): Composition of bronchopulmonary secretions from patients with bronchiectasis. *Thorax,* 35:624–627.
6. Brogan, T. D., Ryley, H. C., Neale, L., and Yassa, J. (1975): Soluble proteins of bronchopulmonary secretions from patients with cystic fibrosis, asthma and bronchitis. *Thorax,* 30:72–79.
7. Clark, E. P., and Collip, J. B. (1925): A study of Tisdall method for the determination of blood/ serum calcium with a suggested modification. *J. Biol. Chem.,* 63:461–466.
8. Clausen, J. (1971): *Immunochemical Techniques for the Identification and Estimation of Macro-molecules.* North-Holland Publishing Company, Amsterdam.
9. Creeth, J. M. (1978): Constituents of mucus and their separation. *Br. Med. Bull.,* 34:17–24.
10. Croft, D. N., and Lubran, M. (1965): The estimation of deoxyribonucleic acid in the presence of sialic acid: Application to analysis of human gastric washing. *Biochem. J.,* 95:612–620.
11. Curtis, H. Ch., and Roth, M. (1974): *Clinical Biochemistry: Principles and Methods,* Walter de Gruyter, Berlin.
12. Gaál, Ö., Medgyesi, G. A., and Vereczkey, L. (1980): *Electrophoresis in the Separation of Biological Macromolecules.* Wiley, Chichester, UK.
13. Girard, F., Tournier, J. M., Polu, J. M., Puchelle, E., Beck, G., and Sadoul, P. (1981): Ultrasonic method of sputum homogenization and its application in the study of the enzymic content of sputum. *Clin. Chim. Acta,* 113:105–109.
14. Harbitz, O., Jenssen, A. O., and Smidsrad, O. (1980): Quantitation of proteins in sputum from patients with chronic obstructive lung disease. *Eur. J. Respir. Dis.,* 61:84–94.
15. Jacquot, J., Tournier, J. M., Carmona, T. G., Puchelle, E., Chazalette, J. P., and Sadol, P.

(1983): Proteines des secretions bronchiques dans la mucoviscidose, role de l'infection. *Bull. Eur. Physiopathol. Respir.*, 19:453–458.

16. Kilbourn, J. P. (1984): Composition of sputum from patients with cystic fibrosis. *Curr. Microbiol.*, 11:19–22.

17. Laine, A., and Hayem, A. (1976): Identification et caracterization des constituants proteiques de la secretion bronchique humaine. *Clin. Chim. Acta*, 67:159–167.

18. Lieberman, J. (1967): *In vitro* evaluation of the mucolytic action of urea. *J.A.M.A.*, 202:694–696.

19. Lieberman, J. (1968): Measurement of sputum viscosity in a cone-plate viscometer. II. An evaluation of mucolytic agents *in vitro*. *Am. Rev. Respir. Dis.*, 97:662–672.

20. Lopez-Vidriero, M. T., Das, I., and Reid, L. (1977): Airway secretion: Source, biochemical and rheological properties. In: *Respiratory Defense Mechanisms*, edited by J. D. Brain, D. F. Proctor, and L. Reid, pp. 289–356. Marcel Dekker, New York.

21. Lopez-Vidriero, M. T., Das, I., and Reid, L. (1979): Bronchorroea—Separation of mucus and serum components in sol and gel phases. *Thorax*, 34:512–517.

22. Lopez-Vidriero, M. T., Das, I., Smith, H. P., Picot, R., and Reid, L. (1977): Bronchial secretion from normal human airways after inhalation of prostaglandin $F_{2\alpha}$, acetylcholine, histamine and citric acid. *Thorax*, 32:734–739.

23. Lopez-Vidriero, M. T., and Reid, L. (1978): Chemical markers of mucous and serum glycoproteins and their relation to viscosity in mucoid and purulent sputum from various hypersecretory diseases. *Am. Rev. Respir. Dis.*, 117:465–477.

24. Lovborg, U. (1984): *Guide to Solid Phase Immuno Assay.* A/S Nunc, Roskilde, Denmark.

25. Lowry, O. H., Rosebrough, N. J., Farr, A. L., and Randall, R. J. (1951): Protein measurement with the folin–phenol reagent. *J. Biol. Chem.*, 193:265–275.

26. Mancini, T. C., Carbonara, A., and Heremans, J. F. (1965): Immunochemical quantitation of antigens by single radial immunodiffusion. *Immunochemistry*, 2:235–254.

27. Mann, C. K., and Yoe, J. H. (1956): Spectrophotometric determination of magnesium with sodium I-azo-2-hydroxy-3-(2,4-dimethylcarboxaniledo)-naphthalene-I'-(2-hydroxybenzene-5-sulfonate). *Anal. Chem.*, 28:202–207.

28. Miller, D. L. (1963): A study of techniques for the examination of sputum in a field survey of chronic bronchitis. *Am. Rev. Respir. Dis.*, 88:473–483.

29. Moretti, M., Giannico, G., Marchioni, C. F., and Bisetti, A. (1984): Effects of methylprednisolone on sputum biochemical components in asthmatic bronchitis. *Eur. J. Respir. Dis.*, 65:365–370.

30. Moretti, M., Marchioni, C. F., Natali, P., Masci, G., and Bisetti, A. (1984): Le traitement préalable des crachats pour l'analyse quantitative des IgA bronchiques (Abstr.). *J. Immunol.* 11:19–20.

31. Moretti, M., Masci, G., Natali, P., Marchioni, C. F., and Bisetti, A. (1986): Effetti favorevoli del 6-metilprednisolone a breve termine sulle S-IgA, sulla lattoferrina e sul lisozima delle secrezioni tracheobronchiali in bronchitici cronici asmatiformi. *G. Ital. Mal. Torace*, 40:417–419.

32. Moretti, M., Natali, P., Masci, G., Penitenti, F., and Marchioni, C. F. (1986): Determinazione del grado di purulenza dell'espettorato: Confronto fra una tecnica fotometrica ed una microscopica. *Lotta Tuber. Mal. Polmon. Soc.*, 56:186–189.

33. Moretti, M., Natali, P., Masci, G., Penitenti, S., Marchioni, C. F., and Bisetti, A. (1986): Trattamento dell'espettorato con ultrasuoni quale metodica preparativa a determinazioni biochimiche non-analitiche. *Lotta Tuberc. Mal. Polmon. Soc.*, 56:183–185.

34. Ohlsson, K., Tegner, H., and Akesson, U. (1977): Isolation and partial characterization of a low molecular weight acid stable protease inhibitor from human bronchial secretion. *Hoppe-Seylers Z. Physiol. Chem.*, 358:583–589.

35. Potter, J. L., Matthews, L. W., Spector, S., and Lemm, J. (1967): Studies on pulmonary secretions. II. Osmolarity and the ionic environment of pulmonary secretions from patients with cystic fibrosis, bronchiectasis and laringectomy. *Am. Rev. Respir. Dis.*, 96:83–87.

36. Puchelle, E., Girard, F., Beck, G., Hayem, A., Bailleul, V., and Laine, A. (1975): Propriétés rhéologiques et biochimique de l'espectoration. Role de l'infection. *Pathol Biol.*, 23:541–545.

37. Puchelle, E., Zahm, J. M., and Havez, R. (1973): Donnees biochimiques et rhéologiques dand l'expectoration. III. Relation des protéines et mucines bronchiques avec les propriétes rhéologiques. *Bull. Physiopathol. Respir.*, 9:237–256.

38. Ritchie, R. F., Alper, C. A., Graves, J., Pearson, N., and Larson, C. (1973): Automated quantitation of proteins in serum and other biologic fluids. *Am. J. Clin. Pathol.*, 59:151–159.

39. Rose, M. C., Voter, W. A., Brown, C. F., and Kaufman, B. (1984): Structural features of human tracheobronchial mucus glycoprotein. *Biochem. J.*, 222:371–377.

40. Ryley, H. C., and Brogan, T. D. (1968): Variation in the composition of sputum in chronic chest diseases. *Br. J. Exp. Pathol.*, 49:625–633.
41. Ryley, H. C., and Brogan, T. D. (1973): Quantitative immunoelectrophoretic analysis of the plasma protein in the sol phase of sputum from patients with chronic bronchitis. *J. Clin. Pathol.*, 26:852–856.
42. Stockley, R. A., Mistry, M., Bradwell, A. R., and Burnett, D. (1979). A study of plasma proteins in the sol phase of sputum from patients with chronic bronchitis. *Thorax*, 34:777–782.
43. Tournier, J. M. (1980): Importance de l'equilibre proteases-antiproteases des secretions bronchiques dans la genese des brochopneumopathies chroniques. *Acts of 24th Session d'enseignement post-universitarie—Nancy*, March 24–28.
44. Voller, A., Bartlett, A., and Bidwell, D. E. (1978): Enzyme immunoassay with special reference to ELISA techniques. *J. Clin. Pathol.*, 31:507–520.
45. Wiggins, J., Hill, S. L., and Stockley, R. A. (1983): Lung secretion sol-phase proteins: Comparison of sputum with secretions obtained by direct sampling. *Thorax*, 38:102–107.
46. Wiggins, J., and Stockley, R. A. (1983): Variability in sputum sol phase protein in chronic obstructive bronchitis. The value of using albumin for standardization. *Am. Rev. Respir. Dis.*, 128:60–64.
47. Zall, D. M., Fisher, D., and Gardner, M. Q. (1956): Photometric determination of chlorides in water. *Anal. Chem.*, 28:1665–1672.

APPENDIX I. CHEMICAL, IMMUNOCHEMICAL, AND INSTRUMENT MANUFACTURERS

Chemicals

Aldrich-Chemie, D-7924 Steinheim, West Germany
BDH Chemical Ltd., Poole, UK
Fluka Chemishe Fabrik, CH-9470 Buchs, Switzerland
Merk, Darmstadt, West Germany
Sigma Chemical Company, P.O. Box 14508, St. Louis, MO 63178, USA

Immunochemicals

Behring Institut–Behringwerke AG, Marburg, West Germany
Bio-Rad, 2200 Wright Ave., Richmond, CA 94804, USA
Dako Patts a/s, P.O. Box 1359, Dk-2600 Glostrup, Denmark
Miles Scientific, 30 W. 475 North Aurora Road, Naperville, IL 60566, USA
Sigma Chemical Company, P. O. Box 14508, St. Louis, MO 63178, USA
Zymed Laboratories, Inc., 52 South Linden Ave., South San Francisco, CA 94080, USA

Equipments for ELISA

Flow Laboratories, P.O. Box 17, Second Avenue, Industrial Estate, Irvine, Ayrshire, Scotland
Nunc, Post Box 280, Kamstrup, OK 4000, Roskilde, Denmark

Equipment and Gel Media for Gel Electrophoresis

FMC, Marine Colloid Division, Rockland, ME 04841, USA
Behring Institut–Behringwerke AG, Marburg, West Germany
LKB Produkter AB, Box 305, S-16126 Bromma, Sweden
Pharmacia Fine Chemicals, Box 175 S-75104, Uppsala, Sweden

Equipment for Nefelometry

Beckman, Rue des Pierres-du-Niton 17, CH-1207 Geneva, Switzerland
Behring Institut–Behringwerke AG, Marburg, West Germany

Sonicators

B. Braun, P.O. Box 346, D-3508 Melsungen, West Germany
MSE, Manor Royal, Crawley, West Sussex, UK
Branson Sonic Power Company, Danbury, CT, USA

APPENDIX II. SINGLE RADIAL IMMUNODIFFUSION (SRID)

Material and Equipment

Agarose medium electroendosmosis (1% in barbital buffer)
Buffer solution, pH 8.6: 41.2 g sodium barbital, 8 g barbital in 1 liter distilled
    water
Specific antiserum and standard antigen solution
10 × 10 cm glass plates

After boiling, mix the liquid agarose with the monospecific antiserum at 56°C in a water bath. The antiserum concentration depends on the test sample dilution and the antibody titer. Pour 10 ml of the solution into a container made of two glass plates held 1.0 mm apart by a U-frame. Punch 2.5 mm holes in the gel, 1.2 cm apart from each other. Fill each well with 5 µl antigen solution; leave three wells for the standards. For low range plates, punch 4 mm holes and fill with 20 µl antigen solution.

Evaluation

Read the precipitation ring diameters after 48 to 72 hr (endpoint method by Mancini et al., 26). The unknown antigen concentration is determined from the calibration curve made by plotting the standard concentration in the abscissa and the respective squared ring diameters in the ordinate.

APPENDIX III. ELECTROIMMUNODIFFUSION (EID)

Material and Equipment

Agarose medium electroendosmosis (1% in barbital buffer)
Specific antiserum and standard antigen solution
Electrophoresis buffer: 41.2 g sodium barbital, 8 g barbital in 1 liter distilled water
Fixing solution: 14 g picric acid in 1 liter distilled water; warm solution to 40°C and then filter it; add 200 ml glacial acetic acid
Staining solution: 5 g Coomassie brilliant blue R, 450 ml ethanol 96%, 100 ml glacial acetic acid, 400 ml distilled water; filter solution
Electrophoresis chamber and supporting plate with cooling coil
Power supply, minimum 300 V and capacity of 150 mÅ per electrophoresis cell
10 × 10 cm or 20 × 11 cm glass plates

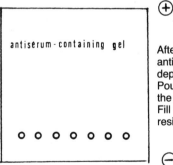

After boiling, mix the liquid agarose with the monospecific antiserum at 56°C in water bath. The antiserum concentration depends on the test sample dilution and the antibody titer. Pour 10 ml or 22 ml warm agarose–antibody solution into the plate; punch holes of 2.5 mm diameter in the gel layer. Fill in the wells with 5 μl antigen solution when the electrophoresis is running; leave three wells for the standards.

Electrophoretic Conditions

Put the barbital buffer in contact with the gel plate in the electrophoresis chambers by double Whatman No. 1 paper bridges

Field strength: 1.5 to 4.0 V/cm
Electrophoresis time: 18 to 24 hr (facultative use of cooling conditions)

Staining

Wash the plate in saline solution for 10 min and then in distilled water; leave the plate in the fixing solution for 15 min. Dry the gel plate under filter paper and blotting paper, pressed by a glass plate weighing 1 kg for 30 min; dry the plate with warm air. Stain with Coomassie brilliant blue solution for 1 hr. Wash out the excessive dye with the solvents of the staining solution three times.

Evaluation

Measure the height of the precipitation peaks between the tip of the rocket precipitate and the upper edge of the well. Measure the antigen concentration by the calibration curve.

APPENDIX IV. LOWRY METHOD OF ESTIMATION OF TOTAL PROTEINS

Reagents

A. 2% Na_2CO_3 in 0.1 N NaOH
B. 0.5% $CuSO_4$ $5H_2O$ in 1% sodium or potassium tartrate
C. The alkaline copper solution is made at the time of use by adding 50 ml of reagent A to 1 ml of reagent B
D. Diluted folin-ciocateus phenol reagent to 1 N in acid

Procedure

1. Add up 0.2 ml of sputum sample diluted 1:200 in distilled water to 1 ml of solution C; mix and let stand for 10 min at room temperature.
2. Add 0.1 ml of reagent D and mix immediately.
3. After 30 min, read the absorbance at 500 nm against blank, or at 750 nm for protein concentration below 25γ per ml of final volume.

The concentration is read from an analytical curve obtained with geometric dilutions of bovine serum albumin ranging between 12.5 γ/ml and 100 γ/ml.

APPENDIX V. ESTIMATION OF DNA

Reagents

Diphenylamine
Acetaldehyde
Glacial acetic acid
Concentrated sulfuric acid
Highly polymerized calf thymus DNA
0.005 N sodium hydroxide
1 N and 0.5 N perchloric acid

Diphenylamine solution. Dissolve 2 g diphenylamine in glacial acetic acid and add 1.5 ml sulfuric acid; make up the mixture to 100 ml with glacial acetic acid. Just before use, add 0.1 ml acetaldehyde solution (2% in distilled water) to each 20 ml diphenylamine solution.

Procedure

Prepare the stock standard DNA solution by adding 4 g of highly polymerized calf thymus DNA to 10 ml 0.005 N NaOH. The various DNA standards are prepared from the stock standard DNA solution in 10 ml test tubes:

Standard DNA (concentration)		Stock standard DNA (ml)		$1 N HClO_4$ (ml)		0.5 N $HClO_4$ (ml)
10 γ/ml	=	0.20	+	0.20	+	7.6
15 γ/ml	=	0.30	+	0.30	+	7.4
25 γ/ml	=	0.50	+	0.50	+	7.0

Dilute the sputum samples in 10 ml test tubes according to the degree of purulence with perchloric acid to bring them into the range of standard DNA solutions:

		Sputum sample (ml)		1 N $HClO_4$ (ml)		0.5 N $HClO_4$ (ml)
Mucoid sputum	=	0.25	+	0.25	+	4.5
Mucopurulent sputum	=	0.10	+	0.10	+	4.8
Purulent sputum	=	0.05	+	0.05	+	4.9

Heat the test tubes at 70°C for 20 min, then cool them in running water; centrifuge the hydrolyzed sputa at 3,000 rpm for 15 min. Add 2 ml aliquots in duplicate for standard and sputum sample to 2 ml diphenylamine solution. The mixture is stirred and then placed at 30°C for 20 hr. Read the sputum sample against blank at 550 nm and 600 nm.

The DNA concentration in the sample is calculated at 600 nm, and at 550 nm any possible interference of the sialic acid is shown. The DNA standard solutions are read at 600 nm. The corrected E'_{600} value for sputum DNA concentration is calculated by:

$$E'_{600} = \frac{1.39 \times E_{600} - 0.72 \times E_{500}}{1 - (1.92 \times E_{550} - 1.04 \times E_{600})}$$

The final E'_{600} for each sample is read from the DNA standard analytical curve.

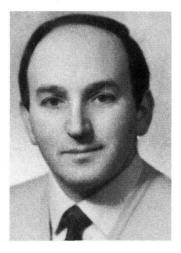

Maurizio Moretti was born in Ancona, Italy, in 1953. He received the M.D. degree in 1977 from the University of Bologna, Italy. He is Hospital Assistant in the Institute of Pneumology, University of Modena, Italy. He is interested in biochemical components and rheological properties of bronchial secretions.

Methods in Bronchial Mucology,
edited by P. C. Braga and L. Allegra.
Raven Press, Ltd. © 1988.

3.2. Surfactant Identification and Investigation

L. Allegra

Istituto di Tisiologia e Malattie, Dell'Apparto Respiratorio, Ospedale Maggiore di Milano, Milano, Italy

Direct methods
Indirect methods
Surfactant and mucociliary transport

For more than three decades, the presence and function of surfactant have been related to the lung alveoli almost exclusively. This can be seen from the commonly used term "alveolar surfactant." However, the material lining the bronchial wall must also be of crucial significance for the mechanical stability of the bronchial system and, therefore, for pulmonary ventilation. A few morphological, histological, and functional findings are reviewed here.

The epithelium of trachea and bronchi includes secretory goblet cells. Their frequency decreases as the bronchial diameter decreases. Within the upper part of the bronchial tree (in the cartilaginous bronchi), secretory cells are arranged in larger groups, which are called "intraepithelial glands." At inside bronchial diameters of less than 0.8 mm, the goblet cells are progressively rare and are always single. They disappear at a diameter of 0.5 mm (inside diameter). With a further decrease in diameter, down to 0.1 to 0.2 mm, a new type of nonciliated cell, the Clara cell, appears. The terminal and respiratory bronchi are characterized by this cell type. The terminal bronchi still have some ciliated cells; the respiratory bronchi do not.

The Clara cells are secretory cells, like the goblet cells, but their secretions are different physicochemically. This was realized by Max Clara himself. He wrote that "no mucus-like substance can be demonstrated by any mucus-specific strains in such cells, so that their secretion is not a mucus-like substance" (11).

The material lining bronchi decreases in viscosity with decreasing bronchial diameter. Within the small bronchi, the fluid is rather watery. This change from watery to viscous lining fluid is a strong argument for the critical roles of the following:

1. The surface forces determining the mechanical stability of small bronchi follow a modified Laplace law, suitable for application to cylindric geometry:

$$P = 2 \gamma/r$$

where P is pressure; γ is surface tension; r is the radius of the cylinder. As a consequence, to separate wetted surfaces distanced in capillary dimensions, requires considerably greater force if the wetting fluid is viscous. With a viscous wetting fluid, the very small bronchi if closed would possibly never again be opened by physiological forces.

2. The cilia-independent transport velocity within and onto the lining surface also is greater in a more watery system because of the greater fluidity.

To consider the relation of surfactant action to transport phenomena, one has to clarify its ultrastructural biochemical and physicochemical nature. At least four distinct ultrastructural types are known: lamellar bodies (LB), tubular myelin (TM), common myelin (CM), and interfacial or surface film (IF). The existence of an amorphous state is theoretically possible but has not been demonstrated. The intracellular LB are the sites of storage and secretion. The TB represents the first step in structural transformation, i.e., the disintegration of LB. The formation of TM may require divalent cations (35). The mode of formation of CM is not known. It might be created from LB directly, from TM, or from both. However, the structural transformation observed in rat fetal pulmonary fluid suggests a sequence LB–TM–CM (Fig. 1).

LB and TM consist of bimolecular phospholipid leaflets. This bimolecular leaflet structure ultimately will become unstable, and small globular micelles of lipid might then be formed if the cholesterol ratio increases in the sheet (19). Rapid uptake and temporary storage of cholesterol in type I but not type II cells has been observed, and there is cholesterol within the extracellular lining layer (14,30). This suggests an extracellular interaction between surfactant phospholipids and cholesterol. A cholesterol-dependent breakdown of bimolecular LB and/or TM leaflets to globular micelles and a rearrangement of the latter to CM structures can be postulated. However, CM structures (Fig. 2) are predominant outside the cells and are found from the alveolar septum to the larger bronchi (22,40). Surface film has been observed at the alveolar surface (38) and at the intrabronchial air–liquid interface (40). It probably originates from the above-mentioned structures or from a hypothetical amorphous surfactant.

Less is known about the contribution of Clara cells to the biochemical and ultrastructural nature of surfactant. They are generally considered to be secretory

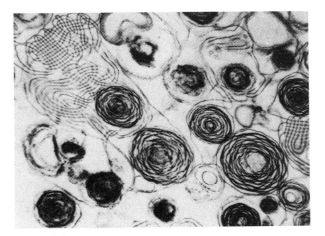

FIG. 1. Lamellar bodies, tubular myelin, and common myelin structures. (From ref. 32.)

cells, and their function is presumably linked to the chemical and physical properties of the lining of small airways, which could behave as a kind of bronchial surfactant limiting airway and lung collapse (39).

The conditions described are the morphological, histological, and ultrastructural background for the concept of surfactant-supported transport phenomena summarized in Fig. 3 (32). Surfactant secretion in the alveoli and the transport along the bronchiolar zone (no glands, no cartilage) produce a concentration gradient toward the trachea. Static and dynamic surface transport must result. The static surface transport is a result of surface film pressure, i.e., the movement of film

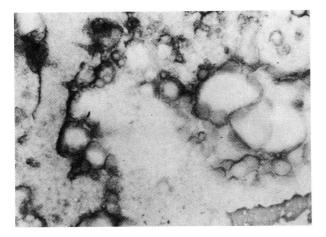

FIG. 2. Common myelin structures in a sample obtained by the alveolar micropuncture rinsing technique (rat lung). (From ref. 32.)

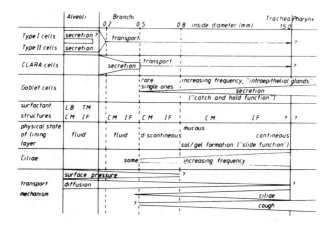

FIG. 3. Histological, ultrastructural, physical, and morphological parameters involved in fluid and mucus transport. (CM) Common myelin; (IF) interfacial or surface film; (LB) lamellar bodies; (TM) tubular myelin. (From ref. 32.)

molecules along the gradient in an open system. The dynamic surface transport during continued compression and decompression of the surface results from surface pressure hysteresis. If film molecules are absorbed from the subphase during decompression, the adsorption kinetics are greater than the kinetics of respreading; the backward movement of particles floating on top of the surface must be less than the forward movement during compression. A net directed movement of particles results. This was demonstrated by Rensch et al. some years ago (33).

Inspiration and expiration are asymmetric changes of the total alveolar area, always beginning at the periphery and progressing to the hili, which is why the movement of the pleura can be compared in this respect with the barrier movement in the trough model. Along the nonmucus zone of airways, surfactant transport within the subphase simply arises from concentration gradients.

The transport of mucus along the bronchial zone (with glands and cartilage) usually is attributed mainly to ciliary function. More recently, the interaction between mucus transport and surfactant has attracted attention. The presence of structured surfactant within the sol phase (lammellar figures) (Fig. 4) and between the sol and gel phases has been demonstrated (22). We do not know whether CM vesicles act directly, like biological ball-bearings, or, more likely, indirectly by donating molecules to surface and interfaces. However, the effect of surfactant on the bronchial wall can be interpreted as a soft soap function, enabling the mucus and/or the sputum to slide on top of the cilia (31).

This would imply also that surfactant is important for an effective cough mechanism (slide-function). In Fig. 5, the adhesive surfaces are represented by zigzag lines and are comparable to an adhesive fastener. If this bronchus should be closed, the wall would very likely stick together because the outer surfaces of these cells are composed of a layer of mucopolysaccharides 200 to 1,000 Å thick (9,17).

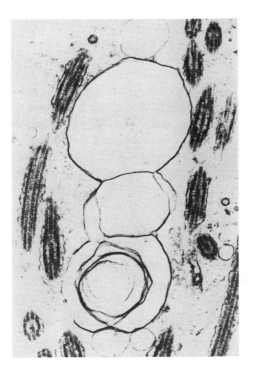

FIG. 4. Foamy aspect of surfactant between cilia (tangential section) in the sol phase of sputum. (From ref. 22.)

This layer of mucopolysaccharides is intimately associated with the cell membrane. Depending on the nature of the molecules, strong adhesive forces may result between the mucopolysaccharide surface of the cells and the mucus. The mucus or the sputum would not slide but would stick to the wall, as they stick to each other.

To investigate surfactant, direct or indirect methods can be used (24,36).

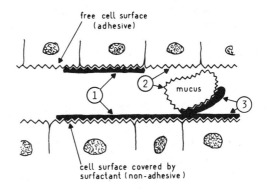

FIG. 5. Schematic representation of interaction among cell surface, surfactant, and mucus. (1 and 3) Surface active substances; (2) cell membranes. (Modified from ref. 32.)

DIRECT METHODS

Chemical Analysis of Surfactant Composition

The first step is to obtain the substances to analyze from mammalian lungs by extraction or washing techniques. The tensioactive substances (surfactant) can be obtained by extraction techniques, which include squeezing (27), micropuncture (30), trituration, and homogenization of bloodless lung fragments, followed by extraction with isotonic solution (20). Surfactant also can be collected mechanically by washing techniques, either endobronchial washing (13) or bronchoalveolar washing with isotonic solution.

Lipids can be obtained by extraction of bronchial lavage or BAL or from alveolar and tissue surfactant in chloroform:methanol (2:1 vol/vol) (15), and phospholipid can be determined by phosphate measurement according to the method of Bartlett (4). Individual phospholipids can be separated by the thin-layer chromatography method of Gilfillan et al. (16), using chloroform:methanol:petroleum either:acetic acid:boric acid (40:20:30:10:1 (vol/vol/vol/vol/wt) as the developing solvent. After removal of the other phospholipid fractions from the thin-layer chromatographic plate, phosphatidylcholine can be treated directly on the plate with 5% osmium tetroxide for separation of unsaturated phosphatidylcholine, using chloroform:methanol:ammonium hydroxide (80:26:6 vol/vol/vol) as the developing solvent.

A second possibility is to perfuse an isolated lung through the pulmonary artery with isotonic solution. Lung accesses are first closed to allow the passage of the solution into the alveoli. The surfactant is collected in the trachea, into which it has been pushed by pulmonary movements induced by a suction-pushing pump (7). Although it has been investigated in mammalians and humans under several experimental conditions, there are still different opinions about the composition of the pool of substances in the lining layer of the alveolus. However, there is agreement about the presence of a watery hypophase containing proteins and the presence of a pool of phospholipids and other kinds of lipids, such as cholesterol, triglycerides, and fatty acids, but in lower concentrations than phospholipids. The β-γ-dipalmitoyl-l-α_2-phosphatidylcholine (a tensioactive substance) is particularly abundant. Other tensioactive phospholipids, such as phosphatidylcholine, phosphatidylethanolamine, phosphatidylserine, phosphatidylglycerol, phosphatidylinositol, and sphingomyelin, are also present in surfactant.

Construction of Area/Surface Tension Curves

This kind of curve is characteristic for the surfactant or for tensioactive substances from lung and can be plotted after using a Wilhelms balance (Fig. 6) to measure

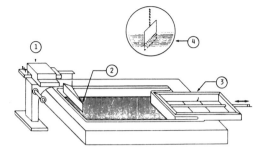

FIG. 6. Wilhelms balance. (1) Force transducer; (2) platinum thin-plate; (3) movable sidewall; (4) meniscus produced by liquid on the thin-plate.

the surface tension. There is a container in which the surfactant forms a layer on a subphase of isotonic or buffered solution. The container also has a thin-plate joined to a force transducer to record the surface tension of the liquid. Using a movable sidewall to adjust the dimensions of the surface where the tensioactive substance is, it is possible to record the changes in the surface tension through the changes in the resulting forces on the thin-plate (12).

By this method, the surface tension of surfactant from mammalian lung is extremely low, approaching 0 dyne/cm, in correlation with the decreasing surface of surfactant. Changing the surfactant area, the surface tension changes from values near 0 at greatest compression to 40 to 50 dyne/cm at greatest expansion. During an expansion–compression cycle, the surface tension has a peculiar hysteresis different from that of other nonbiological tensioactive substances (e.g., detergents) or biological nontensioactive substances (e.g., plasma), thus showing that the elasticity of this material is not perfect (Fig. 7).

FIG. 7. Surface tension (Wilhelms balance) of water, plasma, detergent, and rat pulmonary extract during an expansion–compression cycle. (Modified from ref. 13.)

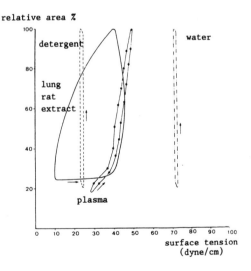

INDIRECT METHODS

Study of Stability of Bubbles from Aerated Lung Fragments

When one observes under the microscope a drop of water into which was squeezed a fragment of lung, a great number of small bubbles of constant dimensions can be seen. The constancy of size could be due to low surface tension at the liquid–gas interface or to the impermeability of the gas through the surface film of the bubbles. This second possibility can be discarded because when air bubbles are produced in boiled water (from which air has been eliminated), the new bubbles disappear within a short time (Fig. 8B), demonstrating that the surface film is not impermeable to air. The stability of the bubbles thus depends on the surface tension and can be correlated with the amount of surfactant (Laplace law: P = 2 γ/r, where P is the pressure of the bubble, γ is the surface tension, and r is the radius of the bubble) (Fig. 8C). In the presence of physiological surfactant, the stability of the bubble is greater because of a better balance between the inside and outside pressures (Fig. 8A) (25,26).

Construction of Quasistatic Pressure–Volume Curves in Isolated Lung

This technique is based on the construction of quasistatic compliance curves during filling and emptying with air or isotonic solution of an isolated and bloodless (2,3,29,37).

In the experimental animal, the lung is made atelectatic and bloodless by giving the animal pure O_2 to breathe for 8 min. Then the trachea is ligated and the abdominal aorta is cut. The lung is isolated, and the trachea is cannulated. The lung is insufflated and desufflated with air, and the pressures corresponding to various degrees of expansion are measured to obtain quasistatic volume–pressure curves (Fig. 9). With this technique, it is possible to reproduce the mechanical

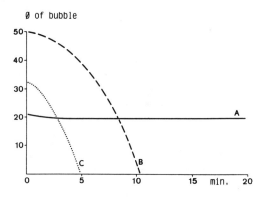

FIG. 8. Modification of bubbles diameter (from a fragment of lung) in relationship to time (A) Bubbles from lung with surfactant; (B) bubbles from lung in boiled water; (C) bubbles from lung lacking surfactant. (Modified from ref. 26.)

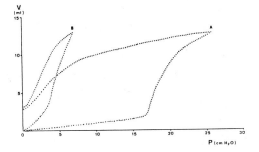

FIG. 9. Volume–pressure curves from atelectatic lungs of rat insufflated with air (A) or saline (B) and then de-sufflated.

conditions of lung, which are related to the tissue elastic forces and to the surface tension. When the air is replaced with an isotonic solution, the surface tension is eliminated, and by comparing the two curves during the recoil phase, it is possible to evaluate the contribution of the surfactant alone to the elasticity of the lung.

Electron Microscopy Investigations

With electron microscopy, intrapneumocytic osmiophilic inclusions (lamellar bodies) or inclusions in the Clara cells, considered to be the site of production of the surfactant (21), can be seen. These bodies also can be seen outside the cells on the alveolar surface or within the cilia. These are TM or CM, considered to be precursors of the surfactant that lines the alveoli (23).

In 1959, there was observed a laminar endoalveolar structure thought to be the surfactant film (10), with images showing continuity between the lumen of the lamellar bodies and the lumen of the alveolus (5).

Fluorescence Microscopy Investigations

Under the microscope with ultraviolet fluorescence, pulmonary tissue shows a clear yellow-green fluorescent line (thickness 1 μm) that is adherent to the alveolar wall in correspondence with the air–tissue interface (18). This line is broken or absent when the surfactant is damaged or surface tension is increased (6).

The Curti and Bracco technique (34) applied to biopsy tissue also gives clear images of the presence of surfactant in the pneumocytes II along the alveolar outline.

SURFACTANT AND MUCOCILIARY TRANSPORT

Addition of surfactant to an *in vitro* model consisting of ciliated mucosa (frog palate) that has no capacity to secrete surfactant can change the rate of mucociliary transport. Measurement of mucociliary clearance to give the rate of mucociliary transport on the mucosa of the frog palate is carried out by the method of Puchelle et al. (28).

The frog is decerebrated, and the palate is excised and kept in a transparent Plexiglas chamber under stable conditions of humidity (95–100%) and temperature (30 ± 0.5°C) from the time of excision to the end of the experiment. This moist chamber is constructed with a double wall to allow circulation of water to control the temperature. The floor and internal walls are covered with pads of wet gauze to increase humidity to the saturation point. The preparation can be observed through a window at the top of the chamber and filmed at low magnification with a stereomicroscope with a micrometric eyepiece to measure mucociliary transport velocity. Manipulation is carried out via glove openings on both sides of the chamber. Shortly after excision of the palate, the initial rate of mucociliary transport is tested by measuring the movement of a small aluminum disk (diameter 0.8 mm, thickness 0.01 mm, weight 0.8 mg). The repeated placement of disks on the palate produces a mechanical depletion of the mucus. In a few hours, the reduction of mucus is such that no motion of the disk can be observed. The aluminum markers are then placed with a drop of mucus freshly obtained from the palate of another frog on an excised palate for control readings.

To test the action of normal surfactant, the palate can be first sprayed (manual spray) either with saline or with surfactant extracted from normal animal or human lung and diluted 1:20 in saline. An aluminum marker and a drop of mucus are then applied, and the transport rate is measured. The volume of saline or surfactant solution applied is 0.25 ml. The ratio of transport rate with saline or surfactant

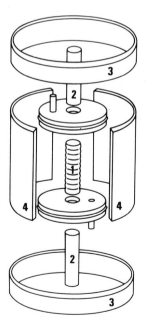

FIG. 10. Portable *in vitro* bath for unsubmerged trachea. (1) Isolated trachea; (2) cannulas; (3) metallic rings to close the chamber; (4) Plexiglas semicylindrical walls.

solution to transport rate with mucus only gives the relative transport rate, in which results are expressed. For each palate, the two materials (saline and surfactant) are each evaluated three consecutive times (in random order), and the means are calculated (1).

The behavior of surfactant activity in a bronchial *in vitro* model can be assessed also in an excised trachea or bronchus placed in a specially designed setting, such as the one devised by Braga and Allegra, shown in Fig. 10 (8). A microscope objective can be placed in this setting and modified to focus on the laminal surface of the bronchus or trachea and to observe ciliary beating and mucociliary transport in the presence or absence of surfactant.

REFERENCES

1. Allegra, L., Bossi, R., and Braga, P. C. (1985): Influence of surfactant on mucociliary transport. *Eur. J. Respir. Dis. (Suppl. 142)*, 67:71–76.
2. Allegra, L., Gioia, V., Monastero, A., and Purpari, L. (1966): La tensione di superficie alveolare in fisiopatologia respiratoria. *Minerva Pneumol.*, 5:216–222.
3. Allegra, L., Gioia, V., and Tocco, G. (1965): Modificazioni dell'elasticità polmonare determinate dalla protamina. *Riv. Sci. Tbc. Mal. Respir.*, 19:277–281.
4. Bartlett, G. R. (1959): Phosphorus assay in column chromatography. *J. Biol. Chem.*, 234:266–272.
5. Bensch, K., Schaefer, V. E., and Avery, M. E. (1964): Granular pneumocytes: Electron microscopic evidence of their exocrinic function. *Science*, 145:1318–1320.
6. Bolande, R. P., and Klaus, M. H. (1964): The morphologic demonstration of an alveolar lining layer and its relationship to pulmonary surfactant. *Am. J. Pathol.*, 45:449–453.
7. Bondurant, S., and Miller, D. A. (1962): A method for producing surface active extracts of mammalian lungs. *J. Appl. Physiol.*, 17:167–172.
8. Braga, P. C., and Allegra, L. (1987): Portable *in vitro* bath for not submerged trachea. (In press).
9. Brandt, P. W. (1962): A consideration of the extraneous coats of the plasma membrane. *Circulation*, 26:1075–1078.
10. Chase, W. A. (1959): The surface membrane of pulmonary alveolar walls. *Exp. Cell Res.*, 18:15–20.
11. Clara, M. (1937): Zur Histologie des Bronchialepitels. *Z. Mikrosk. Anat. Forsch.*, 41:321.
12. Clements, J. A. (1957): Surface tension of lung extracts. *Proc. Soc. Exp. Biol. Med.*, 95:170–174.
13. Clements, J. A. (1962): Surface tension in the lungs. *Sci. Am.*, 207:120–125.
14. Darrah, H. K., and Hedley-Whyte, J. (1971): Distribution of cholesterol in lung. *J. Appl. Physiol.*, 30:78–90.
15. Folch, J., Lees, M., and Sloan-Stanley, G. H. (1957): A simple method for the isolation and purification of total lipids from animal tissues. *J. Biol. Chem.*, 266:497–504.
16. Gilfillian, A. M., Chu, A. J., Smart, D. A., and Rooney, S. A. (1983): Simple phase separation of lung phospholipids including disaturated phosphatidylcholine. *J. Lipid Res.*, 24:1651–1660.
17. Groniowsky, J., and Biscyskowa, Y. (1964): Structure of the alveolar lining film of the lungs. *Nature*, 204:745–749.
18. Hackney, J. D., Rounds, D. E., and Schoen, A. W. (1963): Observation of a lipid lining in mammalian lungs. *Fed. Proc.*, 22:339–342.
19. Haydon, D. A., and Taylor, J. (1963): The stability and properties of bimolecular lipid leaflets in aqueous solution. *J. Theor. Biol.*, 4:281–296.
20. Levine, B. E., and Johnson, R. P. (1964): Surface activity of saline extracts from inflated and degassed normal lungs. *J. Appl. Physiol.*, 19:333–338.
21. Klaus, M. H., Reiss, O. K., Tooley, W. N., Piel, C., and Clements, J. N. (1962): Alveolar epithelial cell mitochondria as source of the surface-active lung lining. *Science*, 137:750–752.

22. Morgenroth, K. (1983): *Bronchitis*. PVG Pharmazentische Verlagsgesellschaft mbH, Munich.
23. Morgenroth, K. (1985): Morphology of the bronchial lining layer and its alteration in IRDS, ARDS and COLD. *Eur. J. Respir. Dis. (Suppl. 142)*, 67:7–18.
24. Pasargiklian, M., and Allegra, L. (1968): *Il Tensioattivo Alveolare in Pneumologia*. Minerva Medica, Torino.
25. Pattle, R. E. (1955): Properties, function and origin of the alveolar lining layer. *Nature*, 175:1125–1126.
26. Pattle, R. E. (1965): Surface lining of lung alveoli. *Physiol. Rev.*, 45:48–52.
27. Pattle, R. E., and Borgess, F. (1961): The lung lining film in some pathological conditions. *J. Pathol. Bacteriol.*, 82:315–319.
28. Puchelle, E., Girard, F., and Zahm, J. M. (1976): Rhéologie des secrétions bronchiques et transport mucociliaire. *Bull. Eur. Physiopathol. Respir.*, 12:771–780.
29. Radford, E. P. Jr. (1954): Method for estimating respiratory surface area of mammalian lungs from their physical characteristics. *Proc. Soc. Exp. Biol. Med.*, 87:58–63.
30. Reifenrath, R. (1973): Chemical analysis of the lung alveolar surfactant obtained by alveolar micropuncture. *Respir. Physiol.*, 19:35–46.
31. Reifenrath, R. (1978): Open airways—An engineering achievement of nature. *Bull. Eur. Physiopathol.*, 14:79–81.
32. Reifenrath, R. (1983): Surfactant action in bronchial mucus transport. In: *Pulmonary Surfactant System*, edited by E. V. Cosmi and E. M. Scarpelli. Elsevier Science Publishers, Amsterdam, New York, Oxford.
33. Rensch, H., Von Seefeld, H., Gebhardt, K. F., Renzow, D., and Sell, P. (1983): Stop and go particle transport in the peripheral airways? A model study. *Respiration*, 44:346–450.
34. Rossi, F. (1974): Ricerca della sostanza tensioattiva dell'induito alveolare umano con metodo istochimico in rilievo bioptico intraoperatorio. In: *Il Lining Alveolare*, edited by A. Mistretta and G. Ascani, pp. 19–25. Minerva Medica, Torino.
35. Sanders, R. L., Hassett, R. J., and Vatter, A. E. (1980): Isolation of lung lamellar bodies and their conversion to tubular myelin figures *in vitro*. *Anat. Rec.*, 198:485–501.
36. Scarpelli, E. M. (1968): *The Surfactant System of the Lung*. Lea & Febiger, Philadelphia.
37. Von Neergaard, K. (1929): Neue Auffassungen über einen Grundbegriff der Atemmechanik. Die Retraktionskraft der Lunge, abhängig von der Oberflächenspannung in den Alvealen, *Z. Ger. Exp. Med.*, 66:373.
38. Weibel, E. R., and Gil, J. (1968): Electron microscopic demonstration of an extracellular duplex lining layer of alveoli. *Respir. Physiol.*, 4:42–40.
39. Widdicombe, J. G., and Pack, R. J. (1982): The Clara cells. *Eur. J. Respir. Dis.*, 63:202–220.
40. Yoneda, K. (1976): Mucous blanket of rat bronchus. *Am. Rev. Respir. Dis.*, 114:837–842.

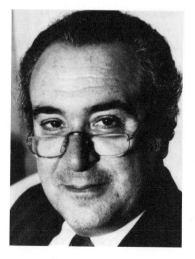

Luigi Allegra was born in 1938 in Palermo, Italy. He received the M.D. degree in 1961 from the University of Palermo, Italy. He is currently Full Professor of Pneumology and Chief of the Division of Pneumology of the University of Milan, School of Medicine, Milan, Italy. Fields of interests are bronchial asthma, chronic bronchitis, mucociliary clearance, and surfactant.

Methods in Bronchial Mucology,
edited by P. C. Braga and L. Allegra.
Raven Press, Ltd. © 1988.

3.3. Defensive Substances Identification

D. Olivieri and P. A. Mori

*Istituto de Clinica e Malattie, Dell'Apparato Respiratorio, Ospedale "G. Rasori,"
Parma, Italy*

Methodological approach
   IgG, IgM, IgE evaluation
   IgA, S IgA evaluation
   Lactoferrin
   Lysozyme
   Complement

The composition of human tracheobronchial secretions has been studied for many years (7,8). Although mucus is produced in both the mouth and the nose, it is possible to identify two functional and histological units: the upper respiratory tract, with the larynx, trachea, and bronchi, and the lower respiratory tract, i.e., the alveolar area. One of the principal problems in studying the mucus in the respiratory apparatus is the relative inaccessibility of native mucus.

METHODOLOGICAL APPROACH

Mucus is difficult to obtain because the quantity of secretion reaching the upper trachea is small. For obtaining mucus from the upper respiratory tract, there are two possibilities. The first method is to collect the sputum, which is a semisolid substance of gelatinous consistency, with characteristics that may change from one patient to another. Since there are always significant differences between the mucus produced in airways and that in the sputum, contamination of sputum by saliva introduces other variables. This has led to some confusion about its protein content. Some of these problems can be solved by using a systematic approach. Lack of homogeneity deriving from upper passage contamination can be avoided by collecting the sputum specimen early in the morning by expectoration following a careful mouthwash with physiological saline. Observations should be made on fresh expectorate in its native state (2).

The second method for obtaining bronchial secretions is to collect the mucus by bronchial aspiration during bronchoscopy, thus avoiding gross admixture of saliva. The bronchoscopy is performed under local anesthesia. When the amount obtained is insufficient, the bronchial tree is washed with 20 ml of prewarmed saline before aspiration.

The collection of both sputum and bronchial aspirations has two negative aspects. The sputum is usually obtained from patients with chronic nonpurulent bronchitis because in the normal subject, the quantity of secretions is very small. However, quantitative and qualitative differences exist between the secretions from normal subjects and those with bronchitis. Specimens obtained during bronchoscopy in subjects without pulmonary disease are not truly representative of the normal state, for bronchoscopy induces a state of hypersecretion in which the composition of secretions is altered.

The sputum samples and the bronchial aspirates should be processed to obtain a sol phase and a gel phase. The sol phase is used for protein analysis. One of the various methods that can be used is ultracentrifugation of the samples at 54,000 g for 90 min. In this way a sol phase is obtained, and it can be stored or immediately analyzed for its protein content (16).

The method used to study the second functional unit, the alveolar area, is bronchoalveolar lavage (BAL), employing a fiberoptic bronchoscope. After the respiratory tract is anesthetized with nebulized lidocaine, the bronchoscope is passed transnasally into a segmental bronchus, generally the lingula or the right middle lobe. One hundred fifty milliliters of sterile normal saline is instilled in three 50-ml portions and recovered by gentle suction. After centrifugation at 80 g for 10 min, the supernatant fluid is removed and stored at $-70°C$ until analyzed. By the use of BAL, we can easily assess the secretions of the alveolar area in control subjects and in various pulmonary diseases.

It is necessary to emphasize that the differential dilution of sputum, bronchial washings, and BAL fluid by sampling techniques makes comparison of protein concentrations in secretions from different levels of the bronchial tree complicated.

IgG, IgM, Ige Evaluation

The immunoglobulins are the most common proteins found in the bronchial mucus. The method usually used for determination of IgG and IgM is single radial immunodiffusion with immunoplates in agarose 1% (Behring) containing antiserum specific for each immunoglobulin. Into each well is placed 20 lt of supernatant. The diameters of the precipitin rings around the antigen wells are measured to within 0.1 mm. The concentration of immunoglobulin is extrapolated from a standard curve. The lower limit of detection for each protein assayed is: IgG 0.8 mg/100 ml and IgM 1.5 mg/100 ml. It is not usually possible with this method to detect IgM in control subjects (5).

In each study, the results are standardized for a standard protein (1). Generally for bronchial fluids, concentrations are expressed as a fraction of a standard protein, albumin. In fact, the immunoglobulins in bronchial mucus can have two sources: they can arise by transudation from the plasma trough, the blood–gas barrier, or they can be locally synthesized. In pulmonary disease, evaluation of immuno-globulin concentration in relation to albumin shows when the alveolar–capillary perme-ability significantly contributes to the increased amount of immunoglobulin. Albumin is not locally produced, and its concentration is a correct index of the permeability of the blood–gas barrier. Single radial immunodiffusion is a simple method, inexpen-sive and standardized, but it has a low sensitivity and it cannot resolve these important problems:

Because of the molecular size (IgM, 900,000 daltons), seepage of plasma proteins across the blood–gas barrier is not usually detected by single radial immunodiffu-sion.

IgE is present in a very low concentration.

Single radial immunodiffusion is not a sensitive and specific assay to assess the levels of IgG subclass proteins in respiratory secretions.

These problems have been resolved by a new method of protein analysis, enzyme-linked immunosorbent assay (ELISA) (6,14). This method provides high sensitivity and accuracy. Another highly sensitive immunoassay, the radioimmunoassay has some disadvantages that ELISA has overcome. The advantages of ELISA are no radiation hazard, relatively inexpensive reagents and equipment, and specific and sensitive assays of wide applicability.

With ELISA, it is possible to measure the concentrations of IgM and IgE in all samples. The immunoglobulins and albumin are measured by a double-antibody ELISA. Flat-bottomed polystyrol 96-well plates are coated overnight with commer-cial antibody (conjugated in alkaline phosphatase) against IgG, IgM, and albumin. Serial dilutions of each sample are made, and wells are filled with each dilution. The plates are incubated at room temperature with P-nitrophenyl phosphate for 30 min. We measure absorbance at 405 nm with a semiautomated ELISA plate reader. A standard curve relating optical density to known protein concentration is constructed for each individual assay by a linear regression. IgE is measured by the ELISA method using a kit obtained commercially (Behring).

In sputum, the concentration of each protein is expressed as a fraction of total protein, which is measured by the Lowry method. The protein levels are 6.04 mg/g for IgG, 0.3 mg/g for IgM, and 65.06 mg/g for albumin.

The concentration of each protein in BAL is expressed as a fraction of albumin. The protein levels are 3.369 mg/100 ml for albumin, IgG/albumin 0.266, IgM/albumin 0.001. IgE is present at a very low concentration in BAL fluid from normal subjects: 0.001 μg/mg of albumin (Table 1).

IgA and S IgA Evaluation

IgA is the predominant immunoglobulin class in lung secretions. Most of the IgA found is in the form of secretory IgA or 11S IgA (2,3). Secretory IgA, which is produced by plasma cells in the lamina propria, comprises two IgA molecules linked by another protein, J chain. which is also synthesized by plasma cells. In addition 11S IgA contains a glycoprotein called "secretory component" (SC), which mediates transport of dimeric IgA as S IgA across the glandular epithelium of the bronchi. IgA-producing plasma cells are more abundant in the glands and lamina propria of major bronchi than in the small bronchi, bronchioles, or alveolar septae. This observation suggests that most 11S IgA production occurs in the upper respiratory tract. In the lower respiratory tract, IgG is the predominant immunoglobulin class, but studies showing that secretory component and IgA with J chain are also located in bronchiolar, nonciliated epithelium and type II alveolar cells suggest that SC-mediated transport of dimeric IgA also could contribute appreciably to 11S IgA in the lower respiratory tract (5).

The single radial immunodiffusion method for determination of IgA, which uses anti-alpha-chain antibody and 7S IgA as a standard, results in a very inaccurate measurement of monomeric IgA, S IgA, and free SC. When assessing the integrity of the secretory IgA system, it is necessary to measure each of these components (4,13). In fact, the IgA in bronchial fluid is not exclusively 11S IgA; approximately 9% of the IgA is monomeric 7S IgA, and unbound SC is detected free and not in association with IgA. To measure the proportions of 11S IgA and 7S IgA, the method of Reynolds (15) is used. It was determined by sucrose density gradient fractionation that 90% of IgA in bronchial fluids is S IgA. The method is complex, and a less complex method developed by Laine et al. (10) can be used. It consists of thin-layer chromatography followed by crossed immunoelectrophoresis to identify

TABLE 1. *Immunoglobulin evaluation by single radial immunodiffusion in bronchoalveolar lavage* (BAL)

	Nonsmokers	Smokers
Albumin mg/100 ml	3.36 ± 3.5	6.56 ± 2.8
IgG/albumin	0.26 ± 0.1	0.32 ± 0.1
IgA/albmumin	0.13 ± 0.1	0.11 ± 0.1

the 11S and 7S IgA components. In this method, separation of monomeric and dimeric IgA can be performed easily (16).

Identification of free SC alone is more complex. The principal technique used to assess the amount of free SC was described by Merril et al. (12). It consists of a competitive double antibody radioimmunoassay. The assay detects antigenic components of SC that are exposed when the protein is free but covered when it is associated with IgA.

Stokley et al. (17) simplified the methods to measure the constituents of the S IgA system. The concentrations of albumin, IgA, and SC, either bound to the 11S IgA or free (FSC), are measured by single radial immunodiffusion with monospecific antisera. The anti-FSC is produced in the laboratory (17). All the other antisera are commercially available. The immunological properties of IgA are assessed by thin-layer chromatography and crossed immunoelectrophoresis.

In a paper by Wiggins et al. (18), results from sputum and BAL are standardized with respect to two proteins, albumin and SC. Using albumin, the intersubject variability in sputum increases significantly, whereas using SC, the opposite effect is observed. The reasons are not clear, but the authors conclude that, for the IgA system, albumin is a poor standardizing protein for sputum and a good protein for BAL. Therefore, standardization techniques for sputum and for Bal should be different. The absolute concentration of components of the IgA system is expressed as a percentage of an appropriate standard. In sputum, Wiggins et al. (18) found these results: albumin 0.58, IgA 17.28, 11S IgA 12.6, 11S IgA (% total IgA) 72.8, FSC 1.31, SC 5.99. In bronchoaspirate secretions, they found: albumin 0.33, IgA 8.14, 11S IgA 0.42, 11S IgA (% total IgA) 13.3, FSC 0.42, FSC 1.08. In BAL fluid, they found: albumin 0.05, IgA 0.49, 11S IgA 0.48, 11S IgA (% total IgA) 72.8, FSC 0.02, SC 0.08 (Table 2).

Lactoferrin

Lactoferrin is produced in bronchial mucosa. This protein can compete for iron ions with some bacteria, thus having bacteriostatic properties. Some fungi and bacteria, especially gram-negative species, show a marked dependence on free iron for growth factor and are greatly inhibited by chelators of free iron, such as lactoferrin.

Lactoferrin is present also in specific granules of neutrophils, and it has been demonstrated that this protein is an important component in the microbicidal activity of neutrophils. Lactoferrin enhances generation of the hydroxyl radical (OH) by human neutrophils during phagocytosis.

The protein content of each sample is determined by the single radial immunodiffusion test (Mancini) using antilactoferrin serum. It is detected normally in the secretions of the upper respiratory tract (9). The sputum concentration of lactoferrin in control subjects is 101 mg/g of protein. In BAL, transferrin is present in a concentration of 0.02 mg/mg of albumin.

TABLE 2. *Albumin, total IgA, 11S IgA, secretory component (SC), and free secretory component (FSC) concentrations (medians with ranges) for seven patients*[a,b]

	Sputum	HS[c]	BAL fluid
Albumin	0.58	0.33	0.05
	(0.37–1.47)	(0.13–0.71)	(0.01–0.19)
IgA	17.28	8.14	0.49
	(3.6–33.0)	(3.18–12.02)	(0.15–18.7)
11S IgA	12.6	0.42	0.48
	(1.35–26.7)	(0.3–7.3)	(0.11–1.55)
11S IgA	72.8	13.3	72.8
(% total IgA)	(28.7–85.6)	(3.3–78.6)	(8.3–97.0)
FSC	1.31	0.42	0.02
	(0.37–3.39)	(0.11–1.49)	(0.01–0.95)
SC	5.99	1.08	0.08
	(0.89–7.81)	(0.80–2.13)	(0.04–1.66)
FSC/SC	0.25	0.40	0.26
	(0.18–0.57)	(0.14–0.73)	(0.06–0.59)
FSC/11S	0.11	0.26	0.09
	(0.05–0.46)	(0.06–3.12)	(0.01–0.61)
FSC/albumin	2.31	0.85	1.0
	(0.64–3.57)	(0.49–4.52)	(0.0.8–5.11)
SC/11S	0.47	1.90	0.35
	(0.26–2.07)	(0.14–5.07)	(0.09–1.07
SC/albumin	9.59	4.22	3.83
	(1.53–13.3)	(1.44–6.21)	(0.46–9.44)

[a] From ref. 18.
[b] Expressed as percentages of the appropriate standards in the upper half of the table and as protein ratios in the lower half.
[c] HS, high secretions; BAL, bronchoalveolar lavage.

Lysozyme

Lysozyme is a common constituent of saliva and bronchial mucus (11). In fact, it is identified also in bronchial secretions uncontaminated by saliva. It can be identified readily by its cathodal electrophoretic mobility on paper.

Although lysozyme is active only against nonpathogenic bacteria when tested *in vitro,* it is possible to exclude its activity in phagolysosome for a wider spectrum of microorganisms. In bronchial secretions, lysozyme may originate from alveolar macrophages and presumably from bronchial glands. The action of lysozyme seems to be synergistic with IgA antibody and complement.

It is a hydrolytic enzyme with a molecular weight of 15,000, which acts specifically on the 1,4-glucosidic linkages of a tetramer of β-acetylglucosamine-β-acetyl-muramic acid, which is a structural unit of the cell walls of many bacteria. This biological property is used to estimate lysozyme by a turbidimetric method. A suspension of *Micrococcus lysodeikticus* is used as substrate, and known concentra-

TABLE 3. *Lactoferrin, lysozyme, C3, and C4 in sputum and bronchiolar lavage*

	Sputum	Bal	Reference
Lactoferrin	104.76[a]	0.02[b]	1, 9
Lysozyme	54.46[a]		9
C3	1.5[a]	2.1[c]	15
C4	0.4[a]	0.7[c]	15

[a] Protein content is calculated in mg/g of protein present in the sample.

[b] Protein content is calculated in mg/mg of albumin present in the sample.

[c] Protein content is calculated in µg/mg of albumin present in the sample.

tions of egg white lysozyme are used as the reference standard. The lysozyme activity is measured by spectrophotometer. The normal concentration is 49.5 mg/g of protein in sputum. The concentration cannot be determined using BAL (Table 3).

Complement

Components of the classic and the alternative pathways of the complement system also have been identified in the bronchial fluid. Levels of C3 and C4 are detected, but they are very low. The origin of this component is unknown, but some local synthesis by cells in the airways is suggested.

The components are measured by the single radial immunodiffusion assay employing immunoplates (1.0% agarose) containing antiserum specific for each component (Behring). The components of complement are normally detected in BAL. The mean concentration in control subjects is 0.7 µg/ml for C4 and 2.1 µg/ml for C3. Like the other proteins in the sputum, the concentration of C3 and C4 can be expressed in mg/g of protein present in the sample. The protein content in each sample is determined according to the method of Lowry; C3 is 1.5 mg/g and C4 is 0.4 mg/g of protein.

REFERENCES

1. Bell, D. Y., Haseman, J. A., Spock, A., McLennan, G., and Hook, G. (1981): Plasma proteins of the bronchoalveolar surface of the lungs of smokers and nonsmokers. *Am. Rev. Respir. Dis.*, 124:72–79.
2. Blasi, A., and Olivieri, D. (1973): Les IgA secretoires dans la defense immunologique de la muqueuse bronchique. Poumon Coeur, 24:383.
3. Blasi, A., and Olivieri, D. (1976): Deficits immunitaires et pathologie bronchopulmonaire (etude

des IgA secretoires chez 10 patients atteints de deficit en IgA serique et alterations broncho-pulmonaires d'origine congenitale). Broncho-pneumologie, 26:462.

4. Blasi, A., and Olivieri, D. (1976): Immunoglobulin A in serum and bronchial secretions (secretory IgA) in chronic lung diseases. *Bull. Int. Union against Tubercolosis* 51:611–615.

5. Burnett, D. (1986): Immunoglobulins in the lung. *Thorax*, 41:337–344.

6. Calhoun, W. J., Christman, J. W., Ershler, W. B., Graham, G. B., and Davis, G. S. (1986): Raised immunoglobulin concentrations in bronchoalveolar lavage fluid of healthy granite workers. *Thorax*, 41:266–273.

7. Chantler, E. N., Elder, J. B., and Elstein, M. (eds.) (1982): Mucus in health and disease. *Advances in Experimental Medicine and Biology*, Vol. II. Plenum Press, New York.

8. Dulfano, M. J. (ed.) (1973): *Sputum. Fundamentals and Clinical Pathology*. Charles C Thomas, Springfield, IL.

9. Gawel, J. (1979): Proteins in bronchial secretion of children with chronic pulmonary diseases. *Scand. J. Respir. Dis.*, 60:63–68.

10. Laine, A., Hayem, A., Lebas, J., and Romon, A. (1977): Determination du rapport IgA7S/IgA11S dans la secretion bronchique humaine par une technique associant la gel-filtration en couche mince a une immunoelectrophorese bidimensionelle. *Clin. Chim. Acta*, 79:541–548.

11. Mason, D. Y., and Taylor, C. (1975): The distribution of muramidase (lysozyme) in human tissues. *J. Clin. Pathol.*, 28:124–132.

12. Merril, W. W., Goodenberger, D., Strober, W., Matthay, R. A., Naegel, G. P., and Reynolds, H. Y. (1981): Free secretory component and other proteins in human lung lavage. *Am. Rev. Respir. Dis.*, 122:156–163.

13. Olivieri, D. (1978): The secretory immune system: Bronchial S IgA in patients with IgA-deficient sera. In: *Developments in Clinical Immunology*, edited by M. Ricci, A. S. Fauci, P. Arcangeli, and P. Torzuoli, p. 161. Academic Press, New York.

14. Rankin, J. A., Naegel, G. P., Scrader, C. E., Matthay, R. A., and Reynolds, H. Y. (1983): Air-space immunoglobulin production and levels in bronchioalveolar lavage fluid of normal subjects and patients with sarcoidosis. *Am. Rev. Respir. Dis.*, 127:442–448.

15. Reynolds, H. Y., and Newball, H. H. (1974): Analysis of proteins and respiratory cells obtained from human lungs by bronchial lavage. *J. Lab. Clin. Med.*, 84:559–573.

16. Stokley, R. A., Afford, S. C., and Burnett, D. (1980): Assessment of 7S and 11S immunoglobulin A in sputum. *Am. Rev. Respir. Dis.*, 122:959–964.

17. Stokley, R. A., Burnett, D., and Afford, S. C. (1981): The immunological measurement of "free" secretory piece and its relationship to local IgA production. *Clin. Exp. Immunol.*, 45:124–130.

18. Wiggins, J., Hill, S. C., and Stokley, R. A. (1984): The secretory IgA system of lung secretions in chronic obstructive bronchitis: Comparison of sputum with secretions obtained during fiberoptic bronchoscopy. *Thorax*, 39:517–523.

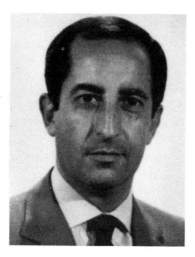

Dario Olivieri was born in Brindisi, Italy, in 1940. He received the M.D. degree in 1964 from the University of Parma, Italy. He is currently Chief of the Institute of Respiratory Diseases, University of Parma, Italy. Fields of interest include immunology, biochemistry, and internal medicine.

Pier Anselmo Mori was born in Parma, Italy in 1957. He received the M.D. degree in 1983 from the University of Parma, Italy. He is currently Hospital Assistant in the Institute of Pulmonary Diseases in the Hospital G. Rasori in Parma, Italy. His field of interest is Bal and biochemistry.

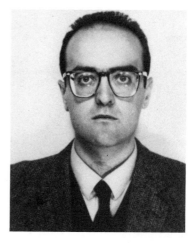

Methods in Bronchial Mucology,
edited by P. C. Braga and L. Allegra.
Raven Press, Ltd. © 1988.

3.4. Enzymes Identification: Protease and Antiprotease

*S. C. Afford and **R. A. Stockley

*Clinical Teaching Block and **Lung Immunobiochemical Research Laboratory,
The General Hospital, Birmingham, United Kingdom

Materials and methods
  Immunological quantitation of neutrophil elastase and α_1-proteinase inhibitor
    in sputum
Functional Assessment of neutrophil elastase and α_1-proteinase inhibitor
Discussion
Appendix

In recent years the protease-antiprotease theory of destructive lung disease (5) has created wide interest in the accurate assessment of enzymes and inhibitors in biological fluids, including lung secretions. Many enzymes, including those derived from macrophages and neutrophils, have been studied, as well as a variety of serum and locally derived inhibitors.

However, neutrophil elastase (NE) and α_1-proteinase inhibitor (α_1PI) have received most attention in relation to the pathogenesis of emphysema. This chapter relates largely to studies of these two proteins in the sputum sol phase (the fluid phase of sputum produced by high speed centrifugation). Nevertheless, the techniques and methodology are broadly applicable to other enzymes and inhibitors in the secretions. In addition, the interactions that occur between NE and α_1PI have been particularly well characterized *in vitro* (12), and this system therefore serves as the best available model for the potential investigator who wants to measure proteinases and proteinase inhibitors in secretions.

The methodological section of this chapter is divided into two parts. The first concentrates on approaches to the immunological quantitation of α_1PI and NE, and the second deals with the most appropriate methods for measurement of enzyme and inhibitor function in sputum.

MATERIALS AND METHODS

Immunological Quantitation of Neutrophil Elastase and α_1-Proteinase Inhibitor in Sputum

The concentration of individual proteins in sputum sol phase or lung lavage is subject to many variable factors. First, the source of the protein is critical, and those derived from the plasma (such as α_1PI) will vary according to the plasma concentrations and the degree of lung inflammation. The concentrations of locally produced proteins depend on the cells of origin and their activity. In addition, the secretion will be diluted to a varying degree by saliva or lavage fluid used to harvest them. Finally, immunochemical alterations within the secretions create problems with obtaining appropriate standards for use in the assays.

The range of concentrations is large, and several dilutions of each sample have to be run with each assay to maximize the likelihood of its falling within the range of standards used. In practice, several assays may have to be run before a result can be obtained, although results can be partly predicted. For a protein, such as α_1PI, the average sputum concentration for a patient with stable chronic bronchitis is of the order of 1 to 2% of the plasma level ($\approx$20–40 mg/liter).

The concentration range of the protein to be measured also affects the choice of assay. For obvious reasons, more sensitive techniques are required for low concentrations (as in lavage fluids), and they are usually more complicated and more expensive and may require inappropriate dilution of sample, such as sputum (where concentrations are higher), giving rise to greater errors. Less sensitive assays may be more appropriate with some secretions.

Because of the dilutional problems (saliva or lavage fluids), it is conventional to express protein concentrations as a ratio of an internal standard (albumin or total protein). In addition, the comparison of plasma/secretion ratios between proteins can be used as a means of identifying proteins that are preferentially concentrated in the lung. Values that exceed that expected for simple diffusion from plasma suggest local production. This indirect method has been used to indicate that much of the inhibitor α_1-antichymotrypsin is locally concentrated or produced in the lung (15).

A major problem in quantitating lung proteins relates to the choice of a suitable standard. Immunoassays are accurate, providing the protein to be measured is physicochemically identical to the standards used. Where differences occur, more critical assessment of the assay is required before the results can be interpreted with confidence. Measurement can also vary with each batch of polyclonal antiserum, and laboratories should either secure large amounts of the same batch of antiserum or fully assess each batch if studies continue over long periods.

Preparation and Storage of Samples

Fresh sputum is collected and centrifuged at 50,000 g (or more) for 90 min at 4°C to remove cell debris and separate the gel phase from the clear supernatant sol phase. After centrifugation, the sol phase is removed and stored in suitable aliquots at -70°C until analysis, and the mucus pellet is discarded.

Quantitation of α_1-Proteinase Inhibitor by Rocket Immunoelectrophoresis (RIEP)

Materials needed are (7) electrophoresis power supply and electrophoresis tanks (LKB), 56°C water bath (Jencons), levelling board (LKB), automatic dispensing pipettes 0 to 200 μl, 200 μl to 1 ml (Jencons), microsyringes 0 to 10 μl, 10 to 100 μl (Fisons), 2 mm well punch (Fisons), disposable polystyrene tubes of 10 or 25 ml capacity (Sterilin), 8 × 8 cm and 8 × 15 cm glass plates (Chance Propper). Suppliers are listed in Appendix I.

The reagents required are monospecific antiserum to α_1PI and calibrated serum standard (BDS Biologicals), in addition to:

Barbitone buffer: 0.05 M, pH 8.6, with sodium azide added to 0.01%
Agarose gel: 1% agarose (w/v) (electran 10 grade, BDH) with 3% polyethylene
  glycol 6,000 (w/v) dissolved in barbitone buffer by boiling at 100°C and cooling
  to 56°C before use
Gel staining solution: 2% Kenacid brilliant blue (BDH) in destaining solution
Destaining solution: 500 ml distilled water, 500 ml methanol (general purpose),
  100 ml glacial acetic acid.

Procedure

Sputum samples together with appropriate standards are placed in wells and electrophoresed into agarose containing monospecific antisera to α_1PI. The areas of the resultant immunoprecipitation peaks are proportional to the concentration of antigen present. The unknowns are measured and compared to the standard diluted plasma. The result may be most conveniently processed by measuring rocket height and using the method of Prince et al. (13).

1. Melt agarose by boiling at 100°C in water bath and cool to 56°C before use.
2. Pipette out molten agarose (0.1–0.15 ml/cm^2) into warmed tubes and add required amount of antibody (depending on manufacturers specifications). Mix

thoroughly and pour onto glass plate on level surface and leave for 5 min to cool.

3. Punch wells in a line 1.5 cm from cathodal end of plate 1 cm in from the edge and 2 mm apart (Fig. 1).

4. Using microdispenser or microsyringes, pipette out 5 μl volumes of diluted standard (as directed by manufacturer) or sample (sputum dilutions usually within range of neat–1:10 in electrophoresis buffer).

5. Electrophorese samples at 2 to 3 v/cm toward the anode (+ve) for 24 hr at room temperature.

6. Remove plates, press dry with filter paper and towels, and stain for 5 min in Kenacid BB followed by destaining until immunoprecipitin rockets are clearly visible.

7. Rockets should be measured to nearest 0.25 mm and related to standards to give the concentration of α_1PI.

Quantitation of Neutrophil Elastase in Sputum Using Radial Immunodiffusion (RID)

This technique (9) requires no electrophoresis equipment. However, in addition to those already mentioned for RIEP, an airtight moist box (sandwich type) and eyepiece graticule marked in 0.01 mm increments (Drifthawk Ltd.) are also required.

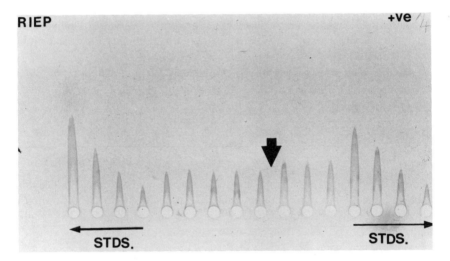

FIG. 1. Typical 8 × 15 cm RIEP plate for α_1PI after staining. Serial dilutions of standard serum are at either end. The samples in this case are fixed amounts of pure α_1PI mixed with increasing amounts of NE. Samples to the left of the black arrow are in inhibitor excess, and those to the right are in enzyme excess. This illustrates the alteration of immunological measurement of α_1PI that has interacted with NE due to the formation of enzyme inhibitor complexes and cleaved α_1PI fragments.

The reagents needed are the same as those used for RIEP with the addition of monospecific antibody to human NE (BDS) and purified NE standard (Elastin Products).

Procedure

Neutrophil elastase is a strongly cationic protein and thus not amenable to quantification by RIEP. Simple radial immunodiffusion is the most convenient method of measuring NE in sputum. This relies on diffusion of the sample into an antibody-containing agarose gel. A circular immunoprecipitation ring is formed, and the square of the diameter is a function of the antigen concentration. Like RIEP, the unknowns are related to a series of standards of known NE concentrations.

1. Agarose gel containing antibody to NE (as directed by manufacturer) is poured onto either 8×8 cm or 8×15 cm glass plates on a level board in the same way as for RIEP.

2. Two mm holes are punched at 1.5 cm equidistances from each other, avoiding curved edges of the gel where antibody distribution is less even (Fig. 2).

3. Five µl serial dilutions of standard NE (2 mg/ml–0.0125 mg/ml) or sputum (neat–1:10) are pipetted into wells with the 10 µl microsyringe.

4. Plates are placed in a moist box for 24 to 48 hr at room temperature, then press dried and stained as for RIEP plates.

5. Immunoprecipitin ring diameters are measured with the eyepiece graticle to the nearest 0.01 mm, and the value is squared. The standards are assessed using linear regression analysis (least squares), and values for the unknowns are obtained by interpolation.

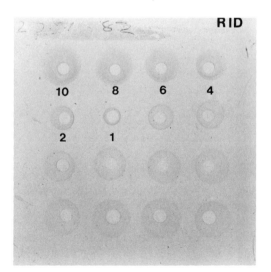

FIG. 2. An 8×8 cm radialimmunodifusion plate for NE after drying and staining. The first six wells are decreasing volumes of pure NE standard (2 mg/ml). The next wells contain a fixed amount of NE with added α_1PI in increasing amounts ranging from enzyme to inhibitor excess, resulting in the formation of increasing amounts of enzyme inhibitor complex.

Quantitation of α₁-Proteinase Inhibitor and Neutrophil Elastase by ELISA

Where large quantities of samples are to be analyzed (particularly at low concentrations), it may be most convenient to use more sensitive methods, such as an ELISA (4). The establishment of an ELISA is initially more complicated and expensive than either RIEP or RID but has the advantages of being more sensitive and conservative of sample and antisera.

It is not possible to give detailed information on setting up a working ELISA within this chapter, and the reader is referred to ref. 8. However, the basic reagents required and the principles of the two most widely adapted ELISA systems are summarized below.

Required materials include an ELISA plate reader with a 492 nm filter (Flow Labs), 50 to 250 μl multichannel pipette (Flow Labs), grade 1 microtiter plates (Gibco), 2 ml polystyrene tubes (Sterilin), 0.4 ml microfuge tubes (Alpha Labs), and 10 to 100 μl microsyringes (Fisons).

The reagents that are needed are monospecific antisera to α_1PI or NE, a calibrated serum standard for α_1PI, horseradish peroxidase (HRP) conjugated sheep anti-α_1PI or NE (for direct binding ELISA, HRP conjugated donkey antisheep IgG (for competitive binding ELISA) (BDS Biologicals), and a pure NE standard (Elastin Products), in addition to:

Carbonate buffer: 0.05 M, pH 9.6, with 0.01% Thiomersil (w/v) added
Phosphate-buffered saline assay buffer (PBSH/T): 1% (v/v) Haemaccel (colloidal gelatin) (Hoescht) with 0.01% (v/v) Tween 20 (polyoxyethylene sorbitan monolaurate) in PBS, pH 7.2
Substrate solution: 0.4% (w/v) orthophenyline diamine (OPD) (Sigma) in citrate buffer, pH 5.0, and activated before use with 20 μl/100 ml H_2O_2 (100 vol)
Stopping solution: 0.5 M citric acid

Procedure

The procedures for both types of ELISA are summarized in Fig. 3. Figure 4 shows standard curves for both types of ELISA.

FUNCTIONAL ASSESSMENT OF NEUTROPHIL ELASTASE AND α₁-PROTEINASE INHIBITOR

The activity of NE can be assessed using a variety of natural or synthetic substrates. However, synthetic substrates assess the amidolytic activity of the enzyme rather than the elastolytic activity. The latter can be assessed only using elastin as a substrate. In principle, the ability of the enzyme or biological fluid to solubilize particulate elastin is quantified by the release of an elastin-bound marker into solution.

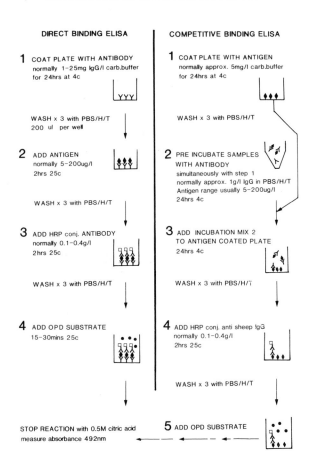

FIG. 3. Flow chart of the procedures for both types of ELISA.

In biological fluids, elastase activity is not necessarily indicative of NE alone, since other enzymes can also digest elastin (cathepsin G from the neutrophil and cathepsin L from the macrophage). The actual function of lung NE can be determined only indirectly as the elastase activity that can be removed by specific antiserum or specific chloromethylketones (methoxysuccinyl-ALA-ALA-PRO-VAL-chloromethylketone for NE).

The most convenient and sensitive elastase assay currently available is based on the solubilization of fluorescein-labeled elastin.

Determination of Elastase Activity Using Elastin Fluorescein Substrate

Materials needed for this determination include fluorimeter fitted with 470 nm excitation filter and 520 emission filter (Perkin Elmer), 37°C incubator (LEEC),

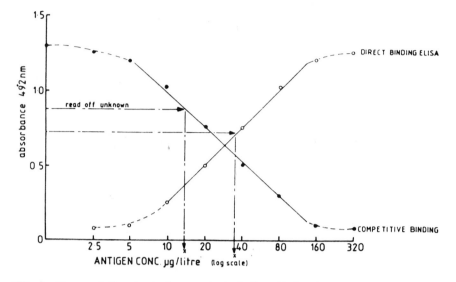

FIG. 4. Representative standard curves for both direct binding (○) and competitive binding (●) ELISA assays. The linear part of curve is used to determine unknowns.

flat well microtiter plates (Sterilin), fluorimetric grade cuvettes (Sarstedt), 200 to 1,000 µl dispensing pipette (Flow), 10 to 100 µl microsyringes, and 0.4 ml microfuge tubes (Alpha Labs).

Required reagents include elastin fluorescein 200 to 400 mesh, pure NE or porcine pancreatic elastase (PPE) standards (Elastin Prods.), and an assay buffer: 0.2 M Tris/HCl, pH 8.6, with 0.1% (v/v) triton × 100.

Procedure:

In principle, insoluble elastin particles coupled with fluorescein isothiocyanate (FITC) are degraded by active NE, and the soluble fluorescent product released is related to the amount of enzyme present. Using this method, it is possible to detect as little as 20 ng active enzyme/ml.

1. Wash a sufficient quantity of the elastin fluorescein (EF) five times in assay buffer and finally in distilled water, to coat the required number of microtiter plates (each well requires approximately 2 mg of EF). The outer rows on each plate are not used, since they are prone to evaporation during the assay. If prolonged incubation times are desirable, this assay is best performed in microfuge tubes to minimize evaporation.

2. Make up the elastin as a suspension of 10 g/liter in distilled water.

3. Gently and continuously stir the suspension to maintain homogenicity. Dispense 200 µl (2 mg EF) per well).

4. Allow EF particles to settle before gentle aspiration of the supernatant. Dry plates overnight at 37°C.

5. Dispense either standards or samples into wells 10 to 100 ng/ml for STD PPE or NE, and sputum sol phase diluted 1:10 to 1:1,000 in a total volume of 200 µl.

6. Incubate the plates for 24 hr at 37°C, gently remove supernatants, and centrifuge if necessary to remove remaining EF particles.

7. Dilute supernatants 1:100 and read on fluorimeter. Relate unknown values to standard curve using linear regression analysis (Fig. 5).

Assessment of Antielastase Inhibitory Capacity of Sputum

The elastin-fluorescein method can be used also to assess the ability of secretions to inhibit a known amount of pure enzyme. Essentially, increasing volumes of secretions are added to a fixed amount of enzyme, and decreasing elastase activity is analyzed by linear regression analysis. However, the assay requires 24 hr incubation with most samples, and since several of the lung inhibitors may function as reversible/competitive inhibitors, enzyme can be released again with time. This may result in an underestimation of the actual inhibitor function.

In view of this problem, short-term assays can be performed using a variety of synthetic peptide substrates coupled to chromogenic or fluorimetric terminal groups (nitroanilides or methylcoumarylamides). It should be reemphasized that activity toward synthetic peptide substrates (although related) may not be an accurate reflection of enzyme activity toward native substrates. In addition, NE and PPE can hydrolyze the synthetic substrate succinyl-L-alanine-L-alanine-L-alanyl para-nitroanilide (SLAPN) when bound to the inhibitor α-macroglobulin while showing no activity toward the larger substrate, elastin, showing disparity between apparent inhibition by both assays.

The major use of the synthetic substrate assay has been to provide a convenient and rapid assessment of the inhibitory capacity of lung secretions. However, a major point to emphasize is that secretions contain several inhibitors of NE, whereas it is likely that $\alpha_1 PI$ is the only inhibitor of PPE present in substantial quantities.

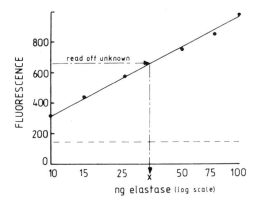

FIG. 5. A standard elastin-fluorescein curve for the 10 to 100 ng elastase range after 24 hr at 37°C. The dotted line shows the background fluorescence and is the mean of multiple blanks ($n = 10$). The y axis shows arbitrary units of fluorescence on the ×2 sensitivity setting.

Thus, inhibition of NE is dependent on the presence and function of several proteins, including α_1PI. It is, therefore, possible by using both enzymes, separately, to determine the function of α_1PI and its contribution to total NE inhibition.

Inhibitory Capacity of Sputum Determined by the Low Molecular Weight Substrate (SLAPN) Assay

Materials required are a microtiter plate reader (as for ELISA reader) with a 405 nm filter, a 37°C incubator, microtiter plates (Sterilin), 50 to 200 µl dispensing pipette, and 10 to 100 µl microsyringes.

Reagents needed are purified NE and PPE, an assay buffer of 0.2 M Tris–HCl, pH 8.6, with Triton X 100 added to 0.012 (v/v), and succinyl trialanyl paranitroanilide (SLAPN) substrate solution (Scientific Marketing Associates) made up to a concentration of 2 mM in assay buffer.

Procedure

The inhibition assay involves preincubating a fixed amount of PPE or NE with increasing volumes of sputum or secretions under carefully controlled conditions of time, temperature, and substrate concentration. It should be emphasized here that the preincubation time should be sufficiently long to allow maximum association of the inhibitors with the enzyme. This and other kinetic phenomena that may give rise to variable results are discussed in detail elsewhere (2). However, the protocol given here was developed in our laboratory and fulfills these criteria under the conditions described.

1. Pipette 100 µl volumes of Tris–HCl assay buffer into microtiter plates.
2. Dispense increasing volumes of sputum 0 to 100 µl neat into the wells using microsyringes, and add sufficient assay buffer to make all volumes to 100 µl.
3. Add either NE (for total elastase inhibitory capacity) or PPE (for α_1PI function) to each tube (approximately 50 pmoles of active NE/well or 10 pmol/well for PPE) and incubate at 37°C for 30 min.
4. Add 100 µl of substrate solutions at time intervals (chosen to relate to subsequent assay reading intervals, e.g., 10–30 sec) and continue incubation for a further 20 to 30 min).
5. Measure absorbance 405 nm using the plate reader, and express results as a percentage of corresponding enzyme alone (control).
6. Plot sputum volume against percentage NE or PPE activity remaining. Extrapolate data using linear regression analysis to give the theoretical volume required to inhibit all of the enzyme present (Fig. 6).

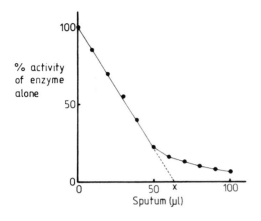

FIG. 6. SLAPN sputum inhibition curve. The linear part of the curve is extrapolated to the axis to give the theoretical volume of sputum required to completely inhibit the known amount of enzyme.

DISCUSSION

The methodology described represents the simplest assays for assessing inhibitors and enzymes in biological fluids. These methods form the basis of such studies, but interpretation of the results requires a detailed knowledge of the artifacts that can occur. Some of these points have been alluded to in the methods and highlighted in the results. However, it seems appropriate to discuss some of the problems that we have encountered while performing these assays in our laboratories.

Immunological Measurements

The agarose gel techniques for quantitative assessment (RIEP and RID) are easy to perform and generally are sensitive to a level of approximately 1 mg/liter depending on the quality of the antiserum available. They both have excellent reproducibility (between batch CV < 5%). However, RIEP is only suitable for measurement of proteins with an anionic mobility in conditions suitable for electrophoresis into antibody-containing agarose gels. This makes it an unsuitable method for measurement of cationic proteins, including such enzymes as NE.

A major problem is physicochemical changes that occur when inhibitors, such as α_1PI, interact with enzymes, such as NE. This may result in a change of the immunological properties of the proteins that affects the assay, depending on the batch of antiserum used (Fig. 7). Thus it is best to secure a large batch of each antiserum, or its performance with relevant forms of α_1PI must be confirmed. In this respect, monoclonal antiserum may prove superior to the polyclonal reagents. However, it must be emphasized that the specificity of monoclonal antisera may also be a weakness, particularly if α_1PI/enzyme interaction alters the relevant epitope so that the antibody no longer binds. Clearly, this is not a problem with polyclonal antisera where multiple epitopes are recognized. Monoclonal antisera cannot gener-

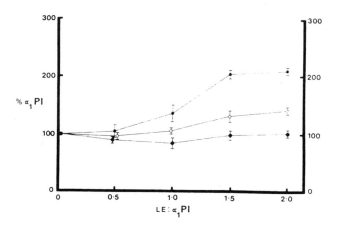

FIG. 7.   Immunological estimation of α_1PI/NE mixtures as in Fig. 1, using three different poly-clonal antisera.

ally be used in gel precipitation techniques but are normally suitable for competitive binding ELISA systems.

Radial immunodiffusion is the simplest method for immunological estimation of enzymes in secretions, although the same reservations regarding immunological changes apply here as with RIEP. In addition, dense nonspecific precipitates may occur within the agarose gel when some sputum samples are analyzed. This may lead to difficulties in protein qualification, since the genuine immunoprecipitation ring may not be visible. This appears to be a particular problem with sputum from patients with active lung infections. One solution is to repeat the assay using less antibody in the gel and less sample in the well. The net effect is to keep the immunoprecipitin ring diameter constant, while reducing the nonspecific ring.

The best alternative if this problem arises is to use ELISA, since they have the additional benefits of sensitivity and speed of assay without the nonspecific precipitations seen in RID. In our laboratory, we use a direct binding ELISA system for measurement of several proteins, including the inhibitors α_1PI, α_1-antichymotrypsin, α_1-macroglobulin, antileukoproteinase, and the enzymes NE and cathepsin G. As with RIEP and RID, it must be remembered that the physicochemical characteristics of the protein to be measured may be altered, and antibody specificity may affect the estimations.

It is possible that the combination of well-characterized monoclonal antibodies (3) raised specifically to the various molecular forms of the proteins to be found in secretions, with an indirect binding ELISA system, may eventually solve many of the technical difficulties associated with immunological estimation of these molecules. In addition, this may dispense with the necessity to perform functional assays. In theory, it should be possible to select antibody clones that will recognize only the protein species of interest, e.g., native, oxidized, complexed, and cleaved α_1PI. However, this is speculative but clearly worth further study.

The direct binding ELISA is the most rapid and convenient form of the assay. However, it may be necessary to develop a competitive binding assay for more detailed studies using monoclonal antibodies. The reason is dependent on the fact that the direct binding ELISA requires two antibody molecules to link to one antigen molecule. When the antigen is captured by the first antibody, epitopic determinants are covered, and this may affect the subsequent binding of the second antibody and hence the estimation of protein. This is indicated by the fact that the concentrations of secondary antibody required in the direct binding ELISA (HRP conj.) are usually higher than those for the primary antibody.

Depending on the reagents used, either form of assay may be subject to higher than expected noise/signal ratio (background). This may normally be eliminated by the inclusion of a blocking step (e.g., 1% haemaccel in PBS Tween for 30 min) between coating the microtiter plate and addition of the second layer. It is advisable to run samples in triplicate, since the greater sensitivity of this technique (<5 µg/liter) means greater inherent variability than that of either RIEP or RID.

Further information about the molecular form of an inhibitor, such as α_1PI can be obtained by several techniques. First, two-dimensional immunoelectrophoresis can be used to visualize α_1PI/NE complex in sputum (17). This is a well-established and simple technique that is possible to perform on sputum with the equipment required for RIEP. More recently, the technique of Western immunoblotting, which essentially combines SDS polyacrylamide gel electrophoresis with electroblotting has been applied to α_1PI. This technique can accurately identify the size of α_1PI molecules in whole secretions. The resolution is sufficient to separate native α_1PI from proteolytically modified and complexed forms. It can also be semiquantitative with the addition of densitometric scanning. This methodology is described in detail elsewhere (16).

Functional Assessment of Enzyme and Inhibitors

The elastin fluorescein assay for measurement of elastase activity or total elastase inhibitory capacity is both sensitive (<20 µg/liter) and reproducible (between batch CV 14%), which makes it comparable with the tritiated elastin radiometric assay (14). In original studies, this assay was described as a test tube method (10). We have developed the assay to be performed in microtiter plates or microfuge tubes to conserve reagents and enable more samples to be measured per assay. It is possible to develop similar fluorimetric assays for collagenase activity. The most common problem with the method is high background fluorescence, which may reflect inadequate washing of elastin or prolongation of incubation time. The fluorescein is released spontaneously from elastin, making the inclusion of multiple blanks necessary. Unsteady readings are usually caused by the presence of insoluble elastin particles that can be removed by further centrifugation.

A wide range of low molecular weight synthetic substrates is available, many of which are highly specific for the target enzyme. The SLAPN assay, when used with PPE, remains the best method for measurement of α_1PI function in sputum. By simultaneous comparison with the NEIC of the sample, it has been possible to assess the contribution made by α_1PI to the total elastase inhibitory screen (18). The nitroanilide substrates are less sensitive than the fluorescent coumarylamides, but nevertheless they are generally adequate for sputum studies. In addition, the assays require basic, relatively inexpensive spectrophotometers for measurement rather than a more costly fluorimeter.

There are several additional problems that may affect results. First, it must be stressed that with any of the functional measurements, the accuracy of the result is wholly dependant on precise knowledge of the specific activity of the enzymes used (and inhibitors for pure protein studies). There are a variety of approaches to titration of enzymes, none of which is singly ideal but, if used in combination, can provide the investigator with a reasonable measure of enzyme function. In our laboratory, we titrate elastase against the substrate to be used, e.g., SLAPN in a carefully controlled Lineweaver–Burk titration. The specific activity can then be derived using the kinetic constants available from the literature (11).

Although this is the easiest method, we compare the results with inactivation of the enzyme of fresh plasma, pure characterized α_1PI, and a specific chlorylmethylketone. Other methods of titration are possible, including the use of active site titrants, such as para-nitrophenol-guanidinobenzoate (NPGB) (20).

Enzyme solutions should be titrated by as many means available at regular time intervals in order that accuracy of results is maintained and assured.

Second, it should be emphasized that several lung inhibitors may behave as reversible/competitive inhibitors, unlike α_1PI, which is generally considered to be noncompetitive due to its rapid rate of association and very slow dissociation. Where association and dissociation rates are similar, however, the inhibitor will behave reversibly. These rates are governed by the concentrations of enzyme, inhibitor, and substrate used in the assay. We have demonstrated that such competitive inhibition occurs in lung secretions and may be obscured when the substrate concentration is sufficiently high (1). In addition, the enzyme will dissociate from inhibitors and interact with substrate as incubation of enzymes and inhibitors continues in the presence of substrate, especially when the inhibitor is of low affinity (reversible).

This presents a problem about the length of incubation time and the choice of substrate concentration. It is important to allow sufficient incubation time before addition of substrate to enable complete association of the proteinase with the inhibitor; for α_1PI and NE a preincubation time of 15 to 30 min is adequate. In order to confirm the time dependency of inhibition, the assay may be performed at different time intervals. If the curve becomes linear with time, the preincubation time should be increased until no further change is noted. If it remains curved, however, it is likely that several inhibitors with different affinities are interacting with the enzyme or that the inhibitor being studied is behaving as a reversible inhibitor (2). All results should be interpreted in the light of these possibilities, and it is thus imperative to define clearly the assay conditions in any experiment, particularly when using biological fluids.

Although this chapter highlights the technical problems encountered in the assays, it should be remembered that this only reflects the current state-of-the-art. Continuing critical appraisal of all assays is imperative, and other artifacts may emerge as the technology advances. Meanwhile, results should be reported with caution.

REFERENCES

1. Afford, S. C., Morrison, H. M., Burnett, D., and Stockley, R. A. (1986): Inhibitory activity of sputum sol phase: Effects of changes in substrate and enzyme concentrations. *Am. Rev. Respir. Dis.*, 133:4:A394.
2. Bieth, J. G. (1980): Pathophysiological interpretation of kinetic constants of protease inhibitors. *Bull. Eur. Physiopathol. Respir.*, 16 (Suppl):183–195.
3. Engvall, E., and Perlmann, P. (1971): Enzyme linked immunosorbent assay (ELISA): Quantitative assay of IgG. *Immunochemistry*, 8:871.
4. Gadek, J. E., Hunninghake, G. W., Fells, G. A., Zimmerman, R. L., Keogh, B. A., and Crystal, R. G. (1980): Evaluation of the protease–antiprotease theory of human destructive lung disease. *Bull. Eur. Physiopathol. Respir.*, 16 (Suppl):27–40.
5. Klanerman, J., Ranger, V., Rynbrandt, D., Sorenson, J., and Powers, J. C. (1980): The effects of a specific elastase inhibitor, alanyl prolylalanine chloromethylketone, on elastase-induced emphysema. *Am. Rev. Respir. Dis.*, 12:381–387.
6. Laurell, C.-B. (1972): Electroimmunoassay. *Scand. J. Clin. Lab. Invest.*, 29:21–37.
7. Maggio, E. T. (1986): *Enzyme Immunoassay.* CRC Press, Boca Raton, FL.
8. Mancini, G., Carbonara, A. O., and Heremans, J. F. (1965): Immunochemical quantitation of antigens by single radial immunodiffusion. *Immunochemistry*, 2:235–254.
9. McGillivray, D. H., Burnett, D., Afford, S. C., and Stockley, R. A. (1981): An evaluation of four methods of measurement of elastase activity. *Clin. Chim. Acta*, 3:289–294.
10. Nakajima, K., Powers, J. C., Ashe, B. M., and Zimmerman, M. (1979): Mapping the extended substrate binding site of cathepsin G and leucocyte elastase. *J. Biol. Chem.*, 254:4027–4032.
11. Ohlsson, K., and Olsson, I. (1979): Neutral proteases of human granulocytes. III. Interaction between granulocyte elastase and plasma protease inhibitors. *Scand. J. Clin. Lab. Invest.*, 34:349–355.
12. Prince, H. P., Burnett, D., and Ramsden, D. B. (1977). Improved statistical method for the calculation of protein concentration by Laurell monorocket immunoelectrophoresis. *J. Chromatogr.*, 143:321–323.
13. Smith, S. F., Guz, A., Cooke, N. T., Burton, G. H., and Tetley, T. D. (1985): Extracellular elastolytic activity in human lung lavage: A comparative study between smokers and non-smokers *Clin. Sci.*, 69(1):17–27.
14. Stockley, R. A. (1984): Measurement of soluble proteins in lung secretions. *Thorax*, 39:241–247.
15. Stockley, R. A., and Afford, S. C. (1984): Qualitative studies of lung lavage α_1-proteinase inhibitor. *Hoppe-Seylers Z. Physiol. Chem.*, 365:503–510.
16. Stockley, R. A., and Burnett, D. (1979): Alpha$_1$-antitrypsin and leucocyte elastase in infected and noninfected sputum. *Am. Rev. Respir. Dis.*, 120(5):1081–1086.
17. Stockley, R. A., Morrison, H. M., Smith, S., and Tetley, T. (1984): Low molecular mass bronchial proteinase inhibitor and α_1-proteinase inhibitor in sputum and bronchoalveolar lavage. *Hoppe-Seylers Z. Physiol. Chem.*, 365:587–595.
18. Twumasi, D. Y., Liener, J. E., Galdston, M., and Levytska, V. (1977): Activation of human leukocyte elastase by α_2-macroglobulin. *Nature*, 267:61–68.
19. Zahnley, J. C., and Davis, J. G. (1970): Determination of the trypsin/inhibitor complex dissociation using the active site titrant p-NPGB. *Biochemistry*, 9:1428–1433.

20. Zhu, X. J. and Chan, S. K. (1986). Distinguishing the tobacco smoke inactivated alpha-1-proteinase inhibitor from the native by the use of a specific monoclonal antibody. In: *Pulmonary Emphysema and Proteolysis,* Vol. II, pp. 351–355, edited by J. C. Taylor and C. H. Mittmann, Academic Press, New York.

ACKNOWLEDGMENT

The authors would like to acknowledge the financial support of the Medical Research Council and the Chest, Heart and Stroke Foundation and the Bicentenary Appeal Fund.

APPENDIX I. SUPPLIERS

Alpha Laboratories, 40 Parkham Drive, Eastleigh, Hants SO5 4NU, UK

BDH Chemicals Ltd., Fourways, Carlyon Ind. Estate, Atherstone, Warwickshire, CV9 1JG, UK

BDS Biologicals Inc., Vincent Drive, University of Birmingham, Edgbaston, Birmingham, B15 2TT, UK

Chance Propper Ltd., Spon Lane, Smethwick, Warley, West Midlands, UK

Drifthawk Ltd., Metal Box Engineering, Crompton Way, Manor Royal, Crawley, RH10 2LE, UK

Elastin Products Company Inc., P.O. Box 147-Pacific, MO 63069

Fisons Scientific Equipment, Bishop Meadow Road, Loughborough, Leicestershire, LE11 ORG, UK

Flow Laboratories, Woodcock Hill, Harefield Road, Rickmansworth, WD3 1PQ, UK

Gibco Ltd., Unit 4, Cowley Mill Trading Estate, Longbridge Way, Uxbridge, Middlesex, UB8 2YG, UK

Hoechst Ltd., Hoescht House, Salisbury Road, Hounslow, TW4 6JH, UK

Jencons (Scientific) Ltd., Cherrycourt Way Industrial Estate, Stanbridge Road, Leighton Buzzard, Bedfordshire, LU7 8UA, UK

LEEC, Private Road 7, Colwick, Nottingham, NG4 2AU, UK

LKB Instruments Ltd., Pharmacia House, Midsummer Boulevard, Milton Keynes MK9 3HP, UK

Perkin-Elmer, Post Office Lane, Beaconsfield, Buckinghamshire HP1 1QA, UK

Sarstedt Ltd., 68 Borston Road, Beaumont-Leys, Leicester LE4 1AW, UK

Scientific Marketing Associates, 37 Mildway Grove, London, N1 4RH, UK

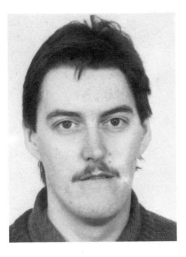

Simon Charles Afford was born in 1957, received the HNC Medical Laboratory Sciences in 1979, F.I.M.L.S. in 1983, and C. Biol., M.I. Biol. in 1984. He received the Thoracic Society Prize for Research in 1980.

Robert Andrew Stockley was born in 1947. He received the M.B. degree in 1971, MRCP in 1973, M.D. in 1978, F.R.C.P. in 1984, and DSc in 1986. He is currently involved in biochemistry of mucus and macromolecular substances identification.

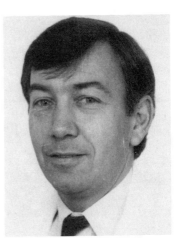

Methods in Bronchial Mucology,
edited by P. C. Braga and L. Allegra.
Raven Press, Ltd. © 1988.

3.5. HISTOCHEMICAL AND OPTICAL METHODS

3.5.1. Histochemical Methods and Light Microscopy

*G. Barbolini, **A. Bisetti, and †M. Moretti

*Istituto di Anatomia e Istologia Patologica Policlinico, Modena, Italy **Cattedra di Tisiologia e Malattie, Apparato Respiratorio, Università di Roma "La Supienza," Istituto C. Forlanini, Rome, and †Istituto di Tisilogia e Malattie, Dell'Apparato Respiratorio, Policlinico, Modena, Italy*

Methods and materials
  Light microscopy
  Histochemistry
  Immunohistochemistry
  Other methods
Results
Discussion
Appendixes

The morphological and functional study of the tracheobronchial mucosa and its secretory modifications—caused by a spectrum of pathological conditions— may be performed by using four different methods; light microscopy, histochemistry, immunohistochemistry, and other methods.

Whatever the selected method may be, an essential prerequisite is identification of the different secretory cytotypes located at different levels: ciliate and mucus-secreting goblet cells of the mucosa, mucus and serous acini of the bronchial glands (main bronchi and intermediate branches), and ciliate, goblet, and Clara cells of bronchioli. According to Reid and Coles (15), another prerequisite is recognition of the remaining cytotypes located in the bronchial wall, mainly basal, neuroendocrine, and neuroepithelial cells. The routine histochemical investigations mainly are of samples from patients with chronic bronchitis. The global results have been evaluated from the viewpoint of progress in methods of clinical chemistry, particularly previous works of traditional histochemistry performed by Reid et al. (11,12,14,15) since 1964.

METHODS AND MATERIALS

The most satisfactory morphological patterns usually are observed on paraffin sections from freshly collected endoscopic or surgical specimens fixed in neutral formalin or in 85 to 95% alcohol.

Light Microscopy

There are two basically reliable methods: buffered hematoxylin & eosin (1) and Kreyberg's alcian green (10) 2Gx method (Fig. 1) (Appendix I).

Histochemistry

These methods are based chiefly on obtaining reactive groups marked by a nondiffusive reaction product revealed by a proper stain (Appendix II).

In terms of traditional histochemistry (13), the most pertinent substances for mucological purposes are (Table 1):

Proteins: SH and SS groups (2)
Neutral mucosubstances: G-mucosubstance (all PAS-positive, periodate-reactive)
Sulfated acid mucosubstances (epithelial sulfomucin, testicular hyaluronidase-resis-

TABLE 1. *Histochemistry of bronchial cytotypes in simple chronic bronchitis*

Stain or reaction	Goblet	Mucus	Serous	Ciliate
SH groups	−	+	±	−
SS groups	±	−	−	−
Alcian green (Kreyberg)	+ +	+ + +	− (±)	−
HID	⎰ + + Black	+ + Black	+ Black	−
	⎱ + + Blue	+ + Blue		−
AB–PAS	+ + + Violet	+ + + Violet	+ + Red	± Red
G-mucosubstance	+ +	+ +	+	±
S-mucin B4.5	+ +	+ +	±	−
GC-mucin	±	+ +	− (±)	−
C-mucin	+ +	+ +	− (±)	−

tant): S-mucin B4.5 (alcohol-resistant azurophilia 0.02% at or above pH 4.5)
Unsulfated acid mucosubstances (epithelial sialomucin): CG-mucin BN (labile to
neuraminidase, PAS-positive, metachromatic with azure A); GC-mucin (stable
to neuraminidase after saponification, PAS-positive); C-mucin (stable to neuraminidase after saponification, PAS-negative)

The remaining mucins tested at the tracheobronchial level showed either negative
or very weak results (S-mucin B2.0, C-mucin N ±) results that were not reproducible
(CG-mucin N ±, S-mucin (Sap) BN). Consequently, they are not listed in Table
1.
Very useful for routine and screening purposes are the alcian blue-PAS reaction
and the high iron diamine-alcian blue stain (HID). The former stains neutral mucosubstances various shades of red and acid mucosubstances blue. With the latter
sulfated mucosubstances are purple-black. The unstained sialomucins are blue after
alcian blue staining (Fig. 2).
The classification by Pearse (13) concerns the following histochemical reactions;

1. Affinity for basic dyes, such as azure A
2. Affinity for alcian blue
3. Lability to testicular hyaluronidase
4. Lability to *Vibrio cholerae* neuraminidase

These properties are expressed by the letters B, A, T, and N, respectively.
The letters G, U, S, and C refer to the presence (or absence) of vic-glycols,
uronic acids, sulfate groups, and sialic acid carboxy, respectively. This classification
is basically histochemical, although it is used to express biochemical status.
Fucose may be well demonstrated by using *Ulex europaeus* I (UEA) lectin,
biotin-labeled, developed by the avidin-biotin complex (ABC) method (6,8).

Immunohistochemistry

In immunohistochemistry, the antigen–antibody reaction is shown by either the
peroxidase-antiperoxidase (PAP) method or the ABC method (7,8) (Appendix III).
Useful results for mucologic studies are obtained with immunohistochemistry for
lactoferrin, α_1-antichimotrypsin, lysozyme, orosomucoid, and S100 proteins.

Other Methods

Other methods may be used to ascertain the concurrent presence of other cytotypes
or substances. In our experience the following stains or reactions have been helpful:

Basal cells. Immunohistochemistry (PAP and/or ABC) for keratin
Neuroendocrine cells. Immunohistochemistry (PAP and/or ABC) for neuronospe-
cific enolase (NSE), argentaffinity (Grimelius)

TABLE 2. *Immunohistochemistry of bronchial cytotypes in simple chronic bronchitis*

Stain or reaction	Goblet	Mucus	Serous	Ciliate	Clara
Fucose	+ +	+ + +	−	−(±)	±/+ +
Lactoferrin	±	−	+ + +	±	−
α_1-Antichimotrypsin	±	−	+ +	−(±)	−(±)
Lysozyme	−	−	+ + +	−	±
Orosomucoid	−(±)	−	±/+ +	−(±)	+/+ + +
S100 proteins	−	−	+ + +	−	−(±)
Keratin	−	−/+ +	−	−(±)	−/+

B lymphocytes and plasmocytes. Immunohistochemistry (PAP) for IgG, light chains
K and λ
Amyloids: Congo red, pagoda red (3)

RESULTS

Light Microscopy

The different cytotypes show basically the same histochemical and immunohisto-chemical pattern at different bronchial levels (main and intermediate bronchi, bron-chioli) (Tables 1 and 2).

Ciliate cells are practically devoid of secretion. Serous and mucus cells differ greatly in their products of secretion, whereas mucus cells and mucus-secreting goblet cells show a common spectrum of secretion (Fig. 1).

Histochemistry and Immunohistochemistry

Mucus cells (Figs. 2, 3, 4) present a very strong reaction for fucose, a medium-strength reaction for epithelial sulfomucin and sialomucin and for neutral mucosub-stances, and a negative reaction for lactoferrin. Goblet cells differ from mucus

---

FIG. 1. Kreyberg's alcian green method. Mucus and goblet cells are stained green. Ciliate and basal cells are not alcianophilic. Serous cells contain some cyanophilic granules of secretion. ×320.

FIG. 2. Mucus and goblet cells contain sulfomucin (purple-black) and sialomucin (blue). The weak reaction of serous cells is more marked toward the apical segment. HID. ×320.

FIG. 3. Mucus-secreting goblet cells exhibit a positive reaction for S-mucin B4.5. Scattered mast cells and cartilage are also reactive. Azure A. ×320.

FIG. 4. A positive reaction for fucose is shown by mucus and goblet cells and by endothelia. Serous cells are not reactive. UEA 1. ×320.

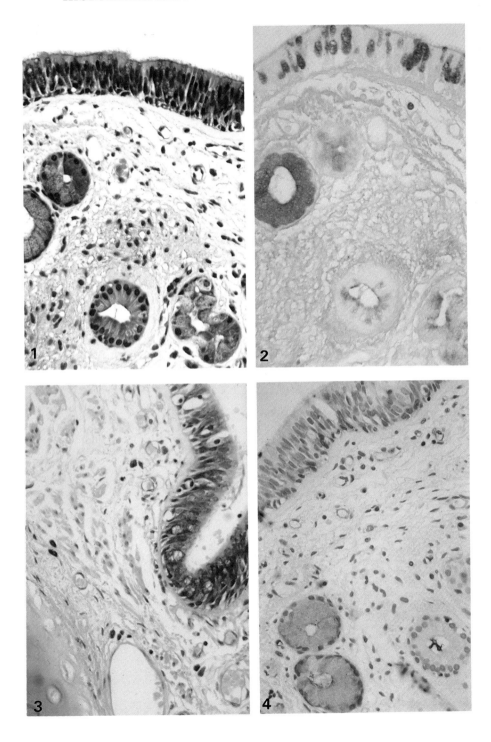

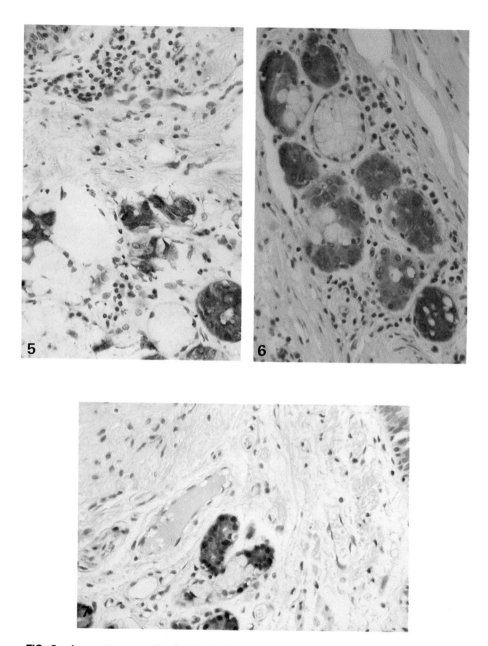

FIG. 5. A very strong reaction for lactoferrin in serous cells and traces of stain in ciliate and goblet cells are noticeable. Mucus acini are negative. ×320.

FIG. 6. Immunohistochemistry for lysozyme is sharply positive in serous acini and in scattered neutrophils.

FIG. 7. Serous acini and bronchial nerve endings are positive for S100 proteins. Scattered neuroepithelial and cartilage are also reactive. ×320.

cells owing to weaker reactions for fucose and GC-mucin and weak reactions for lactoferrin (Fig. 5) and α_1-antichimotrypsin.

Serous cells exhibit a very strong reaction for lactoferrin, lysozyme, and S100 proteins (Figs. 5, 6, 7), a medium-strength reaction for α_1-antichimotrypsin and orosomucoid, and a negative reaction for fucose.

Clara cells are characterized by positive reactions for orosomucoid and fucose.

Other Methods

Basal cells are sharply demonstrated by a strong reaction for keratin. Mucus cells, too, affected by squamous metaplasia, show a positive but frequently weaker reaction.

DISCUSSION

Chronic bronchitis is characterized mainly by hypertrophy, hyperfunction, and hyperplasia of mucus cells. These cells have the strongest reaction for fucose and present a morphological basis that explains the findings of clinical chemistry: increase of fucose and of the fucose/sialomucin ratio. On the other hand, the well-known increase of lactoferrin may have, at least in part, a bronchial origin at the serous cell level.

Ciliate cells do not show clearly the presence of secretion. However, the release of a glycoconjugate for these cells has been suggested (15), and it could explain the traces of stain recorded for them in Tables 1 and 2.

According to Reid et al. (9,11,12,14), mucus-secreting goblet cells and mucus acini of bronchial glands secrete neutral and acid (sulfomucin, sialomucin) glycoproteins. Our results suggest that goblet cells are mainly secretive of S-mucin B4.5 (Fig. 3) and of PAS-negative sialomucin (C-mucin).

Moreover, the figures recorded for SH and SS groups (Table 1) could be related to a different function of cysteine and cystine for goblet (mucus) and serous cells concerning a different production of epithelial sulfomucin. Actually, serous acini have a weak but not negative reaction for sulfomucin (Fig. 2).

Our results with lactoferrin and lysozyme stress the previous ultrastructural findings of Bowes and Corrin (5) and of Bowes et al. (4).

Finally, the same substances studied in patients affected by simple chronic bronchitis may be found in patients affected by pulmonary adenocarcinoma and used for differentiation of oncotypes (Table 3).

REFERENCES

1. Barbolini, G., Saviano, M. S., and Menozzi-Tucci, F. (1973): Conception structurale nouvelle de la caséose. *Poumon Coeur,* 29:95–99.
2. Barbolini, G., Trentini, G. P., Botticelli, A. R., and Pagnotta, W. (1965): Istochimica dei cosiddetti corpi amilacei:prostata, polmone e midollo spinale. *Arch. Vecchi Anat. Patol.,* 46:607–637.

3. Battaglia, S., Barbolini, G., Botticelli, A. R., and Trentini, G. P. (1985): Apoptotic amyloid: A study on prostatic amyloidosis with particular reference to corpora amylacea. *Appl. Pathol.*, 3:105–114.

4. Bowes, D., Clark, A. E., and Corrin, B. (1981): Ultrastructural localization of lactoferrin and glycoprotein in human bronchial glands. *Thorax*, 36:108–105.

5. Bowes, D., and Corrin, B. (1977): Ultrastructural immunocytochemical localization of lysozyme in human bronchial glands. *Thorax*, 32:163–170.

6. Halthöfer, H., Virtanen, I., Kariniemi, L., Hormia, H., Linder, E., and Miettinen, A. (1982): *Ulex europaeus* I lectin as a marker for vascular endothelium in human tissues. *Lab. Invest.*, 47:60–66.

7. Hsu, S. M., Raine, L., and Fanger, M. (1981): A comparative study of the peroxidase–antiperoxidase method and an avidin–biotin complex method for studying polypeptide hormones with radioimmunoassay antibodies. *Am. J. Clin. Pathol.*, 75:734–738.

8. Hsu, S. M., Raine, L., and Fanger, H. (1981): Use of avidin–biotin–peroxidase complex (ABC) in immunoperoxidase techniques. *J. Histochem. Cytochem.*, 29:577–580.

9. Jones, R., and Reid, L. (1978): The effect of pH on alcian blue staining of epithelial acid glycoprotein. II. Human bronchial submucosal gland. *Histochem. J.*, 5:19–27.

10. Kreyberg, L. (1981): Méthode de coloration combinée de la kératine et des substances mucoïdes. In: *Types Histologiques des Tumeurs du Poumon*, 2nd ed. pp. 37–38. Organisation Mondiale de la Santé, Genève.

11. Lamb, D., and Reid, L. (1970): Histochemical and autoradiographic investigation of the serous cells of the human bronchial glands. *J. Pathol.*, 100:127–138.

12. McCarthy, C., and Reid, L. (1964): Intracellular mucopolysaccharides in the normal human bronchial tree. *Q. J. Exp. Physiol.*, 49:85–94.

13. Pearse, A. G. E. (1968): Carbohydrates and mucosubstances. In: *Histochemistry: Theoretical and Applied*, 3rd ed., pp. 294–380. Churchill, London.

14. Reid, L. (1968): Bronchial mucus production in health and diseases. In: *The Lung*, pp. 87–108. Williams & Wilkins, Baltimore.

15. Reid, L. M., and Coles, S. J. (1984): The bronchial epithelium of humans. Cytology, innervation and functions. In: *The Endocrine Lung in Health and Disease*, edited by K. L. Becker and A. F. Gazdar, pp. 56–78. Saunders, Philadelphia.

APPENDIX I: LIGHT MICROSCOPY

Buffered Hematoxylin & Eosin
(From ref. 1)

Method

1. Cut sections at 5 μm.

2. Bring sections to a water faucet.

3. Stain for 10 to 15 min with 0.1% heamtoxylin buffered at pH 4.0 with 0.2 M phosphate.

4. Wash in running water for 30 min.

5. Immerse sections in 1% eosin, buffered at pH 6.0 with 0.2 M NA$_2$HPO$_4$ and 0.1 M citric acid.

6. Wash in distilled water.

7. Dehydrate, clear, and mount in a synthetic resin medium.

Histological and cytological details are more evident than by routine hematoxylin & eosin.

TABLE 3. *Histochemical and immunohistochemical differential diagnosis of lung adenocarcinoma*

Oncotype	Marker
Poorly differentiated adenocarcinoma	Fucose
Acinar adenocarcinoma	α_1-Antichimotrypsin, fucose, orosomucoid
Papillary adenocarcinoma	α_1-Antichimotrypsin
Bronchioloalveolar carcinoma	Alcian green, HID, lysozyme, S100 proteins

Kreyberg's Alcian Green Method
(From ref. 10)

Preparation of Solutions

1. Celestin blue solution. Dissolve 5 g iron alum in 100 ml distilled water by letting it stand overnight at room temperature. Add 0.5 g celestin blue and boil for 3 min. Filter when cool and add 14 ml glycerol. The solution lasts for several months.

2. Alcian green (2Gx) solution. To 50 ml 1% alcian green add 50 ml 1% acetic acid and 2 mg thymol.

3. Saffron solution. Add 4 g of saffron (Sigma, S-8381) to a flask containing 100 ml absolute ethanol. Stir and boil under reflux in a water bath. Allow to cool, add 100 ml absolute ethanol and boil for 1 hr. Repeat the procedure five times. Filter all the collected supernatant. The dark yellow solution lasts for several months.

Method

1. Bring sections to a water faucet.
2. Stain nuclei for 5 min with celestin blue solution. Rinse in water. Stain for 5 min with Mayer's hemalum. Rinse in water.
3. Differentiate in 0.5% hydrochloric acid.
4. Wash carefully in running water.
5. Stain for 5 min in 1% aqueous erythrosin.
6. Rinse briefly in distilled water.
7. Differentiate quickly in 96% ethanol.
8. Rinse briefly in distilled water.
9. Stain for 5 min with alcian green solution.
10. Rinse in distilled water.
11. Dehydrate quickly in 96% ethanol.
12. Immerse for 5 min in saffron.

13. Dehydrate in two changes of absolute ethanol.

14. Clear in xylene and mount in synthetic resin medium.

Nuclei are deep blue, acid mucopolysaccharides are green, connective tissue is yellow-orange, keratin is red, and other structures are different shades of red.

APPENDIX II. HISTOCHEMISTRY

DDD Reaction for SH Groups
(From ref. 2)

Method

1. Bring paraffin sections to a water faucet.

2. Incubate for 1 hr at 50°C in a solution containing 35 ml 0.1 M veronal acetate buffer (pH 8.5) and 15 ml absolute ethanol in which 25 mg of the DDD reagent has been dissolved. Some of the reagent may remain in suspension.

3. Cool to room temperature.

4. Rinse sections briefly in distilled water.

5. Wash for 10 min in two changes of distilled water acidified to pH 4 to 4.5 with acetic acid. This step converts the sodium salt of the reagent and of the unwanted reaction product (6-thio-2-naphthol) to free naphthols.

6. Extract the free naphthols by passage through a graded series of alcohols and wash twice in absolute either for 5 min in each wash.

7. Rinse in distilled water.

8. Stain for 2 min at room temperature in a freshly prepared solution of 50 mg tetrazotized diorthoanisidine (fast blue B salt) in 50 ml 0.1 M phosphate buffer at pH 7.4.

9. Wash in running tap water.

10. Dehydrate in alcohols, clear in xylene, and mount in Permount, DPX, or other suitable medium.

Blue staining indicates a high concentration of SH groups; red staining areas contain lower concentrations.

DDD Reaction for SH and SS Groups

If it is necessary to demonstrate SH and SS groups together, sections are first treated with thioglycollate. If SS groups alone are to be shown, it is necessary to block existing SH groups with iodoacetate or N-ethylmaleimide and then to reduce the SS groups to SH with a reagent that will not unblock the original SH groups. Potassium cyanide is suitable for this purpose.

Iodoacetate Block (SH)

Treat sections for 20 hr at 37°C with 0.1 M iodoacetic acid titrated to pH 8 with 0.1 N NaOH.

Maleimide Block (SH)

Treat sections for 4 hr at 37°C with 0.1 M *N*-ethylmaleimide in 0.1 M phosphate buffer at pH 7.4. Follow this by washing in 1% acetic acid and then in tap water.

High Iron Diamine-Alcian Blue Stain (HID)
(From ref. 13)

Prepare a fresh solution containing 120 mg *N,N*-dimethyl-*m*-phenylenediamine dihydrochloride and 20 mg *N,N*-dimethyl-*p*-phenylenediamine hydrochloride in 50 ml distilled water.

When the reagents are dissolved, pour the solution into a Coplin jar containing 1.4 ml 62% $FeCl_3$ (anhydrous).

$FeCl_3$ Solution

Add very slowly under aspiration 62 g $FeCl_3$ (anhydrous) to 100 ml distilled water. Allow to cool, then filter.

Method

1. Bring sections to a water faucet.
2. Stain overnight (18 hr) in the dark with the reagent.
3. Wash for 5 min in running water.
4. Stain for 40 min in 1% alcian blue in 3% acetic acid.
5. Wash for 5 min in running water. Rinse in distilled water.
6. Dehydrate, clear, and mount in synthetic resin.

Sulfated mucosubstances stain purple-black. Uronic acid-containing mucosubstances and sialomucins are unstained (blue after alcian blue).

Alcian Blue-PAS Procedure
(From ref. 2)

Method

1. Bring sections to a water faucet.
2. Rinse briefly in 3% aqueous acetic acid.

3. Stain for 2 hr in 1% alcian blue 8GX in 3% acetic acid.

4. Rinse briefly in water and then in 3% acetic acid, running water, and distilled water.

5. Oxidize for 10 min in 1% periodic acid (aqueous) at room temperature.

6. Wash in running water for 5 min.

7. Immerse in Shiff's reagent for 10 min.

8. Wash in running water for 2 min.

9. Rinse in three changes of 0.5% sodium bisulfite, 1 min for each rinse.

10. Wash in running water for 5 min.

11. Dehydrate, clear, and mount.

This procedure stains periodate-unreactive, alcianophilic mucosubstances blue, periodate-reactive and alcianophilic components bluish purple, and periodate-reactive, nonalcianophilic components red. Acid mucosubstances stained blue by this procedure include hyaluronic and sialomucins, and all but the most strongly acidic sulfated mucosubstances stain blue or bluish purple.

Periodic Acid-Schiff (PAS) Technique

Proceed as in alcian blue-PAS procedure through steps 1 and 5 to 11.

Periodic Acid-Paradiamine Method (PAD)
(From ref. 13)

Reagents

Add 50 mg *N,N*-dimethyl-*p*-phenylenediamine HCl, just before use, to 50 ml citrate-phosphate buffer (0.1 M citric acid 4.8 ml, 0.2 M disodium phosphate 7.2 ml, distilled water 38 ml). Alternatively, dissolve 100 mg paradiamine in 50 ml distilled water and adjust pH to 5.0 with 0.4 M Na_2HPO_4.

Method

1. Bring slides to a water faucet.

2. Oxidize in 1% periodic acid for 10 min.

3. Rinse in running water for 10 min.

4. Immerse in paradiamine solution for 7, 24, or 48 hr.

5. Differentiate in 1% HCl in 70% alcohol for 8 sec (after 24-hr stain) or for 10 sec (after 48-hr stain).

6. Wash in water for 5 min.

7. Dehydrate through the alcohols, clear in xylene, and mount in a synthetic medium.

Neutral mucopolysaccharides stain brown, periodate-reactive polymers are purple or gray-brown, and periodate unreactive mucosubstances are black.

Azure A Staining Procedure

Solution pH *4.5*

Dissolve azure A 1:5,000 as follows: 48 ml 1:5,000 azure A, 1.1 ml 0.1 M citric acid; 0.9 ml 0.2 M Na$_2$HPO$_4$.

Method

1. Bring sections to water.
2. Stain in pH 4.5 solution for 30 min.
3. Dehydrate in alcohols and in alcohol-xylene.
4. Clear in xylene and mount in synthetic resin.

S-mucin B 4.5-containing epithelial sites stain metachromatically (they are also testicular hyaluronidase resistant).

Sialic Acid-Rich Mucosubstances Procedures

Saponification

Barium hydroxide 1% in 70% ethanol, 45 min at room temperature.

Neuraminidase

Vibrio cholerae neuraminidase 100 units/ml for 18 hr at 39°C. (Material labile to neuraminidase shows a decrease in basophilia toward azure A and alcian blue.)

GC Mucin Stable to Neuraminidase after Saponification, PAS-positive.

C Mucin Stable to Neuraminidase after Saponification, PAS-negative.

Lectins. Fucose-Lectin (ABC) Method
(From ref. 8)

Reagents

Biotinylated *Ulex europaeus* agglutinin I (UEA) (Vector, E-10651), protease XIV, pronase (Sigma, P-5147).

Method

The avidin–biotin–peroxidase complex (ABC) method by Hsu et al. (8) was slightly modified as follows.

1. Bring sections to a water faucet.
2. Immerse for 15 min in phosphate-buffered saline (PBS), pH 7.4 at 37°C.
3. Incubate at 37°C for 15 min in 0.05% pronase in PBS, pH 7.4.
4. Wash in three changes of PBS.
5. Treat for 30 min at room temperature with 0.5% H_2O_2 in methanol to block the endogenous peroxidase activity.
6. Wash in running water and in distilled water.
7. Preincubate for 30 min at room temperature with normal swine serum diluted 1:3 to reduce the nonspecific background.
8. Incubate for 60 min at room temperature in UEA diluted 1:200 in 0.5 M PBS, pH 7.4.
9. Wash in three changes of PBS.
10. Incubate for 60 min at room temperature with the ABC complex.
11. Wash in three changes of PBS.
12. Demonstrate peroxidase activity with 3,3'-diaminobenzidine-tetrahydrochloride (DAB), 0.5 mg/ml, 2 to 5 min at room temperature. DAB is dissolved in PBS by adding 0.02% H_2O_2.
13. Wash in running water 5 min.
14. Counterstain, if desired, with hematoxylin.
15. Wash in running water 15 min.
16. Dehydrate, clear, and mount in synthetic resin.

Endothelia and fucose-containing sites stain sharply brown.

APPENDIX III. IMMUNOHISTOCHEMISTRY

ABC Method
(From ref. 8)

Reagents

1. Lactoferrin: Rabbit immunoglobulins to human lactoferrin (Dako, A-186), diluted 1:2,000 in 0.5 M PBS, pH 7.4.
2. α_1-Antichimotrypsin: Rabbit immunoglobulins to human α_1-antichimotrypsin (Dako, A-022), diluted 1:1,000 in 0.5 M PBS, pH 7.4.
3. Lysozyme: Rabbit immunoglobulins to human lysozyme (muramidase) (Dako, A-099), diluted 1:2,000 in 0.5 M α_1 PBS, pH 7.4.
4. Orosomucoid: Rabbit immunoglobulins to human orosomucoid (Dako, A-011) diluted 1:2000 in 0.5 M PBS, pH 7.4.

5. S100 proteins: Rabbit immunoglobulins to cow S100 (Dako, Z-311), diluted 1:200 in 0.5 M PBS, pH 7.4.

6. Biotinylated antirabbit IgG made in goat (Vector, BA-1000).

7. ABC reagent (vectastain, ABC Kit, Standard, Vector, PK-4000). Reagent A: avidin DH, 2 ml; reagent B: biotinylated horseradish peroxidase H, 2 ml. Add exactly 2 drops of reagent A to 10 ml 0.5 M PBS, pH 7.4, and mix. Then add exactly 2 drops of reagent B to the same mixing bottle. Mix immediately and allow to stand for about 30 min before use.

8. Protease XIV: Pronase (Sigma, P-5147).

The commercial names cited indicate only that the reagents have been tested by the authors, with satisfactory results. Obviously, many other products may be used.

Method

1. Bring sections to a water faucet.

2. Immerse for 15 min in PBS, pH 7.4, at 37°C.

3. Incubate at 37°C for 15 min in 0.05% pronase in 0.5 M PBS, pH 7.4.

4. Wash in three changes of PBS.

5. Treat for 30 min at room temperature with 0.5% H_2O_2 in methanol to block the endogenous peroxidase activity.

6. Wash in running water and in distilled water.

7. Preincubate for 30 min at room temperature with normal (goat) nonimmune serum, diluted 1:4 in 0.5 M PBS, pH 7.4.

8. Incubate overnight at 0 to 4°C in the specific rabbit reagent (1 through 5 in reagents list).

9. Wash in three changes of PBS.

10. Incubate for 30 min at room temperature in 0.5% biotinylated antirabbit IgG (made in goat) in 0.5 M PBS, pH 7.4.

11. Wash in three changes of PBS.

12. Incubate for 60 min at room temperature in ABC reagent.

13. Wash in PBS.

14. Demonstrate peroxidase activity with 3,3'-diaminobenzidine tetrahydrochloride (DAB), 0.5 mg/ml, 2 to 5 min at room temperature. DAB is dissolved in PBS by adding 0.02% H_2O_2.

15. Wash in running water 5 min.

16. Counterstain, if desired, with hematoxylin.

17. Wash in running water, 10 to 15 min.

18. Dehydrate, clear, and mount in synthetic resin.

The sites corresponding to reagents 1 through 5 are sharply brown.

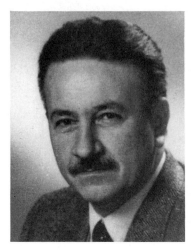

Giuseppe Barbolini was born in Modena, Italy, in 1934 and received the M.D. degree in 1958 from the Modena University, Italy. He is full Professor of Pathology in the University of Modena, School of Medicine, Italy. His research interests are concentrated in lung pathology, medical informatics (SNOMED), and prostate gland.

Alberto Bisetti was born in 1927 in Paris. He received the M.D. degree in 1953 from Rome University, Italy. He is Full Professor in Lung Diseases and Director of the Institute of Pneumology of the Rome University, Italy. His interest is lung pathology.

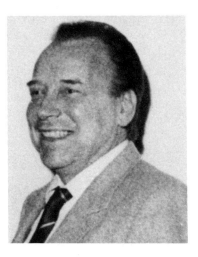

Methods in Bronchial Mucology,
edited by P. C. Braga and L. Allegra.
Raven Press, Ltd. © 1988.

3.5.2. Electron Microscopy Investigation of Mucus

J. M. Sturgess

Parke-Davis, Scarborough, Ontario, Canada

Methods
    Electron microscopy of mucous blanket
    Electron microscopy of mucus
Results
    Mucous blanket *in situ*
    Mucous glycoproteins
Discussion

The existence of an extracellular fluid lining of the airways was based originally on light microscopic studies, using frozen sections. These studies have demonstrated the thickness of the mucous layer to be about 5 μm in large airways, decreasing progressively in more distal airways to 1 μm in bronchioles and less than 0.1 μm in terminal bronchioles. However, our understanding of the organization and continuity of the mucous blanket has been gained by electron microscopy. Scanning electron microscopy has been applied to investigate the surface topography of the bronchial mucosa and the overlying fluid and mucous layers (13,16–20). By transmission electron microscopy, further information has been derived for cellular elements in sputum (11), on the mucus layers in major bronchi (10), and on the extracellular fluid layers in the bronchioles (4,9). The fine structure of mucins purified from bronchial secretions has been evaluated using scanning electron microscopy (7,8) and transmission electron microscopy (12).

These approaches have provided some important information on the structural organization of the viscous mucous blanket that protects the bronchial epithelium. This complex mixture has proved difficult to analyze because of its biochemical heterogeneity. Electron microscopy also has provided insight into the ultrastructure and, particularly, the biphasic nature of the extracellular lining of the airways in health and disease.

METHODS

Electron Microscopy of Mucous Blanket

Scanning Electron Microscopy

For scanning electron microscopy, careful fixation, dehydration, and coating techniques are essential to preserve mucus. To study mucus *in situ,* samples of bronchial wall overlying cartilage, approximately 1 cm^2, are resected from the major airways, including the trachea, main bronchus, and lobar bronchus, washed gently by immersion in phosphate-buffered saline (PBS) pH 7.4, and then fixed in 1% glutaraldehyde in 0.1 M sodium phosphate buffer, 350 mOsm and pH 7.4, at 4°C for 4 to 5 hr. After fixation, the tissue samples are protected by wrapping loosely in lens paper to maintain the structural relationship between the mucus blanket and the underlying tissues during processing. Tissues are then placed in stainless steel mesh baskets, dehydrated in graded acetone solutions, and then dried with carbon dioxide, using the critical point method (10). The dried samples are mounted on aluminum stubs and coated with approximately 20 nm of gold in a high vacuum rotary evaporator. Samples are examined in a scanning electron microscope at 13 to 20 kV, and micrographs are recorded on 120 mm film.

To investigate the continuity of the mucus layer, cryofracture techniques have been used in conjunction with scanning electron microscopy (13). Samples of trachea or bronchi are fixed in 2% glutaraldehyde by vascular perfusion and postfixed in ruthenium red–osmium tetroxide–cacodylate solution (13,14). The tissues are dehydrated in ethanol, cryofractured, and then critical point dried using carbon dioxide. The ethanol–cryofracture technique allows study of the organization and depth of the mucous layer. In the rat lung, these techniques have demonstrated a biphasic mucous blanket, with a thin hypophase and an epiphase of up to 5 μm thickness.

Transmission Electron Microscopy

For transmission electron microscopy, samples of trachea and mainstem bronchus are fixed in 3% glutaraldehyde in 0.1 M sodium phosphate buffer, rinsed in 0.1

M sodium phosphate buffer, and postfixed in 1% osmium tetroxide in veronal acetate buffer. After *en bloc* staining with uranyl acetate, samples are dehydrated in a graded series of ethanol solutions and then embedded in Epon-Araldite epoxy resin and allowed to polymerize. Ultrathin sections are stained with lead citrate and uranyl acetate and examined by transmission electron microscopy at 60 kV and recorded on 35 mm film.

Other approaches to examine extracellular lining layers of the airways include vascular perfusion (9,13) and vapor fixation (20) at −8 cm water using 25% glutaraldehyde followed by 2% osmium tetroxide in cacodylate buffer for 1 hr. Perfusion and nebulization of fixative into the bronchial tree are alternative methods that stabilize the mucous layer of the respiratory tract (10). These approaches have allowed quantification of the thickness of the mucus layer by transmission electron microscopy and characterization of the biphasic nature of the mucus blanket.

Enhancement of respiratory tract secretions for transmission electron microscopy may be achieved cytochemically using ruthenium red for glycoproteins (14) and using a tricomplex salt mixture containing lead nitrate and potassium ferricyanide for lipid-rich secretions (5). Monoclonal antibodies have been prepared against mucous and serous glycoproteins from rabbit and monkeys (1,15) and used to localize secretions to epithelial cells. Similar techniques may provide valuable new approaches to the study of distinct types of glycoproteins in mucous secretions by electron microscopy. Cellular constituents of bronchial mucus may be demonstrated after fixation with phosphate-buffered osmium tetroxide. Such fixation provides good preservation of cell architecture for diagnostic purposes (11).

Electron Microscopy of Mucus

Mucous glycoproteins are isolated from rat or human bronchial secretions as described by Forstner et al. (8). The techniques for isolation and reconstitution of mucus have been developed to maintain composition, molecular interactions, and functional side groups as closely as possible to the native state. The isolated mucins have been characterized by viscosity, sedimentation, and biochemical analyses.

For electron microscopy of purified mucus glycoproteins, samples of purified mucus at a concentration of about 0.1% are either (a) freeze-dried from liquid carbon dioxide or dried by the critical point technique or (b) fixed rapidly in 1% glutaraldehyde, dialyzed against distilled water, and then rapidly frozen and dried. The specimens are coated with 7 mm gold in a high vacuum evaporator and examined immediately in a scanning electron microscope.

To evaluate ultrastructural changes after the interactions of mucus with ions and proteins, samples of mucous glycoprotein are incubated with various molarities of salts or other agents in an M-Tris HCl buffer, pH 7.4. Control samples in buffer at equivalent osmolarity are prepared in parallel with each test sample.

RESULTS

Mucous Blanket *In Situ*

By scanning electron microscopy, the mucous blanket in the respiratory tract forms a continuous sheet, although discontinuities may exist in the large airways. The characteristic features of the mucous layer are determined by complex glycoproteins that make up about 1% of the mucus. In the normal human lung, the mucus blanket forms a continuous lining and closely follows the contours of the epithelial surface. The extracellular lining layer varies in thickness from 5 to 10 μm in the larger airways to 1 to 4 μm in the bronchioles to 0.1 μm in the terminal bronchioles.

In the trachea, mucus forms a smooth, cohesive layer overlying the tips of the ciliated and mucus-secreting epithelial cells (Figs. 1, 2). Occasional gaps in the

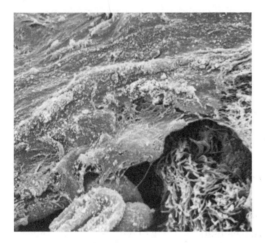

FIG. 1. Mucous blanket in normal trachea, showing smooth layers of mucous glycoproteins situated over the tips of the ciliated epithelium.

FIG. 2. Scanning electron micrograph of mucus in patient with chronic obstructive pulmonary disease. The mucous blanket is thick, with dense layers of mucus, often appearing in ropelike strands, and cellular debris.

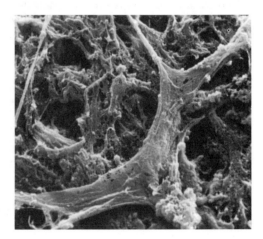

mucous blanket reveal the underlying epithelial cells. The smooth mucous blanket in the trachea is often characterized by series of overlapping layers or plaques, which may be smooth in appearance or may be fenestrated with holes 0.1 to 2 mm in diameter.

In the mainstem bronchi, the mucous blanket exhibits a more elaborate, overlapping, layered structure, with few smoother mucous sheets and more elaborate fibrillar networks and perforated sheets, superimposed and interconnected with fibers. (Fig. 3). In lobar bronchi, the mucous blanket becomes thinner and is characterized by open networks of fine fibrils and narrow interfibrillar spaces (Fig. 4). There are few smooth sheets or plaques in the lining layer in more distal airway generations.

Mucus secretions discharged from epithelial cells show an expanded network of fine fibers. Examination of stereopairs and scanning electron microscopy demon-

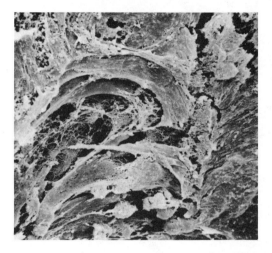

FIG. 3. Mucous blanket showing characteristic features and three-dimensional arrangement of glycoprotein layers in the major bronchi. Mucus is organized in layers, with smooth overlapping sheets and networks of interconnecting fibrils.

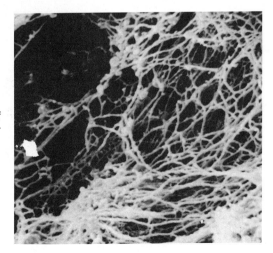

FIG. 4. Detail of fibrillar networks of mucus in lower layers of mucus blanket.

strate similar open fibrillar structures close to the epithelial cell surface and more densely packed fibers and sheets toward the airway lumen. These observations reflect the changes in the mucous glycoproteins in the respiratory tract, presumably caused by interactions with fluid, electrolytes, and other macromolecules after release into the airway.

Removal of the mucous lining reveals epithelial cell surfaces. There is little evidence of any macromolecular material under the macromolecular glycoprotein

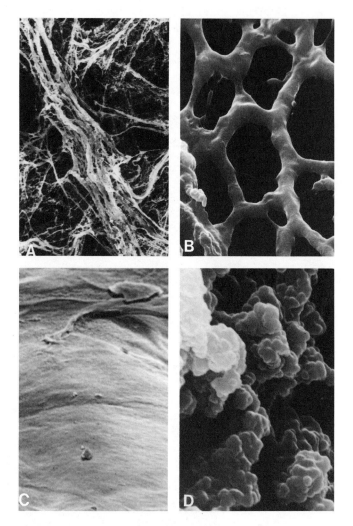

FIG. 5. Mucous glycoproteins, purified and examined by electron microscopy. **A:** Control mucous glycoprotein showing fine fibrillar networks. **B:** Detail of glycoprotein fibrils. **C:** After removal of sialic acid, mucus forms smooth sheets. **D:** With divalent cations (Ca^{2+}), mucous fibers thicken and clump into dense aggregates.

layer. These observations support earlier cytochemical studies that have indicated that little or no acidic glycoproteins are present under the mucous layer.

Transmission electron microscopy of mucus in the bronchial tree in experimental animal has confirmed the separation of the extracellular lining into an epiphase, rich in mucous glycoproteins, and an underlying hypophase. The upper layer is electron dense, with a dense fibrillar appearance, whereas the hypophase has a dispersed granular appearance. A thin osmiophilic layer is seen overlying both layers and resembles the material lining the bronchioles. Osmiophilic structures with whorl–like myelin figures, 4 nm in diameter, are often observed in the hypophase (20).

In hypersecretory states, the epiphase becomes significantly thicker, with more densely packed sheets of mucus and fibrils, whereas the hypophase diminishes in thickness (10). These ultrastructural changes correlate with increasing viscosity and elasticity of bronchial secretions. The changes in the mucous blanket result in penetration of mucous glycoproteins among the epithelial cilia.

Mucous Glycoproteins

Mucous glycoproteins, purified from bronchial mucus or intestinal mucus, form three-dimensional networks of interlacing fibrils. The morphological characteristics of the mucous glycoproteins may be modified by change in concentration and by the presence of monovalent or divalent cations. Changes in the mucus affect the diameter of the fibrils and of the interfibrillar spaces (Fig. 5).

Purified mucous glycoproteins form a loose web of random or parallel orientated fibers, interlinked with thinner fibers or filaments, to form a layered network. Increasing concentrations of sodium or calcium ions cause shortening and thickening of fibrils and a reduction in size of the interstices and volume of the interfibrillar spaces. Increasing the concentration of cations causes thickening and aggregation of fibrils, with decreased hydration, viscosity, and solubility (7).

DISCUSSION

The highly hydrated nature of mucus presents a major challenge in preservation of structure for electron microscopy. Mucus contains approximately 98% water, so that freezing and drying techniques may result in significant artifacts. Furthermore, mechanical stress developed during drying may cause alignment of filaments in the direction of shear or flow, thus influencing the apparent organization of mucus molecules.

Despite these limitations, different procedures of rapid freeze-drying, using fixed and unfixed mucus, critical point drying, and substitution techniques have demonstrated similar ultrastructure and organization of mucus. The mucous glycoproteins, purified from intestinal and bronchial secretions, show similar structural characteristics, with different diameters of fibrils, varying from 50 to 500 mm in diameter. The fibrils form a three-dimensional arrangement of layers and interconnecting structures.

The preservation of extracellular lining layers in the respiratory tract has been achieved by immersion fixation, vapor fixation, and vascular perfusion. In general, vascular perfusion provides good preservation of alveolar and bronchiolar lining layers (4,10). However, the intricate vascular supply of the major bronchi renders this approach less effective for large airways. Vapor fixation or careful instillation of fixative is necessary to examine the mucus layer of the large airways.

Although mucus secretions are heterogeneous in nature and composition, there are remarkable similarities in chemical and structural organization, regardless of cellular orgin. Mammalian mucus from the gastrointestinal tract, cervix, or respiratory tract shares similar ultrastructural characteristics. The chemical and physical properties of mucus substances from marine animals also show similarities (6). In these species, mucus forms regular uniform filaments, 10 to 20 mm thick, in expanded networks with regular lattice arrangement. The open fibrillar network of glycoproteins has been thought to reflect a mechanism for selective filtration of material in different species.

Human endocervical mucus has been studied by scanning electron microscopy (2), which revealed long thick fibers (300–600 mm in diameter) interconnected by regular arrays of thinner fibrils (50–100 mm). The structural organization of cervical mucus changes as a reflection of glycoprotein composition during the ovulatory cycle, reflecting changes in chemical composition and rheological properties. The ultrastructural changes are considered in cervical mucus to provide a selective barrier to restrict passage of materials and of sperm.

In the respiratory tract, the variation in structural organization reflects changes in composition and hydration of bronchial secretions (16–18). The thicker, cohesive layers in the trachea reflect a protective barrier, with tightly linked mucous macromolecules and other proteins and electrolytes. With progressive airway branching, the mucous layer becomes more expanded and hydrated, providing less of a mechanical barrier and more of a hydrated expanded network of glycoproteins.

ACKNOWLEDGMENT

This research was supported by the Medical Research Council of Canada and the Canadian Cystic Fibrosis Foundation. The excellent technical assistance of Ms. Erma Minaker and Nina Czegledy-Nagy is acknowledged.

REFERENCES

1. Basbaum, C. B., Mann, J. K., Chow, A. W., and Finkbeiner, W. E. (1984): Monoclonal antibodies as probes for unique antigens in secretory cells of mixed exocrine organs. *Proc. Natl. Acad. Sci. USA,* 81:4419–4423.

2. Chretien, I. C., Gernigon, C., David, G., and Psychoyos, A. (1973): The ultrastructure of human cervical mucus under scanning electron microscopy. *Fertil. Steril.,* 24:746–757.
3. Czegledy-Nagy, E., and Sturgess, J. M. (1978): Mucus-secretion in the lung. In: *Scanning Electron Microscopy/1978, Vol. II,* pp. 1083–1088. SEM Inc., Chicago, IL.
4. Ebert, R. V., and Terracio, M. J. (1975): Observations of the secretion on the surface of the bronchioles with the scanning electron microscope. *Am. Rev. Respir. Dis.,* 112:491–496.
5. Finlay-Jones, J. M., and Papadimitriou, J. M. (1972): Demonstration of pulmonary surfactant by tracheal injection of tricomplex salt mixture for electron microscopy. *Stain Technol.,* 47:59–63.
6. Flood, P. R. (1981): On the ultrastructure of mucus. *Biomed. Res.,* 2 (Suppl.):49–53.
7. Forstner, G., Forstner, J., and Sturgess, J. M. (1976): Physical changes induced in mucin by calcium: Implications for the obstructive complications of cystic fibrosis. *Proc. VII Int. Cystic Fibrosis Congress,* Paris, pp. 31–37.
8. Forstner, G., Forstner, J., and Sturgess, J. M. (1977): Malfunction of intestinal mucus and mucus production. *Adv. Exp. Biol. Med.,* 89:349–369.
9. Gil, J., and Weibel, E. R. (1971): Extracellular lining of bronchioles after perfusion fixation of rat lungs for electron microscopy. *Anat. Rec.,* 169:185–194.
10. Hulbert, W. C., Forster, B. B., Laird, W., and Walker, D. C. (1982): An improved method for fixation of the respiratory epithelial surface with the mucus and surfactant layers. *Lab. Invest.,* 47:354–363.
11. Kory, R. C., Pendharker, M. B., Siegesmund, K. A., Pederson, H. J., and Boren, H. G. (1970): Electron microscopy of sputum. *Am. Rev. Respir. Dis.,* 101:385–394.
12. Lamblin, G., Lhermitte, M., Degand, P., and Roussel, P. (1979): Chemical and physical properties of human bronchial mucus glycoproteins. *Biochimie,* 61:23–43.
13. Luchtel, D. L. (1978): The mucus layer of the trachea and major bronchi in the rat. *Scan. Electron Microsc.,* 2:1089–1094.
14. Luft, J. H. (1971): Ruthenium red and violet. I. Chemistry, purification, methods of use for electron microscopy and mechanisms of action. *Anat. Rec.,* 171:347–359.
15. St. George, J. A., Cranz, D. L., Zicker, S. C., Etchison, J. R., Dungworth, D. L., and Plopper, C. G. (1985): An immunohistochemical characterization of rhesus monkey respiratory secretions using monoclonal antibodies. *Am. Rev. Respir. Dis.,* 132:556–563.
16. Sturgess, J. M. (1977): The mucous lining of major bronchi in the rabbit lung. *Am. Rev. Respir. Dis.,* 115:819–827.
17. Sturgess, J. M. (1977): Bronchial mucus secretion in cystic fibrosis. *Mod. Probl. Pediatr.,* 19:129–140.
18. Sturgess, J. M. (1979): Mucous secretions in the respiratory tract. *Pediatr. Clin. North Am.,* 26:481–501.
19. Van As, A., and Webster, I. (1974): The morphology of mucus in mammalian pulmonary airways. *Environ. Res.,* 7:1–12.
20. Yoneda, K. (1976): Mucous blanket of rat bronchus. An ultrastructural study. *Am. Rev. Respir. Dis.,* 114:837–842.

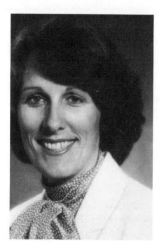

Jennifer M. Sturgess was born in 1944 and received the B.Sc. (Hons. Microbiology) in 1966 from the University of Bristol, Bristol, England, and the Ph.D. (Pathology) in 1970 from the University of London, England. She is currently the Director for Scientific Affairs, Warner-Lambert, Canada, and Associate Professor, Department of Pathology, University of Toronto, Canada.

4. Biological Methods of Analysis

Methods in Bronchial Mucology,
edited by P. C. Braga and L. Allegra.
Raven Press, Ltd. © 1988.

4.1. CILIARY MOTION

4.1.1. *In Vitro* Observation and Counting Methods for Ciliary Motion

P. C. Braga

Department of Pharmacology, University of Milan, Milan, Italy

Methods
  Obtaining the specimen
  Maintenance
  Observation
  Counting
Discussion

The word "cilia," first used in 1786 by F. O. Muller (54), identifies a particular type of hairlike cell structures (Fig. 1) that project from the free surfaces of cells and were first described in 1684 by Anton de Heide (54). Cilia, which are found in nearly all phyla of the animal kingdom, perform some vital functions, such as locomotion, feeding, digestion, excretion, reproduction, sensory perception, respiration, and cleansing of surfaces (55).

Mammalian cilia are, on the average, 6 to 7 μm in length and densely distributed (3–11/μm^2), with a tip-to-tip spacing of 0.2 to 0.6 μm, which is about twice the diameter of the cilia at the base, 0.2 to 0.25 μm (23,39) (Fig. 1). Microvilli protrude from the surface between the cilia. The cilia oscillate with a fast, rigid, effective stroke in the forward direction that occupies about one fourth to one third of the cycle and a slow, limp, recovery stroke in the recoil direction that lasts the remainder, at frequencies ranging generally between 10 and 20 Hz (600–

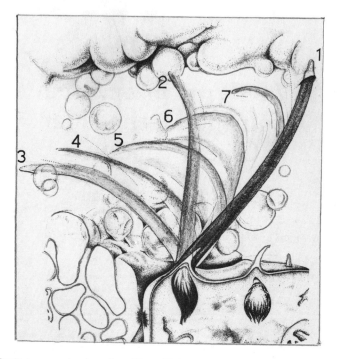

FIG. 1. Oscillatory mechanics of a cilium. Rigid effective stroke (1,2,3) and recoil phase (4,5,6,7). (Courtesy of L.I.R.C.A. Synthelabo, Italy.)

recoveystroke

(From P. Braga .L. Alleyra 1988 pg 258)

1,200 beats/min). This means that the period of oscillation is asymmetrical, since the recoil phase is longer than the rigid phase.

The mechanics of ciliary movement (3,7) have been investigated with particular interest because studying them provides immediate visual control of the ciliated cell's behavior in different environmental, physiological, or pathological situations. Pneumologists are particularly interested in studying cilia because the beat of the cilia on the respiratory tree mucosa is considered to be the biological engine that continuously moves physiological or pathological bronchial mucus secretions (2, 4,46).

Function has been investigated by evaluating the cilia and mucus as a whole system, i.e., using different kinds of markers to visualize the movement of the mucus induced by cilia, and also by examining ciliary activity on its own by measuring the rate of ciliary beating.

METHODS

Many studies of ciliary motion have been performed with protozoa, such as *Paramecium, Opalina, Stentor,* and *Chamydomonas,* or with *Lamellibranchia*

(3,53–55). These observations of motility during basal conditions or after drug administration are interesting to the pneumologist mainly from the point of view of the kinds of techniques used to investigate amphibian or mammalian ciliated tissue. There are some differences in dimension, number, and kinds of distribution of cilia or flagella and in their functions from those of mammalian tracheal cilia.

Investigation of *in vitro* ciliary motion requires a combination of different kinds of technique to obtain the biological specimen, to maintain it in the best physiological condition, to observe it in the best microscopic conditions, and to measure its activity (Fig. 2).

Obtaining the Specimen

A modern technique for obtaining ciliated cells is simply to brush the epithelia of respiratory airways. This can be done during routine fiberoptic bronchoscopy, using a disposable cytological brush (Medi-Tech, BTI/58/140, Medi-Tech, Inc., Watertown, MA) with soft nylon bristles 1 mm long distributed over 1 cm. The brush is housed in a small flexible Teflon tube; the bristles come into contact with the epithelium only very briefly, i.e., when the brush is pulled out of the

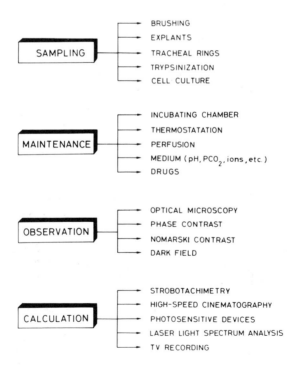

FIG. 2. Schematic description of the successive steps and related techniques or instruments in the study of ciliary motility.

tube at the point from which the sample is to be taken. An easier noninvasive technique is to obtain samples from the tissue between the inferior turbinate and the anterior wall of the nose from conscious, unmedicated subjects. The step-by-step sequence is shown in Fig. 3A (5). By releasing and withdrawing the brush once or twice, it is possible to remove small fragments or single ciliated cells that remain immersed in the culture medium into which the brush had been dipped before sampling. The material is then removed, sampled, and placed in a perfusion chamber (Fig. 3A) (5). This technique has been used for humans (33,48,49) but can also be applied to animals (37,38). Two modifications are to use a biopsy forceps to obtain explants (20,65) or punches (14) from epithelial islets or to scrape the middle part of the inferior turbinate (nose) with a sharp 2-mm spoon (curette) (42,43,47).

A technique for investigation of ciliary beat frequency (CBF) uses cross-sectional tracheal rings, which are generally obtained from small laboratory animals. Chick embryo tracheal rings are removed aseptically from embryos 19 to 20 days old and placed in screw-capped tissue culture tubes containing 1 ml of Eagle's basal medium (each milliliter contains 100 units of penicillin G, 100 μg streptomycin,

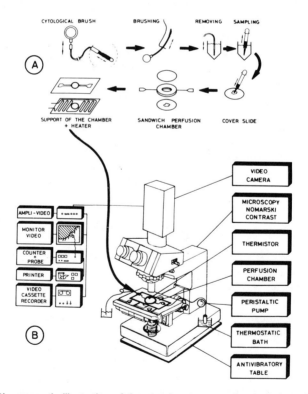

FIG. 3. A: Diagrammatic illustration of the step-by-step sampling technique. **B:** Schematic view of the experimental setup.

and 0.25 μg amphotericin B). The ring sections are incubated on a roller drum (15 rph) at 35°C (8,9). With similar techniques, tracheal ring cultures have been prepared from New Zealand-Dutch white rabbits that were 2 weeks old (9). Even rats (51) and hamster (1) tracheal rings or fragments of trachea from larger animals, such as ram (26), have been used to study CBF.

Another approach is to use explants of ciliated epithelium. New Zealand White rabbits can be used as donors. Under pentobarbital anesthesia, the trachea is aseptically removed and thoroughly washed with basal Eagle's medium (pH 7.4). The epithelia are microdissected with a sterilized scalpel. The mucosal sheets are then rinsed with medium, transferred to a sterile watch glass, and divided into 15 to 20 pieces, 1 to 3 mm^2, which are placed in Falcon 30 ml culture flasks and incubated in 3 ml of Eagle's medium supplemented 10% with 1% fetal calf serum, 200 mM L-glutamine, penicillin (50 U/ml), and streptomycin (50 μg/ml). Explanted epithelial sheets are incubated at 37°C and kept alive for a week (10,12,22).

Tissue culture of single ciliated cells or cellular aggregates is a subsequent step to explant techniques. Sheets of ciliated cells or pieces of excised trachea are digested with protease for 24 hr at 4°C to obtain a cell suspension. Then the protease activity is neutralized, and lavage and centrifugation are carried out. Standard cell culture techniques are applied. Ciliated cell cultures have been performed with human (13,61), dog (11), rabbit (59,63), frog (62), newt (60,27), hamster (35), and mouse (41) cells.

Maintenance

After the biological specimen of ciliated cells has been obtained, the next step in the procedure is to apply the now well-standardized maintenance techniques. We put the materials (brushing, explant rings, isolated cells) into an adapted incubation chamber to maintain a controlled environment, thermostated (37°C for mammalian cells, 25°C for amphibian cells) with continuous medium perfusion and controlled pH, Pco_2, ions, and so on. There are many types of incubation chambers (Table 1) (44). The basic idea for an incubation chamber is a glass support on which to deposit the materials and another thin glass cover to maintain the transparency. The space between the two glasses is maintained by a rigid, usually metallic, structure, through which the liquid medium can be perfused without loss. Perfusion can be performed with a laboratory fluid pump, such as a peristaltic pump, and the medium can be prewarmed. The chamber temperature can be regulated in an air stream incubator monitored by a telethermometer or on a temperature-controlled, warmed microscope stage.

Observation

When the incubation chamber is placed on an XY stage of a microscope, one can observe the beating of the cilia. High magnification, usually greater than

TABLE 1. Comparison of perfusion chamber designs[a]

Chamber and Materials[b,g]		Shape of field	Viewing area (mm²)	Chamber depth minimum (mm)	Distance[c] (mm)	Distance[d] (mm)	Thickness of chamber (mm)	Volume of chamber (ml)	Type of seal[e]
1. Pomerat	(1951) A	□	484	0.5	0	0.63	12	0.24	W/PR
2. Mackaness	(1952) A	○	284	1.5	0.23	1.86	2.2	0.43	W/PR
3. Christiansen	(1953) A	○	227	0.6	0	0.73	6.5	0.14	W/PR
4. Buchsbaum	(1951) SS	○	314	1.0	1.0	2.13	3.3	0.31	W/PR
5. Rose	(1954) SS	○	573	Up 3.6	3.6	7.33	11.1	1.9	Gasket
6. Richter	(1955) Cd	□○	480	Up 1.8	1.27	3.2	4.3	0.95	Gasket
7. Powell	(1955) SS	○	177	3.0	0	3.0	7.0	0.53	W/PR + Gasket
8. Balducci	(1957) SS	⬭	110	3.0	6.0	9.13	15.3	0.33	Gasket
9. Toy	(1958) A	○□	284/412	1.0	0.8	2.0	3.0	0.28	W/PR
10. Cruickshank	(1959) A	○	314	0.75	4.25	5.0	5.0	0.24	W/PR
11. Sykes	(1959) B/SS	○	284	Up 3.6	0.8	4.53	6.5	0.70	O-ring
12. Shadomy	(1963) SS	○	800	1.0	6.0	8.0	10.2	0.28	Gasket
13. Thomas	(1966) A	○	754	1.8	3.6	5.53	9.3	1.21	Gasket
14. White	(1966) SS/A	○	192	Up 1.5	0.05	6.10	7.5	Up 9.4	W/PR + O-ring
15. Poyton	(1970) SS	□	400	Up 1.0	0.8	1.98	4.1	Up 0.63	W/PR + O-ring
16. Dvorak[f]	(1971) SS	○	630	0.5	1.0	2.2	8.9	0.45	O-ring

[a] Modified from ref. 44, where references can be found.

[b] A, aluminum; B, brass; Cd, cadmium; SS, stainless steel.

[c] Distance from bottom coverslip to microscope stage.

[d] Distance from top coverslip to microscope stage.

[e] W/PR, wax or plastic resin.

[f] Dvorak et al. (1971): *Exp. Cell Res.*, 68:144–148.

[g] Usable with interference microscope: Nos. 1, 2, 3, 4, 9, 15, 16. Usable with cellophane strip technique (Rose et al., 1958: *J. Biochem. Cytol.*, 4:761): Nos. 5, 6, 8, 13, 14, 15, 16. Commercially available: No. 5 (Wahlberg-McCreary Inc., 212 Pease Ave., Houston, TX); No. 10 (Sterilin Ltd., 9–11 The Quadrant, Richmond, Surrey, UK); No. 11 (Bellco Glass Inc., 340 Ednudo Rd, Vineland, NJ); No. 15 (Scientific Instrument Co, 348 6th St., San Francisco, CA); No. 16 (Nicholson Precision Instrument Inc, Bethesda, MD).

×500, is used. Microscopic fields in which the ciliary crown of the cell groups or a single cell appears tangent to the cell body are selected to show the largest ciliary axis (Fig. 3B), and the entire beat cycle is in the plane of focus. Microscopes generally are equipped with phase contrast optics. The use of a Nomarski differential interference contrast optical system can improve observation of the cilia. In darkfield, there is an interesting picture in which cilia are white luminous filaments, but the high magnification required for better observation needs a special darkfield immersion condenser that is not available for all kinds of microscope. The quality of the images obtained is obviously influenced by the quality of the microscope's optics. High quality planar apochromatic optics should be used. Cold light is a necessity to avoid interference by a hot spot of light concentrated by the condenser on the cilia.

Counting

Various methods with different advantages and disadvantages have been used to estimate the frequency of ciliary activity and to test the effects of various substances. When individual cilia movements can be observed in detail, as in the techniques previously described, there are some counting techniques that have been found to be useful.

Strobotachymetry is one of the earlier methods used and consists of adjustment of the stroboscopic flash frequency to that of the light reflected (flickering) from the beating cilium (1,16,25,36,60). The results are available immediately, but the ciliary movements are not exactly periodic so that it is difficult to obtain exactly the freezing of movement. Moreover, the rate of flashes is disagreeable to the operator and can be epileptogenic (28). This method is useful for investigation of mussels, e.g., in which the cilia are large and well separated and the frequency is low (17,29).

High-speed cinematography is a high-speed motion picture recording that needs a special camera with frame rates of up to 500 to 700 frames/sec for fast black and white film. After the film is developed, it is viewed at low speed (2–24 frames/sec), which makes it possible to count the flicker activity by direct vision (15,16) or to count the number of ciliary beats (10,45,62). This method, when used with a very precise time marker, is accurate. The disadvantages are those due to the high frame velocity and the very brief period of time that can be measured. It is expensive for experiments lasting longer than a few minutes, because of using a large quantity of film. Developing the film is laborious, and there is a time lag between the filming and the time-consuming collection of data from the developed film.

A number of photoelectronic techniques have been developed along two lines: those that use the principle of monitoring reflected light (Chap. 4.1.2.) and those that analyze the images obtained by transmitted light. Initially, photosensitive cells were used to detect changes in light intensity due to ciliary movements (correlated with their frequencies) across the aperture of a pinhole, and the results were displayed in several numerical or graphic ways (18,21,28,64). More recently, photomultipliers have been used (32,42,43,48,49), which have the advantages of relatively good precision, depending on the diameter of the pinhole and the continuous monitoring frequency. However, they are sensitive to vibrations and are rather expensive. Flash saturation of the photomultiplier with excess light can lead to variable recovery times in the system and, if extreme, will damage the tube permanently. The resulting measure can be considered as an average or a mass effect of the movements of an area in which cilia can move or not and can have different frequencies.

A recent method directs a laser light beam to the moving cilia. The resulting scattering of light can be detected with a photomultiplier, and the spectrum of its intensity fluctuation can be analyzed to give quantitative information (33,58,59). This method, previously used to analyze the motility of sperm (19,30,52), is accurate, but its devices and extraction of data are very complicated.

Fast Fourier transform and autocorrelation analysis has been used in conjunction with photoelectric techniques (31,33,34,57,59). The results of these analyses are interpreted as a distribution or spectrum of ciliary beat frequencies from which a dominant beat frequency is determined. Computer-assisted recording and analysis has been proposed (24,50).

An additional method is modernization of the cinematographic method, i.e., recording the activity by a television camera on a videotape recorder with the option of slow motion and then counting directly from the screen. In this case, the method is accurate but time consuming, and the data are not available in real time. A new method is to shoot the selected microscopic field with a black and white (B/W) television camera equipped with a 1 inch Plumbicon tube, with which it is possible to visualize the rapid movement of the cilia without any trail phenomenon. The signals from the television camera are fed to a B/W 14-inch 400-line monitor in parallel with a videorecorder (6) (Fig. 4). Using appropriate microscope magnification (100× objective and 10× ocular), the length of the cilia seen on the monitor screen is about 3 cm, with proportional diameters. These dimensions make it possible to count the CBF by means of an instrument with a digital readout purposely designed to receive and count the signals from a phototransistor (visual field of 2 degrees) placed directly on the protective screen of the monitor in exact correspondence with the point of passage of the back and forth movements of the cilium selected (Fig. 5) (6). The final count is the number of passages in front of the phototransistor of the dark area, representing the ciliary body on the light background, in a predetermined time. The results are given in both digital and analog form. The sensitivity of the phototransistor is adjusted for each experiment according to a scale of shades of gray. With this method of counting in real time, a high degree of accuracy and easy reproduction can be achieved. The difference in rates between this technique and those of a slow-motion technique was 8%. This method is less expensive, there is no need for complicated instruments,

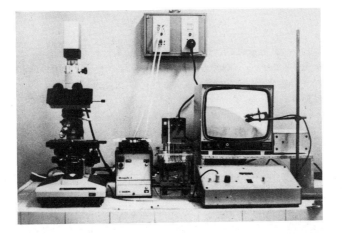

FIG. 4. Arrangement of instruments, with the probe positioned on the television monitor screen.

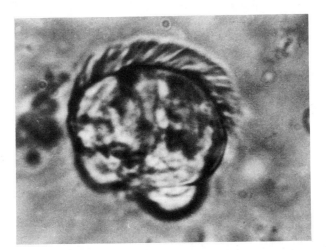

FIG. 5. Photomicrograph of living ciliated cell showing ciliary crown. ×1,000.

and there is the possibility of precisely studying the behavior of only one or two or up to five cilia. A potential disadvantage is the analysis of CBF approaching 50 Hz because of the 50 Hz television scan rate. However, human cilia beat *in vitro* at a rate less than 50 Hz (56). A method similar to that just described that uses a photodiode as a probe and fast Fourier transform analysis to perform a real time spectral study of beating cilia has been proposed (56).

DISCUSSION

The great interest of researchers in investigating the mechanics of ciliary movement has provided pneumologists with many techniques for studying the behavior of ciliated airway epithelium in physiological or pathological conditions or after drug administration.

The logical sequences of the steps of these methods have been described. For every step, there are several different technical approaches to orientate the researcher who needs to set up an instrumental complex to record CBF.

Single specific technical details must obviously be determined according to the availability of the different kinds of incubating chambers, microscopes, photoelectric counter devices, and so on, and according to economic limitations.

The techniques described have been standardized and well validated, are not particularly difficult, and do not require any specific background. The current good state-of-the-art is indicated by the progressively increasing number of articles dealing with ciliary motility.

REFERENCES

1. Adalis, D., Gardner, D. E., and Miller, F. J. (1978): Cytotoxic effects of nickel on ciliated epithelium. *Am. Rev. Respir. Dis.*, 118:347–354.
2. Barton, C., and Raynor, S. (1967): Analytical investigation of cilia induced mucous flow. *Bull. Math. Biophysiol.*, 29:419–428.
3. Blake, J. R., and Sleigh, M. A. (1974): Mechanics of ciliary locomotion. *Biol. Rev.*, 49:85–125.
4. Blake, J. R., and Winet, H. (1980): On the mechanics of mucociliary transport. *Biorheology*, 17:125–134.
5. Braga, P. C., Bossi, R., and Allegra, L. (1986): A method for maintaining *in vitro* TV monitoring and counting ciliary beat frequency of samples from human ciliated respiratory epithelial brushing. *Methods Find. Exp. Clin. Pharmacol.*, 8:321–326.
6. Braga, P. C., Dall'Oglio, G., Bossi, R., and Allegra, L. (1986): Simple and precise method for counting ciliary beats directly from the TV monitor screen. *J. Pharmacol. Meth.*, 16:161–164.
7. Brennen, C., and Winet, H. (1979): Fluid mechanics of propulsion by cilia and flagella. *Annu. Rev. Fluid Mech.*, 9:339–398.
8. Cherry, J. D., Roden, V. J., Rejent, A. J., and Dorner, R. W. (1971): The inhibition of ciliary activity in tracheal organ cultures by sera from children with cystic fibrons and control subjects. *J. Pediatr.*, 6:937–942.
9. Cherry, J. D., and Taylor-Robinson, D. (1970): Large-quantity production of chicken embryo tracheal organ cultures and use in virus and mucoplasma studies. *Appl. Microbiol.*, 19:658–663.
10. Cheung, A. T. W., and Jahn, T. L. (1976): High-speed cinematographic studies on rabbit tracheal (ciliated) epithelia: Determination of the beat pattern of tracheal cilia. *Pediatr. Res.*, 10:140–144.
11. Coleman, D. L., Tuet, I. K., and Widdicombe, J. H. (1984): Electrical properties of dog tracheal epithelial cells grown in monolayer culture. *Am. J. Physiol.*, 264 (*Cell Physiol.*, 15):C355–C359.
12. Conover, J. H., Bonforte, R. J., Hathaway, P., et al. (1973): Studies on ciliary dyskinesia factor in cystic fibrosis. I. Bioassay and heterozygote detection in serum. *Pediatr. Res.*, 7:220–225.
13. Corssen, G., and Allen, C. R. (1958): A comparison of the toxic effects of various local anesthetic drugs on human ciliated epithelium *in vitro. Texas Rep. Biol. Med.*, 16:194–202.
14. Corssen, G., and Allen, C. R. (1959): Acetylcholine: Its significance in controlling ciliary activity of human respiratory epithelium *in vitro. J. Appl. Physiol.*, 14:901–904.

15. Dalham, T. (1955): A method for determination *in vivo* of the rate of ciliary beat and mucous flow in the trachea. *Acta Physiol. Scand.*, 33:1–5.
16. Dalhamn, T. (1956): Mucous flow and ciliary activity in the trachea of healthy rats and rats exposed to respiratory irritant gases. *Acta Physiol. Scand.*, 36 (Suppl. 136):1–161.
17. Dalhamn, T. (1970): Ciliary motion studies. *Arch. Intern. Med.*, 126:424–427.
18. Dalhamn, T., and Rylander, R. (1962): Frequency of ciliary beat measured with a photosensitive cell. *Nature*, 196:592–593.
19. Dubois, M., Jouanne, T. P., Berge, P., and David, G. (1974): Spermatozoa motility in human cervical mucus. *Nature*, 252:711–713.
20. Dulfano, H. J., Lk, C. K., Beckage, M., and Wooten, O. (1981): Ciliary beat frequency in human respiratory explants. *Am. Rev. Respir. Dis.*, 123:139–140.
21. Eckert, R., and Murakami, A. (1972): Calcium dependence of ciliary activity in the oviduct of the salamander *Necturus*. *J. Physiol.*, 226:699–711.
22. Farrel, P. N., Fox, G. N., and Spicer, S. S. (1976): Determination and characterization of ciliary ATPase in the presence of serum from cystic fibrosis patients. *Pediatr. Res.*, 10:127–135.
23. Fawcett, D. W., and Porter, K. R. (1954): A study of the fine structure of ciliated epithelia. *J. Morphol.*, 94:221–281.
24. Glazzard, A. N., Hirous, M. R., Mellor, J. S., and Holwill, M. E. J. (1983): The computer-assisted analysis of television imaging as applied to the study of cell motility. *J. Submicrosc. Cytol.*, 15:305–308.
25. Gray, J. (1930): The mechanism of ciliary movement. VI. Photographic and stroboscopic analysis of ciliary movement. *Proc. R. Soc. Lond. (Biol.)*, 107:313–332.
26. Guillerm, R., Badre, R., Hec, J., and Pibarot, R. (1965): Une nouvelle méthode de mesure de l'activité ciliaire: La photo-oscillographie. *J. Physiol. (Paris)*, 57:725.
27. Hard, R., and Cypher, C. (1987): Reactivation of newt lung cilia: Evidence for a possible temperature- and MgATP-induced conformational change controlling beat frequency. *J. Cell. Biol.*, (in press)
28. Hee, J., and Guillerm, R. (1973): Influence des facteurs de l'environnement sur l'activité ciliaire et le transport du mucus. *Bull. Physiopathol. Respir.*, 9:377–393.
29. Jennison, M. W., and Bunker, J. W. (1934): Analysis of the movement of cilia from che clam (*Mya*) by high-speed photography with stroboscopic light. *J. Cell. Comp. Physiol.*, 5:189–197.
30. Jouannet, P., Volochine, B., Deguent, P., Serres, C., and David, G. (1977): Light scattering determination of various characteristic parameters of spermatozoa motility in a series of human sperm. *Andrologia*, 9:36–49.
31. Kennedy, J. R., and Duckett, K. E. (1981): The study of ciliary frequency with an optical spectrum analysis system. *Exp. Cell Res.*, 135:147–156.
32. Kennedy, J. R., and Ranyard, J. R. (1983): Morphology and quantitation of ciliated outgrowths from cultured rabbit tracheal explants. *Eur. J. Cell Biol.*, 29:200–208.
33. Lee, W. I., and Verdugo, P. (1976): Laser light scattering spectroscopy. A new application in the study of ciliary activity. *Biophys. J.*, 16:1115–119.
34. Lee, W. I., and Verdugo, P. (1977): Ciliary activity by laser light scattering spectroscopy. *Ann. Biomed. Eng.*, 5:248–259.
35. Lee, T. C., Wu, R., Brody, A. R., Barrett, J. C., and Nettesheim, P. (1984): Growth and differentiation of hamster tracheal epithelial cells culture. *Exp. Lung Res.*, 6:27–45.
36. Lucas, A. M. (1931): Dissection of ciliary movement in the nasal cavity of Macaca rhesus. *Trans. Am. Laryngol. Otol. Rhinol.*, 37:172–176.
37. Maurer, D. R., Schor, J., Sielczak, M., Wanner, A., and Abraham, W. M. (1982): Ciliary motility in airway anaphylaxis. *Cell Motil.*, (Suppl. 1):67–70.
38. Maurer, D. R., Sielczak, M., Oliver, W. Jr., Abraham, W. M., and Wanner, A. (1982): Role of ciliary motility in acute allergic mucociliary dysfunction. *J. Appl. Physiol.*, 52:1018–1023.
39. Miller, C. E. (1968): The kinematics and dynamics of ciliary fluid systems. *J. Exp. Biol.*, 49:617–629.
40. Nakhosteen, J. A., Wichtmann, G., Petro, W., and Konietzko, N. (1980): Beeinflusst ipratropium-bromid die mukoziliaire klarfunktion. *Prax. Klin. Pneumol.*, 34:570–574.
41. Olsen, I., and Jonsen, J. (1979): Effect of cadmium acetate copper sulfate and nickel chloride on organ cultures of mouse trachea. *Acta Pharmacol. Toxicol.*, 44:120–127.
42. Pedersen, M. (1983): Specific types of abnormal ciliary motility in Kartagener's syndrome and analogous respiratory disorders. *Eur. J. Respir. Dis.*, 64 (Suppl. 127):78–90.
43. Pedersen, M., Sakakuro, Y., Winther, B., Brofeldt, S., and Mygind, N. (1983): Nasal mucociliary

transport, number of ciliated cells and beating pattern in naturally acquired common colds. *Eur. J. Respir. Dis.*, 64 (Suppl. 128):355–364.

44. Poyton, R. O., and Branton, D. (1970): A multipurpose microperfusion chamber. *Exp. Cell Res.*, 60:109–114.

45. Proetz, A. W. (1932): Motion picture demonstration of ciliary action and other factors of nasal physiology. *Trans. Am. Laryngol. Assoc.*, 54:264–273.

46. Ross, S. M., and Corrsin, S. (1974): Results of an analytical model of mucociliary pumping. *J. Appl. Physiol.*, 37:333–340.

47. Rossman, C. M., Forrest, J. B., Lee, R. K. W., and Newhouse, M. T. (1930): The dyskinetic cilia syndrome. Ciliary motility in immotile cilia syndrome. *Chest*, 74:580–582.

48. Rutland, J., Griffin, W. M., and Cole, P. (1981): Nasal brushing and measurement of ciliary beat frequency. *Chest*, 80:865–867.

49. Rutland, J., Griffin, W. M., and Cole, P. (1982): Human ciliary beat frequency in epithelium from intrathoracic and extrathoracic airways. *Am. Rev. Respir. Dis.*, 125:100–105.

50. Sanderson, M. J., and Dirksen, E. R. (1985): A versatile and quantitative computer assisted photoelectronic technique used for the analysis of ciliary beat cycles. *Cell Motil.*, 5:267–292.

51. Scudi, J. V., Kimura, E. T., and Reinhard, J. F. (1951): Study of drug action on mammalian ciliated epithelium. *J. Pharmacol. Exp. Ther.*, 102:132–137.

52. Shimizu, H., and Matsumoto, G. (1977): Light scattering study on motile spermatozoa. *IEEE Trans. Biomed. Eng.*, 25:153–157.

53. Sleigh, M. A. (1961): An example of mechanical co-ordination of cilia. *Nature*, 191:931–932.

54. Sleigh, M. A. (1962): *The Biology of Cilia and Flagella.* Plenum Press, Oxford.

55. Sleigh, M. A. (1962): Some aspects of the comparative physiology of cilia. *Am. Rev. Respir. Dis.*, 93:16–31.

56. Teichtahl, H., Wright, P. L., and Kirsner, R. L. G. (1986): Measurement of *in vitro* ciliary beat frequency: A television-video modification of the transmitted light technique. *Med. Biol. Eng. Comput.*, 24:193–196.

57. Toremalm, N. G., Hakansson, C. H., Mercke, U., and Dahlerns, B. (1974): Mucociliary wave pattern: An analysis of surface light reflection. *Acta Otolaryngol.*, 781:247–252.

58. Verdugo, P., Hinds, T. R., and Vincenzi, F. F. (1979): Laser light-scattering spectroscopy: Preliminary results on bioassay of cystic fibrosis factor(s). *Pediatr. Res.*, 13:131–135.

59. Verdugo, P., Johnson, N. T., and Tarn, P. Y. (1980): β-Adrenergic stimulation of respiratory ciliary activity. *J. Appl. Physiol.*, 48:868–871.

60. Weaver, A., and Hard, R. (1985): Isolation of newt lung ciliated cell models. Characterization of motility and coordination thresholds. *Cell. Motil.*, 5:355–375.

61. Widdicombe, J. H., Coleman, D. L., Finkbeiner, W. E., and Tuet, I. K. (1985): Electrical properties of monolayers cultured from cells of human tracheal mucosa. *J. Appl. Physiol.*, 58:1729–1735.

62. Wilson, G. B., Jahn, T. L., and Fonseca, J. R. (1975): Studies on ciliary beating of frog pharingeal epithelium *in vitro*. I. Isolation and ciliary beat of single cells. *Trans. Am. Microsc. Soc.*, 94:43–57.

63. Wu, R., and Smith, D. (1982): Continuous multiplication of rabbit tracheal epithelial cells in a defined hormonic-supplemented medium. *In Vitro*, 18:800–812.

64. Yager, J. A., Chen, T. M., and Dulfano, M. J. (1978): Measurement of ciliary beat frequency on human respiratory epithelium. *Chest*, 73:627–633.

65. Yager, J. A., Ellman, H., and Dulfano, M. J. (1980): Human ciliary beat frequency at three levels of the tracheobronchial tree. *Am. Rev. Respir. Dis.*, 121:661–665.

Methods in Bronchial Mucology,
edited by P. C. Braga and L. Allegra.
Raven Press, Ltd. © 1988.

4.1.2. *In Vivo* Observation and Counting Methods for Ciliary Motion

P. C. Braga

Department of Pharmacology, University of Milan, Milan, Italy

Methods
  Kinds of preparations
  Observation techniques
  Measuring techniques
Discussion

Curiosity about tracheal ciliary activity *in vivo* began over 100 years ago, when the first scientific studies were performed with reptiles, amphibians, birds, and mammals (9,10,26,29). In Chapter 4.1.1., technical methods of investigation of ciliary motion *in vitro* are described. Some of these methods can be applied also for *in vivo* studies, in which the same target is investigated under another biological condition. In articles dealing with this subject, there is confusion between "ciliary activity *in vivo*" and "mucus transport." Although some techniques can be used to investigate both aspects, the two parameters are different, since observation of the transport of mucus (with markers) by ciliated epithelia is an indirect method of investigating ciliary motion. Specific mucus transport techniques are described in Chapters 4.2.1. and 4.2.2. Here we consider mainly the techniques for direct observation of ciliary movement.

The logical sequence of steps for *in vivo* studies is the same as that for *in vitro* studies. Observation and measuring techniques in the two conditions overlap, with only small modifications. The main difference is in the biological material to be observed, which in this case is the trachea *in toto* and generally *in situ*.

METHODS

Kinds of Preparations

There is a dichotomy in the experimental models for amphibian and mammalian preparations. One commonly used ciliated epithelial preparation is the excised frog palate (or esophagus). Since this is an excised preparation, including it in the *in vitro* methods would seem more correct. Generally speaking, *in vitro* studies of ciliary beat frequency (CBF) are performed with biological materials of cellular dimensions. However, in view of the dimensions of the frog palate and its peculiar ability to remain vital for hours after excision, this preparation has been included in the *in vivo* chapter. The same considerations are valid for submerged or air-exposed, excised mammalian trachea.

The ciliated epithelium of the frog palate has been used extensively as a model for evaluating mucociliary transport and ciliary activity. The frog is pithed (Fig. 1) and then decapitated, and the head with palate exposed (or the palate mucosa dissected) is placed in a Plexiglas thermostated moist chamber in which the tempera-

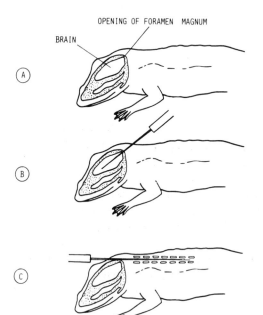

OPENING OF FORAMEN MAGNUM

BRAIN

(A)

(B)

(C)

FIG. 1. Procedure for the pithed frog preparation. **A:** Bend the head downward. **B:** Needle insertion into cranium through the opening of the foramen magnum to destroy the brain. **C:** Same procedure with needle inserted into vertebral column to destroy spine. **B** and **C:** Double pithed frog.

ture (30°C) and humidity (100%) remain constant (23,25,30) (Fig. 2). Esophagus and pharynx also have been used (4,13). Figure 3 shows the results obtained with this technique (3). An alternative is to use the excised trachea of such mammals as the mouse (28), the rabbit (12,17), or the dog (31) either in a moist chamber, like that for the frog, or submerged.

A second possibility is to investigate the ciliary activity in the trachea *in situ*. The animal is anesthetized, and by blunt dissection the trachea is exposed and a small hole, like a window, is opened in the cartilaginous rings to observe the underlying ciliated epithelium. This type of study can be done with rats (7) placed in a moist chamber (31–35°C, humidity 95–97%). In this case, the rat no longer breathes through the upper respiratory tract but through the lower part of the trachea. More physiological conditions can be obtained by connecting the microscope to the exposed trachea by a rubber bellows fitted around the objective. By preventing air escape by accurate suturing of the tissue, physiological breathing can be obtained (6,7). A heating coil warming the objective prevents condensation on the lens at the point where it comes into contact with the warm, moist air in the trachea (Fig. 4). Ciliary activity has been observed under these condtions in rabbits and cats (2,7).

Using air-tight windows, tracheal ciliary activity *in vivo* can be observed in

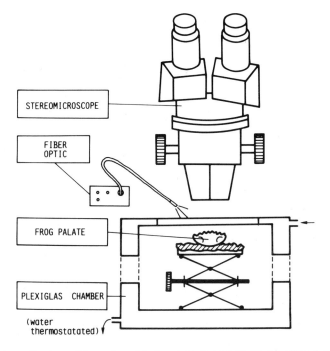

FIG. 2. Schematic view of the setup of instruments to investigate the ciliated epithelium of the frog palate.

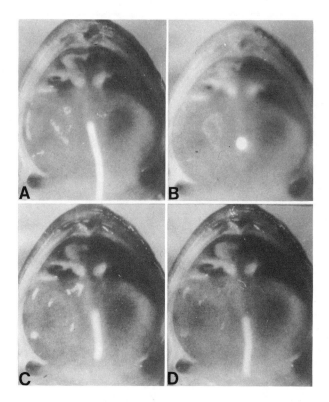

FIG. 3. Observation of mucociliary transport in the frog's palate. Using a calibrated long film exposure, it is possible to show the progressive travel, in a predetermined time, of the marker (a small fluorescent disk) caused by the vibratile cilia of the frog's palate. The length of the clear strip left by the fluorescent disk against the background of the frog's palate indicates the rate of mucociliary transport. **A:** Basal rate of mucociliary transport. **B:** No motion of the disk indicates that the mucus depletion has been obtained. **C:** Relative rate of transport of samples of mucus taken from bronchopulmonary patient before treatment with sobrerol. **D:** Relative rate of transport of sample of mucus taken from the same patient after treatment with sobrerol. Travel increased 23%.

any animal, e.g., the turtle or the duck (21), the only limiting factor being the tracheal dimensions.

To study ciliary activity in the intrapulmonary airways of the rat with preserved anatomical continuity, a method that involves more difficult surgery than preparing a simple tracheal window has been proposed (14,15). The pleura and the overlying lung tissue are removed, and the bronchial tree is exposed from the terminal bronchioles to the lobes. In this preparation, ciliary movement can be observed through the bronchial wall from the side of the basement membrane by incident light microscopy, and the frequency, amplitude of beat, coordination, and direction of effective stroke under normal and pathological conditions can be observed (16). Transparent (plastic) windows can be inserted, after the mucosa is exposed, via a trepination hole of about 2 × 8 mm in the lateral wall of the frontosuperior part

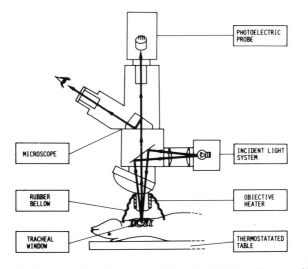

FIG. 4. Schematic drawing of a microscope with incident light system, positioned on the tracheal window.

of the maxillary sinus of the anesthetized rabbit to study the ciliary activity of the mucous membrane under more nearly physiological conditions (18–20).

Observation Techniques

With the biological preparations described, no transmitted light can be used because, owing to the thickness of the samples and the *in vivo* conditions, transillumination (except in the intrapulmonary technique) is not possible. Reflected light is used to obtain incident light illumination of the field. This is obtained with a microscopy lamp (parallel light beam) positioned for lateral illumination of the field with respect to the microscope axis or, preferably, with a microscope equipped for reflected light observation. (The Leitz Ultrapak system was used extensively in the past, but now it is not on the market.)

In *in vivo* observations, the activity of a single cilium cannot be investigated; since the cilia are closely packed, high magnifications are not needed. In addition to microscopes with low power objectives, stereomicroscopes can be used. A further reason for using relatively low magnifications is the measuring technique for ciliary activity *in vivo*, which is based on the flickering of the light beam on the reflecting surface.

Measuring Techniques

The incident light illuminating the exposed ciliated epithelium is reflected from the cilia packed together and from the thin layer of mucus covering the cilia.

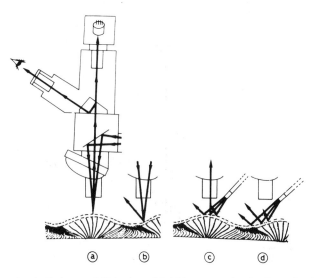

FIG. 5. Measuring techniques of flickering of light beam on the *in vivo* reflecting surfaces. **a:** Setup with incident light passing through the microscope. The light spot is reflected into the microscope to the measuring system. **b:** The light falls outside the frontal lens of the microscope when cilia change their angle. **c:** Setup with fiber light. Cilia position as **a**. **d:** Setup with fiber light. Cilia position as **b**.

This reflection is cyclic, i.e., its direction changes according to the movements of underlying cilia. At a certain angle during their stroke, the cilia reflect the incident light into the microscope, and the area of that group of cilia appears as a light spot. Some fraction of seconds later, the cilia change their angle and the light falls outside the frontal lens of the objective and this area appears dark (Fig. 5). These rhythmic changes of flaring and fading intensity are assumed to represent ciliary activity (of a group of cilia), and each cycle of light fluctuation corresponds to a beat cycle (5,12,21,22,24).

With this flickering phenomenon, the CBF can be recorded directly stroboscopically (1,5,11), photographically (high-speed cinecamera) (5,11,21), or photoelectrically (8,21,25,27). The distribution function of the CBF can be obtained by the fast Fourier transform technique, either online with a spectrum analyzer or offline feeding the data into a digital computer (25).

DISCUSSION

The *in vitro* and *in vivo* methods for detecting ciliary motion overlap in some of the techniques used, and, like the *in vitro* techniques, the *in vivo* techniques have some advantages and some disadvantages.

The *in vivo* techniques allow direct observation of the phenomenon under good physiological conditions (tissue temperature, air moistness, secretion, blood supply intact) for periods of time, depending on the kind of preparation, that generally last some hours. On the other hand, the investigation of cilia mechanics is not as deep as it is *in vitro*, which permits observation of ciliated cells or single cilia. Moreover, *in vitro* studies can be used for mass studies for longer periods of time.

In *in vivo* studies, a relatively large tissue area is observed (~0.1 mm diameter). This means that many cells and cilia are involved, and since there is variation in the individual ciliary strokes and in the subsequent synchronization in methachronous wave, a mucociliary wave frequency rather than a CBF is measured.

The choice of *in vivo* or *in vitro* methods depends on what the pneumologist or the researcher is investigating and what kind of information is being sought.

REFERENCES

1. Ballanger, J. J., and Orr, M. F. (1963): Quantitative measurements of human ciliary activity. *Ann. Otolaryngol.*, 72:31–38.
2. Blair, A. M. J. N., and Woods, A. (1969): The effects of isoprenaline, atropine and disodium cromoglycate on ciliary motility and mucous flow measured *in vivo* in cats. *Br. J. Pharmacol.*, 35:379P–380P.
3. Braga, P. C. (1981): Macrophotographic evidence of the activity of sobrerol on mucociliary transport in the frog's palate. *Clin. Trials J.*, 18:30–38.
4. Carson, H. E., and Robbins, J. (1974): Effects of hormones and nucleotides on ciliary beating on frog esophagus and guinea pig trachea. *Life Sci.*, 14:2413–2418.
5. Dalhamn, T. (1956): Mucus flow and ciliary activity in the trachea of healthy rats and rats exposed to respiratory irritant gases. *Acta Physiol. Scand.*, 36 (Suppl. 123):1–161.
6. Dalhamn, T. (1960): The determination *in vivo* of the rate of ciliary beat in the trachea. *Acta Physiol. Scand.*, 44:242–250.
7. Dalhamn, T. (1964): Studies on tracheal ciliary activity. Special reference to the effect of cigarette smoke in living animals. *Am. Rev. Respir. Dis.*, 89:870–877.
8. Dalhamn, T., and Rylander, R. (1962): Frequency of ciliary beat measured with a photosensitive cell. *Nature*, 196:592–593.
9. Gosselin, M. (1851): Sur la durée des mouvements vibratiles ciliares chez un supplicié. *C. R. Soc. Biol. (Paris)*, 3:57.
10. Gray, J. (1928): *Ciliary Movement.* Cambridge University Press, Cambridge, England.
11. Gray, J. (1930): The mechanism of ciliary movement. VI. Photographic and stroboscopic analysis of ciliary movement. *Proc. R. Soc.*, 167:313–319.
12. Hakansson, C. H., and Toremalm, N. G. (1965): Studies on the physiology of the trachea. I. Ciliary activity indirectly recorded by a new light beam reflex method. *Ann. Otol. Rhinol. Laryngol.*, 74:954–969.
13. Inch, T. D., and Brimblecombe, R. W. (1971): Acetylcholine-like action of atropine on the ciliary epithelium of the frog esophagus during the warmer months. *J. Pharm. Pharmacol.*, 23:815–819.
14. Iravani, J. (1967): Flimmerbewegung in den intrapulmonalen Luftwegen der Ratte. *Pflugers Arch.*, 297:221–237.
15. Iravani, J. (1969): Koordination der Flimmerbewegung im Bronchialepithel der Ratte. *Pflugers Arch.*, 305:199–209.
16. Iravani, J., and Melville, G. N. (1975): Factors affecting ciliary activity in the intrapulmonary airways. *Can. J. Physiol. Pharm.*, 50:354–359.
17. Kensler, C. J., and Battista, S. P. (1963): Components of cigarette smoke with ciliary-depressant activity. Their selective removal by filters containing activated charcoal granules. *N. Engl. J. Med.*, 269:1161–1172.
18. Lierle, D. M., and Moore, P. M. (1935): Further study of the effects of drugs on ciliary activity: A new method of observation in the living animal. *Ann. Otol.*, 44:671–684.

19. Lindberg, S., and Mercke, U. (1985): Substance P antagonists and mucociliary activity in rabbit. *Naunyn. Schmiedeberg. Arch. Pharmacol.*, 329:376–381.
20. Lindberg, S., and Mercke, U. (1986): Capsaicin stimulates mucociliary activity by releasing substance P and acetylcholine. *Eur. J. Respir. Dis.*, 68:96–106.
21. Lucas, A. M. (1933): Principles underlying ciliary activity in the respiratory tract. I. A method for direct observation of cilia *in situ* and its application. *Arch. Otolaryngol.*, 18:516–524.
22. Lucas, A. M., and Douglas, L. C. (1935): Principles underlying ciliary activity in the respiratory tract. *Arch. Otolaryngol.*, 20:285–296.
23. Miani, P., and Piragine, F. (1962): Studi sugli epiteli vibratili delle prime vie aeree. I. Metodi in uso per lo studio del movimento ciliare. *Clinica O.R.L.*, 3–4:143–171.
24. Proetz, A. R. (1933): Studies on nasal cilia in the living mammals. *Ann. Otol. Rhinol. Laryngol.*, 42:778–789.
25. Puchelle, E., Zahm, J. M., and Sadoul, P. (1982): Mucociliary frequency of frog palate epithelium. *Am. J. Physiol.*, 242 (*Cell Physiol.*: 11):C31–C35.
27. Rylander, R. (1966): Current techniques to measure alteration in the ciliary activity to intact respiratory epithelium. *Am. Rev. Respir. Dis.*, 93:67–85.
28. Scheppy, C. A., and Elter, J. C. (1976): Technique nouvelle pour l'expérimentation *in vitro* de préparations nasales sur les cils vibratiles de la trachée de la souris. *Pharm. Acta Helv.*, 51:362–367.
29. Sharpey, W. (1835): Cilia. In: *Cyclopedia of Anatomy and Physiology*, edited by R. B. Todd, Vol. 1, pp. 606–638. Longman, Braon, Green, Longman and Roberts, London.
30. Suzuki, N. (1966): Motor control of the ciliary activity in the frog's palate. *J. Fac. Sci. Hokkaido Univ. Sez. VI Zoology*, 16:67–71.
31. Yanaura, S., Inanura, N., and Misawa, M. (1981): Effects of expectorants on the canine tracheal ciliated cells. *Jpn. J. Pharmacol.*, 31:957–965.

Methods in Bronchial Mucology,
edited by P. C. Braga and L. Allegra.
Raven Press, Ltd. © 1988.

4.2. MUCUS MOVEMENTS

4.2.1. Mucus Transport *Ex Vivo*

E. Puchelle and J. M. Zahm

INSERM U314, Faculté de Médecine, 51095 Reims, France

It was initially suggested by Sade et al. (5) and by King et al. (2) that the depleted frog palate was an appropriate model for studying the mucociliary transport velocity of mucus systems and analyzing the role of mucus as a mechanical coupler. After pithing and dissecting the head of the frog, the palate is introduced into a transparent box in which a relative humidity of 100% and a temperature of 30°C are maintained. Under these experimental conditions, it is assumed that the ciliary activity of the excised frog palate remains constant for a period of about 24 hr. The mucus transport velocity can be determined easily by depositing tracer particles on the palate and measuring the time required for traveling a given distance. The range of mucociliary transport velocity of the freshly excised frog (8–14 mm/mn) is similar to that of human tracheal mucus transport velocity. Then, the transport progressively decreases with time and stops when the secretion of endogenous mucus is exhausted. At the depletion stage, a drop of mucus collected from the edge of a freshly excised frog palate is capable of restoring the transport of the tracer particle.

Mucus from different sources (dog tracheal mucus, cow cervical mucus, mucus scraped from fish scales) as well as non–mucus systems, such as egg white or guaran gels, also can restore the initial transport velocity of the tracer. All these systems possess a common property, that of being viscoelastic. The mucociliary transport cannot, however, be restored by adding purely viscous substances, such as oil. These results demonstrate that the elastic properties of mucus play a fundamental role in the mucociliary transport mechanism.

Using this model, it has been shown that an intermediate range of viscosity (close to 12 Pa) and elastic modulus close to 1 Pa are optimal for an efficient mucociliary transport (1,4). The ciliary transport rate of respiratory mucus is correlated to its spinability: the higher the spinability, the faster the transport rate even if the elasticity is abnormally low (3). The interdependence between the rheological properties of mucus, the ciliary beat frequency (CBF), and the ciliary transport of mucus have been studied (4). The CBF was analyzed in the presence of mucus by monitoring the variations of the light intensity due to the ciliary beating and reflected by the mucus. We, therefore, analyzed consecutively on the same depleted frog palate model the mucociliary frequency and mucus transport rate in the presence of respiratory mucus samples whose rheological properties also had been determined. Two important features are:

1. A significant and close positive correlation relates the mucociliary frequency and transport rate.
2. The lower the viscosity, the higher the mucociliary frequency.

For pathological mucus with a viscosity higher than 12 Pa, the mucociliary frequency and transport rate decrease in parallel. Therefore, the frog palate model can be considered as a valuable model for analyzing the transport capacity of mucus and assessing the efficiency of respiratory mucoactive drugs.

REFERENCES

1. Chen, T. M., and Dulfano, M. J. (1978): Mucus viscoelasticity and mucociliary transport rate. *J. Lab. Clin. Med.,* 91:423–443.
2. King, M., Gilboa, A., Meyer, F. A., and Silberberg, A. (1974): On the transport of mucus and its rheologic stimulants in ciliated systems. *Am. Rev. Respir. Dis.,* 110:740–744.
3. Puchelle, E., Zahm, J. M., and Duvivier, C. (1983): Spinability of bronchial mucus. Relationship with viscoelasticity and mucus transport properties. *Biorheology,* 20:239–249.
4. Puchelle, E., Zahm, J. M., and Quemada, D. (1987): Rheological properties controlling mucociliary frequency and respiratory mucus transport. *Biorheology,* 24:557–563.
5. Sade, J., Eliezer, N., Silberberg, A., and Nevo, A. C. (1970): The role of mucus in transport by cilia. *Am. Rev. Respir. Dis.,* 102: 48–52.

Methods in Br
edited by P. (
Raven Press,

4.2.2. Mucus Transport *in* .

A. Wanner

*University of Miami, Division of Pulmonary Disease,
Miami, Florida 33101*

Methods and technical details
Results
Discussion

The mucosa lining the tracheobronchial tree is covered by a liquid that is produced primarily by mucus cells and active epithelial water transport. In normal airways, this surface layer extends from the larynx to the terminal bronchioles. In the large airways, the liquid lining is considered to be stratified, consisting of a periciliary fluid layer (sol) covered by a mucus layer (gel). This concept, first developed by Lucas and Douglas (1), forms the basis for the currently favored mechanism of mucociliary interaction, i.e., the cephalad transport of mucus by the tips of beating cilia making contact with the underface of the mucus layer. The depth of the surface liquid is, therefore, determined by the net mucosal secretory rate and ciliary clearance of the surface liquid. Theoretically, a mismatch between these two processes leads to depletion or accumulation of the surface liquid. Thus, mucus transport, in addition to clearing inhaled or aspirated material from the conducting airways, contributes in an important way to the defense of the normal depth of the liquid that lines the tracheobronchial tree. Under normal conditions, peripheral airways lack mucus-producing structures, and only a single liquid layer (periciliary fluid) seems to be present. The sources of surface liquid and the mechanism and rate of its transport in these airways are uncertain. In the trachea, the presence of a mucus layer and periciliary fluid layer has been clearly demonstrated in several animal species (2). However, the mucus layer, which is 5 to 10 μm

...p, may be discontinuous, forming a blanket in some areas and small foci ...oating on the periciliary fluid in other areas (3).

Surface particle transport by ciliated epithelium has been shown to fail in the absence of mucus but can be restored by placing autologous or heterologous mucus on the epithelium (4). Thus, mucus could move as an entire blanket or as a small island. With respect to the latter mechanism, it has even been suggested that mucus is absent in the unstimulated airway and is only secreted in response to the local irritant effect of an inhaled particle or vapor, which would be trapped in or chemically bound to the mucus and then cleared from the airway (3). Between the trachea and the terminal bronchioles, there must be a gradual transition from the two layers (or the potential to form two layers) to a single layer.

There are three principal methods that have been used extensively for the measurement of surface liquid transport in the airways. One method is based on the clearance of inhaled radioaerosols and provides information on peripheral and central airways (5). In the second technique, the airway clearance of insufflated radiopaque tantalum powder is determined; this permits a semiquantitative assessment of liquid transport in large and intermediate size airways (6). The third method involves the placement of discrete markers or solutions onto the airway epithelium. For technical reasons, this method is generally limited to central airways. The following discussion focuses on methods that use the last principle and, by virtue of assessing mucus clearance in central airways, examine the integrity of mucociliary interaction. The other two methodologies are addressed in Chapters 5.1.4., 5.2.1. and 5.2.2.

METHODS AND TECHNICAL DETAILS

The techniques for *in vivo* measurement of mucus transport rates involve the placement of an optically, radiographically, or scintigraphically detectable solid or liquid marker on the mucosa. By measuring the distance traveled by the marker per unit time by observing it with the naked eye, by a microscope, a fluoroscopy unit, or scintillation counters, a mucus transport rate or mucus velocity can be calculated. A variety of markers has been used, including India ink (7), lamp black (8), carbon lycopodium (9), barium sulfate (10), methylene blue solution (11), ^{99m}Tc pertechnetate solution, ^{99m}Tc-labeled resin beads and macroaggregates of albumin (12–14), Teflon disks with or without bismuth impregnation (15,16), or simply cellular debris (17).

Dalhamn (17) described a method to observe mucus transport directly through an incision or window in the rat trachea; this technique was later adapted for cats (18). Transillumination of the exposed intact cat trachea for the measurement of particle transport was described by Goldhamer et al. (19) and was extensively used by Laurenzi et al. (20,21). Another *in vivo* technique ues the temporary exteriorization of the mobile chicken trachea for the direct observation of particle transport (22). Iravani (23) described a method by which bronchi of rats and hamsters are surgically freed of lung parenchyma so that both ciliary beat frequency

(CBF) and the transport of mucus and debris can be observed through the bronchial wall.

Injection of barium sulfate (10,24) or solutions of radioisotopes (13,25) into the airway requires an X-ray unit or scintillation detectors to measure mucus transport rates. In contrast to particle transport techniques, which allow averaging of individual particle transport rates, these methods determine the frontal movement of a solution or suspension.

Finally, endoscopy has been employed by various investigators in combination with cinematography, fluoroscopy, and scintillation detection. Sackner et al. (15) first described the measurement of particle transport in the trachea of intact animals and human subjects by means of fiberoptic bronchoscopy. Since standard fiberoptic bronchoscopic techniques are used, the method is applicable in unanesthetized animals and human subjects using topical anesthesia (26,27). Standardized Teflon disks are blown through the inner channel of the fiberoptic bronchoscope onto the tracheal mucosa, and their cephalad motion is filmed. Because of considerable variability in individual particle transport rates due to the anatomical and functional characteristics of the respiratory mucosa, 10 to 20 particles distributed circumferentially around the airway lumen are analyzed. As the disks approach the distal lens of the fiberoptic bronchoscope, they appear larger. By standardizing the disk size, film projection factor, and filming speed, velocities can be computed from image size and frame number. Because fiberoptic bronchoscopy is invasive, the method was subsequently improved by impregnating the Teflon disks with bismuth trioxide to render them radiopaque (16). The motion of the radiopaque Teflon disks can be followed by a fluoroscopic image intensifier, and tracheal mucus velocity can be calculated by recording both the fluoroscopic image and the time on videotape. Because the Teflon disks can be blown into the airway through the vocal cords without having to intubate the trachea with the endoscope, topical anesthesia in the trachea is not required. Chopra et al. (28) used the fiberoptic bronchoscope to deposit a 0.04 to 0.1 ml droplet of indium-133m ([133m]In) or ^{99m}Tc-labeled albumin microspheres at the carina. The motion of the marker was then observed by an external scintillation counter, and from the distance traveled by the marker per unit time, a mucus velocity was calculated.

RESULTS

The different techniques used to measure mucus transport rates *in vivo* have yielded divergent values in the same species and among different species. In mammals, normal tracheal mucus transport rates have been reported as low as 2.7 mm/min (guinea pigs) and as high as 20 mm/min (cats) (Table 1). In general, a relatively large intersubject variability has been found. For example, coefficients of variations of 36% and 41% have been reported for unanesthetized rats and human subjects, respectively (16,33). In the human subjects, tracheal mucus velocity ranged between 6.9 and 19.4 mm/min (16). In those studies in which intrasubject

TABLE 1. *Normal in vivo tracheal mucus transport rates in mammals*

Reference[a]	Species	Anesthesia	Technique	Marker	Mean transport rate (mm/min)
Berke and Roslinski (10)	Rat	General	Radiographic	Barium sulfate suspension	6–10
Dalhamn (17)	Rat	General	Microscopy (incised trachea)	Debris	13.5
Iravani (29)	Rat	General	Microscopy (exposed intact airway)	Debris and mucus	11
Felicetti (33)	Rabbit	None	Scintillation detector	^{99m}Tc-labeled macro-aggregated albumin	2.7
Kilburn and Salzano (34)	Guinea pig	None	Scintillation detector	^{99m}Tc-labeled albumin microspheres	2.7
Goldhamer et al. (19)	Cat	General	Transillumination (microscope)	Carbon lycopodium	13
Laurenzi et al. (20)	Cat	General	Transillumination (microscope)	Carbon lycopodium	20
Kensler and Battista (9)	Cat	General	Tracheal window	Debris	10.5
Hilding (30)	Dog	None	Bronchoscopy	India ink	14–15
Giordano and Holsclaw (12)	Dog	General	Scintillation detector	^{99m}Tc-pertechnetate solution	10
Sakkakura and Proctor (13)	Dog	General	Scintillation detector	^{99m}Tc-labeled resin beads	10.5
Marin and Morrow (31)	Dog	General	Scintillation detector	^{99m}Tc-O$_4$ solution	16
Wanner et al. (32)	Dog	General	Cinebronchoscopy	Teflon disks	13.5
Chopra et al. (28)	Dog	General	Scintillation detector	^{99m}Tc-labeled albumin microspheres	19.2
Landa et al. (26)	Sheep	General	Cinebronchoscopy	Teflon disks	17.5
Weissberger et al. (46)	Sheep	None	Radiography	Teflon disks	11.5
Friedman et al. (16)	Man	Local[b]	Radiography	Radiopaque Teflon disks	10
Yeates et al. (14)	Man	None	Scintillation detector	^{99m}Tc-labeled albumin microspheres	3.5

[a] Representative references.
[b] Topical anesthesia in upper airway, not in trachea.

reproducibility was assessed, its variation has been considerably less than that of the intersubject variability.

Many *in vitro* studies have demonstrated a progressive increase in the rate of mucus transport from the small to the large airways. Kilburn and Salzano (34) found that mucus velocity in frogs, cats, rabbits, dogs, and humans was 10 to 25% lower in the smaller airways than in the trachea. Barclay and Franklin (7) and Morrow et al. (5) saw a 4-fold increase in the transport velocity in cats from the bronchioles to the trachea and a 14-fold increase in humans in the same areas. Asmundsson and Kilburn (35) reported the following mucus velocities in fresh dog lungs: 12.6 mm/min in the trachea, 8.3 mm/min in the lobar bronchi, 4 mm/min in the segmental bronchi, and 1.6 mm/min in the distal bronchi. In a rat preparation in which the bronchi are dissected free of surrounding lung tissue but

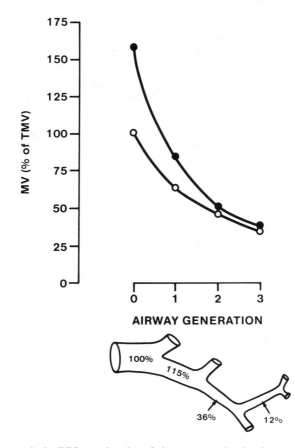

FIG. 1. Mucus velocity (MV) as a function of airway generation (trachea = 0) in anesthetized dogs. MV expressed as percent of tracheal mucus velocity (TMV). Baseline values (○) and values after 4 mg/kg i.v. aminophylline (●). Percent ciliation of airway epithelium relative to trachea shown at the bottom. (From Wanner (1985): In: *Bronchial Asthma,* 2nd ed., edited by E. Weiss, M. S. Segal, and M. Stein, pp. 270–279. Little, Brown, Boston.)

are otherwise intact, Iravani and Van As (36) observed mean transit velocities of 11.5 mm/min in the trachea and of 0.4 mm/min in distal bronchioles. In anesthetized, intubated, intact dogs, Serafini et al. (37) found mucus velocities to decrease by 38% from the trachea to the main bronchi, by 55% to the lobar bronchi, and 66% to the segmental bronchi. They also found a positive correlation between mucus velocity and the percentage of ciliated cells in those airways (Fig. 1). As stated, the currently available techniques for the measurement of mucus transport by discrete markers are not capable of measuring axial transport velocities in the most peripheral conducting airways. However, the liquid lining these small bronchioles is probably transported cephalad at a very low rate. An increase in transport velocity from peripheral to central airways is believed to account, at least in part, for the failure of airway secretions to accumulate in large airways.

Although the general direction of mucus transport is toward the larynx, specific mucociliary streaming patterns have been described in mammalian airways. Hilding (30) observed whirlpool formations and areas of stasis at the sites of airway divisions, and Iravani (38) found focal derangements of metachronous coordination, ciliary activity, reversal of transport direction, and an abnormal pattern of mucus production in normal rat bronchi. Many investigators have reported spiral mucociliary pathways in mammalian tracheas, including human subjects (7,35,39,40). The direction of transport appears to be clockwise when viewed from the larynx, at least in the northern hemisphere. Between such pathways, areas of stasis have been demonstrated even in intact normal tracheas.

DISCUSSION

The *in vivo* tracheal mucus transport rates listed in Table 1 compare well with *in vitro* measurements made mainly in frog palates and esophagi or in mammalian tracheas (41–44). Giordano et al. (45) determined the transport velocity of a radioisotope solution in the canine trachea *in vivo* and of tracheal secretions from the same dogs on the frog palate *in vitro*. Mean mucus velocity was 12.4 mm/min *in vivo* and 13.7 mm/min *in vitro;* this small difference was statistically not significant.

Several explanations have been offered for the considerable variability in mucus transport rates reported by different laboratories. Choice of species, age, site of deposition of transport marker, general or local anesthetics, or the physicochemical properties of the marker itself have all been thought to influence mucus transport velocity. Most of these factors have been assessed, and some appear to be more important than others.

Species

A superficial inspection of the mean transport rates in Table 1 does not reveal a systematic difference among different mammalian species. However, differences in technique render an objective comparison difficult. Felicetti et al. (33) measured the transport velocity of a ^{99m}Tc-labeled macroaggregated albumin solution deposited at the carina of four animal species in the unanesthetized state. The leading edge velocity in rats, guinea pigs, rabbits, and dogs was 1.9, 2.7, 3.2, and 9.8 mm/min, respectively. On the other hand, the mean tracheal mucus velocity determined by the radiographic Teflon disks method appears to be similar in unanesthetized sheep and human subjects, with values of 11.5 and 10 mm/min, respectively (16,46). Thus, the application of the identical technique brings out interspecies differences in normal mucus transport rates depending on the marker used. This indicates that the species-related variability in mucus transport is as significant as the variability introduced by the choice of marker.

Age

Goodman et al. (47) investigated the effect of aging on mucociliary transport in normal nonsmokers. Mean tracheal mucus velocity (5.7 mm/min) was significantly slower in elderly subjects 56 to 70 years of age than in young healthy subjects 19 to 28 years of age (9.7 mm/min). All particles in the young subjects showed cephalad motion, whereas 10% of deposited particles in the elderly subjects failed to show any movement at all. This age-related decrease in mucociliary transport was subsequently confirmed by others using a radioaerosol clearance technique (48). This phenomenon of aging mandates the use of proper age-matched controls when examining the influence of airway disease, inhalants, and pharmacological agents on airway mucociliary clearance.

Location of Marker

Since the mucus streaming pattern along the surface of the large airways is not homogeneous and areas of rapid mucus motion can be found in the vicinity of stagnant mucus, the site where a given marker is deposited plays a critical role. This inhomogeneous pattern of mucus transport is of minor importance if a large number of markers are deposited and their mean velocity is calculated. However, a single solid marker or a single small droplet of a liquid marker is subject to a larger variability in transport velocity depending on where the marker is deposited. In dogs, sheep, humans, and possibly other species, the fastest axial transport velocity is observed in the membranous part of the trachea. Therefore, a marker deposited at the posterior wall of the carina will be transported consistently at a higher velocity than the mean transport rate of markers distributed around the entire circumference of the trachea. Indeed, a comparison between the roentgenographic Teflon disk method and the ^{99m}Tc macroaggregated albumin method has confirmed this expected difference (49). In that study, which was carried out in dogs, both methods were reproducible. However, the mean velocity of 10 to 15 1-mm Teflon disks was 3.7 mm/min, whereas the advancing front of a drop of the radiolabeled albumin solution (individual particle size 6–30 μm) deposited at the carina was 5.5 mm/min (ratio 1:1.5). When the particles and the solution were placed at the same location, the velocity of the two markers was identical.

Anesthesia

Many experimental conditions involving the measurement of *in vivo* mucus transport require the use of general anesthesia. Marin and Morrow (31) failed to demonstrate an effect of intravenously administered barbiturates on tracheal mucociliary transport in dogs. More recent studies, however, strongly suggest a depressant effect of general anesthetics on mucociliary transport. Thus, mucociliary transport in the trachea as determined by the motion of a radioactive tracer was found to cease during deep pentobarbital or thiamylal anesthesia, whereas some motion was observed during light anesthesia with the same barbiturates (50). In intact sheep in which tracheal mucus velocity can be determined without sedation or topical anesthesia of the airways, i.v. administration of 30 mg of pentobarbital or thiamylal/kg of body weight decreased tracheal mucus velocity by 35% from the preanesthesia control value (26). Similar observations have been made in rats (51). It appears, therefore, that the systemic administration of barbiturates impairs mucociliary transport in several animal species.

Topical anesthetics are given to conscious animals and human subjects when endoscopic methods are used to determine mucus transport in the lower airways. Most local anesthetics, when placed on the mucosa, depress mucus transport, presumably by interfering with ciliary activity (52). Lidocaine is an exception. The application of 4% lidocaine to the nose in human subjects or 2% lidocaine to the trachea of sheep has been shown not to affect mucociliary transport (53,54). It is not known why lidocaine differs from other local anesthetics in this regard.

Physicochemical Properties of Marker

Physical and chemical characteristics of solid and liquid markers may influence their transportability. For example, the weight of large solid markers, such as bismuth-impregnated Teflon disks (0.6 mg, 1 mm in diameter), may depress or stimulate mucociliary interaction. This, however, is unlikely, according to Stewart (55), who investigated the weight-carrying capacity of ciliated epithelium. He found that up to a weight of 20 mg/mm^2, there was no decrease in test particle transport and that no acceleration of particle transport occurred with lighter weights. The Teflon disks weigh approximately 1.3 mg/mm^2. Another difference among various markers may be their ability to penetrate the airway liquid layers. For example, a liquid marker would be expected to sink deeper into the surface liquid of the mucosa than a large solid marker. Again, this does not apparently influence transport velocity, as demonstrated by Ahmed et al. (56), who found that in a canine tracheal preparation, the advancing front of a drop of methylene blue moved at the same rate as a Teflon disk placed at the same location. Yet there are other physicochemical properties of markers that might influence the transportability of the markers. For example, the shape (amorphous versus spherical) or electrical charge of the particles may play an important role. Thus, anion and cation exchange resin particles and macroaggregates of albumin (neutral) have been shown to be transported at similar velocities, but both are transported consistently slower than sulfur colloid (negative charge) (57,58). Finally, the radioactivity of the marker has been suggested to influence its transportability (59). In this study, the transport velocity of inert Teflon particles in the sheep trachea was found to be increased by 93% and 87% with the concomitant administration of ^{99m}Tc-labeled macroaggregated albumin or ^{99m}Tc-pyrophosphate, respectively. The dose of local radioactivity was about 40 times higher than what has been used by other investigators using the radioactive droplet method. Therefore, the question if ionizing radiation emitted by radioactive markers stimulates mucus transport remains unanswered. If there is such an effect, it would be expected to be more significant for instilled radioactive solutions than inhaled radioaerosols, which are distributed over a much greater surface area.

Despite these technical differences among the various techniques that have been used to measure lower airway mucus transport *in vivo*, all of the methodologies can be put to good use as long as their limitations are recognized. The degree of reproducibility and sensitivity in detecting spontaneous changes or experimentally induced perturbations of mucociliary interaction clearly is the most important criterion by which a given technique should be judged.

REFERENCES

1. Lucas, A. M., and Douglas, L. C. (1934): Principles underlying ciliary activity in the respiratory tract. *Arch. Otolaryngol.*, 20:518–541.
2. Nowell, J. A., and Tyler, W. S. (1971): Scanning electron microscopy of the surface morphology of mammalian lungs. *Am. Rev. Respir. Dis.*, 103:313–328.
3. Van As, A. (1977): Pulmonary airway clearance mechanisms: A reappraisal. *Am. Rev. Respir. Dis.*, 115:721–726.
4. Sade, J., Eliezer, N., Silberberg, A., et al. (1970): The role of mucus in transport by cilia. *Am. Rev. Respir. Dis.*, 102:48–52.
5. Morrow, P. E., Gibb, F. R., and Gazioglu, K. M. (1967): A study of particulate clearance from the human lungs. *Am. Rev. Respir. Dis.*, 96:1209–1221.
6. Wood, P. B., Nagy, E., Pearson, F. G., and Rae, S. (1973): Measurement of mucociliary clearance from the lower respiratory tract of normal dogs. *Can. Anaesth. Soc. J.*, 20:192.
7. Barclay, A. E., and Franklin, K. J. (1968): The rate of excretion of India ink injected into the lungs. *J. Physiol.*, 90:482–484.
8. Hill, L. (1928): The ciliary movement of the trachea studied *in vitro*. *Lancet*, 215:802.
9. Kensler, C. J., and Battista, S. P. (1966): Chemical and physical factors affecting mammalian ciliary activity. *Am. Rev. Respir. Dis.*, 93:93.
10. Berke, H. L., and Roslinski, L. M. (1971): The roentgenographic determination of tracheal mucociliary transport rate in the rat. *Am. Ind. Hyg. Assoc. J.*, 32:174.
11. Hilding, A. C. (1971): Laryngotracheal damage during intratracheal anesthesia. *Ann. Otol. Rhinol. Laryngol.*, 80:565.

12. Giordano, A., and Holsclaw, D. S. (1976): Tracheal resection and mucociliary clearance. *Ann. Otol. Rhinol. Laryngol.*, 85:631.

13. Sakkakura, Y., and Proctor, D. F. (1972): The effect of various conditions on tracheal mucociliary transport in dogs. *Proc. Soc. Exp. Biol. Med.*, 140:870.

14. Yeates, D. B., Aspin, N., Levinson, H., Jones, M. T., and Bryan, A. C. (1975): Mucociliary tracheal transport rates in man. *J. Appl. Physiol.*, 39:487.

15. Sackner, M. A., Rosen, M. J., and Wanner, A. (1973): Estimation of tracheal mucous velocity by bronchofiberscopy. *J. Appl. Physiol.*, 34:495–499.

16. Friedman, M., Stott, F. D., Poole, D. O., et al. (1977): A new roentgenographic method for estimating mucous velocity in airways. *Am. Rev. Respir. Dis.*, 115:67–72.

17. Dalhamn, T. (1956): Mucous flow and ciliary activity in the trachea of healthy rats and rats exposed to respiratory irritant gases. *Acta Physiol. Scand.*, (Suppl.) 36:1.

18. Carson, S., Goldhamer, R., and Carpenter, R. (1966): Mucus transport in the respiratory tract. *Am. Rev. Respir. Dis.*, 93:86.

19. Goldhamer, R. E., Barnett, B., and Carson, S. (1964): A method for studying mucus flow in the intact animal. Food and Drug Research Laboratory Publication, New York.

20. Laurenzi, G. A., Yin, S., Collins, B., and Guarneri, J. J. (1967): Mucus flow in the mammalian trachea. *Aspen Emphysema Conference*, No. 10, p. 27. American College of Chest Physicians, Chicago.

21. Laurenzi, G. A., Yin, S., and Guarneri, J. J. (1968): Adverse effect of oxygen on tracheal mucus flow. *N. Engl. J. Med.*, 279:333.

22. Battista, S. P., and Kensler, C. J. (1970): Mucus production and ciliary transport activity. *Arch. Environ. Health*, 20:326.

23. Iravani, J. (1967): Flimmerbewegung in den intrapulmonalen Luftwegen er Ratte. *Pfluegers Arch.*, 297:221.

24. Baetjer, A. M., and Bates, L. M. (1966): Measurement of ciliary activity in the intact trachea. *Am. Rev. Respir. Dis.*, 93:79.

25. Baetjer, A. M. (1967): Effect of ambient temperature and vapor pressure on cilia–mucus clearance rate. *J. Appl. Physiol.*, 23:498.

26. Landa, J. F., Hirsch, J. A., and Lebeaux, M. I. (1975): Effects of topical and general anesthetic agents on tracheal mucous velocity of sheep. *J. Appl. Physiol.*, 38:946.

27. Santa Cruz, R., Landa, J., Hirsch, J., and Sackner, M. A. (1974): Tracheal mucous velocity in normal man and patients with obstructive lung disease: Effects of terbutaline. *Am. Rev. Respir. Dis.*, 109:458.

28. Chopra, S. K., Taplin, G. V., Simmons, D. H., and Elam, D. (1977): Measurement of mucociliary transport velocity in the intact mucosa. *Chest*, 71:155–158.

29. Iravani, J. (1971): Physiologie und Pathophysiologie der zilientaetigkeit und des Schleimtransportes im tracheobronchialbaum. *Pneumologie*, 144:93.

30. Hilding, A. C. (1957): Ciliary streaming in the bronchial tree and the time element in carcinogenesis. *N. Engl. J. Med.*, 256:634.

31. Marin, M. G., and Morrow, P. E. (1969): Effect of changing inspired O_2 and CO_2 levels on tracheal mucociliary transport rate. *J. Appl. Physiol.*, 27:385.

32. Wanner, A., Hirsch, J. A., Greneltch, D. E., Swenson, E. W., and Forrest, T. (1973): Tracheal mucous velocity in beagles after chronic exposure to cigarette smoke. *Arch. Environ. Health*, 27:370–371.

33. Felicetti, S. A., Wolff, R. K., and Muggenburg, B. A. (1981): Comparison of tracheal mucous transport in rats, guinea pigs, rabbits, and dogs. *J. Appl. Physiol.*, 51:1612–1617.

34. Kilburn, K. H., and Salzano, J. V. (1966): Symposium on structure, function and measurement of respiratory cilia. *Am. Rev. Respir. Dis.*, 93 (Suppl):1–184.

35. Asmundsson, T., and Kilburn, K. H. (1970): Mucociliary clearance rates at various levels in dog lungs. *Am. Rev. Respir. Dis.*, 102:388–397.

36. Iravani, J., and Van As, A. (1972): Mucous transport in the tracheobronchial tree of normal and bronchitic rats. *J. Pathol.*, 106:81–93.

37. Serafini, S. M., Wanner, A., and Michaelson, E. D. (1976): Mucociliary transport in central and intermediate size airways: Effect of aminophyllin. *Bull. Eur. Physiopathol. Respir.*, 12:415–422.

38. Iravani, J. (1975): Mucociliary abnormalities underlying impaired mucus elimination. *Bull. Eur. Physiopathol. Respir.*, 9:397.

39. Hirsch, J. A., Swenson, E. W., and Wanner, A. (1975): Tracheal mucous transport in beagles after long-term exposure to 1 ppm sulfur dioxide. *Arch. Environ. Health,* 30:249–253.

40. Sackner, M. A., Landa, J., Hirsch, J., and Zapata, A. (1975): Pulmonary effects of oxygen breathing: A 6-hour study in normal men. *Ann. Intern. Med.,* 82:40.

41. Lierle, D. M., and Moore, P. M. (1934): Effects of drugs on ciliary activity of mucosa of upper respiratory tract. *Arch. Otolaryngol.,* 19:55.

42. Scudi, J. V., Kimura, E. T., and Reinhard, J. F. (1951): Study of drug action on mammalian ciliated epithelium. *J. Pharmacol. Exp. Ther.,* 102:132.

43. Boyd, E. M., Clark, J. W., and Perry, W. F. (1941): Estrogens and their effect on ciliated mucosa. *Arch. Otolaryngol.,* 33:909.

44. Hill, J. R. (1957): The influence of drugs on ciliary activity. *J. Physiol.,* 139:157.

45. Giordano, A., Jr., Shih, C. K., Holsclaw, D. S. Jr., Khan, M. A., and Litt, M. (1977): Mucus clearance: *In vivo* canine tracheal vs. *in vitro* bullfrog palate studies. *J. Appl. Physiol.,* 42:761–766.

46. Weissberger, D., Oliver, W. Jr., Abraham, W. M., and Wanner, A. (1981): Impaired tracheal mucous transport in allergic bronchoconstriction: Effect of terbutaline pretreatment. *J. Allergy Clin. Immunol.,* 67:357–362.

47. Goodman, R. M., Yergin, B. M., Landa, J. F., Golinvaux, M. H., and Sackner, M. A. (1978). Relationship of smoking history and pulmonary function tests to tracheal mucous velocity in non-smokers, young smokers, ex-smokers, and patients with chronic bronchitis. *Am. Rev. Respir. Dis.,* 117:205–214.

48. Puchelle, E., Zahm, J.-M., and Bertrand, A. (1979): Influence of age on bronchial mucociliary transport. *Scand. J. Respir. Dis.,* 60:307–313.

49. Wolff, R. K., and Muggenburg, B. A. (1979): Comparison of two methods of measuring tracheal mucous velocity in anesthetized beagle dogs. *Am. Rev. Respir. Dis.,* 120:137–142.

50. Bridger, G. P., and Proctor, D. F. (1972): Mucociliary function in the dogs' larynx and trachea. *Laryngoscope,* 82:218.

51. Cralley, L. V. (1942): The effect of irritant gases upon the rate of ciliary activity. *J. Ind. Hyg. Toxicol.,* 24:193.

52. Kilburn, K. H. (1968): Theory and models for cellular injury and clearance failure in the lung. *Yale J. Biol. Med.,* 40:339.

53. Ewert, G. (1967): The effect of two topical anesthetic drugs on the mucus flow in the respiratory tract. *Ann. Otol.,* 76:359.

54. Rossman, C. M., and Newhouse, M. C. (1977): Effect of lidocaine on nasal mucociliary in normals and smokers. *Am. Rev. Respir. Dis.,* 115 (Suppl.):239.

55. Stewart, W. C. (1948): Weight-carrying capacity and excitability of excised ciliated epithelium. *Am. J. Physiol.,* 152:1.

56. Ahmed, T., Januszkiewicz, A. J., Brown, A., Chapman, G. A., and Landa, J. F. (1980): *In vitro* estimation of tracheal mucous velocity: Comparison of a solid and a liquid marker. *Bull. Eur. Physiopathol. Respir.,* 16:533–538.

57. Lee, T. K., Man, S. F. P., Connolly, T. P., and Noujaim, A. A. (1980): Simultaneous comparison of canine tracheal transport of anion exchange resin particles to albumin macroaggregates and sulfur colloid. *Am. Rev. Respir. Dis.,* 121:487–494.

58. Connolly, T. P., Nujaim, A. A., and Man, S. F. P. (1978): Simultaneous canine tracheal transport of different particles. *Am. Rev. Respir. Dis.,* 118:965–968.

59. Ahmed. T., Januszkiewicz, A. J., Landa, J. F., et al. (1979): Effect of local radioactivity on tracheal mucous velocity of sheep. *Am. Rev. Respir. Dis.,* 120:567–575.

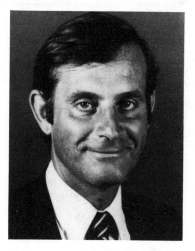

Adam Wanner was born in 1940 in Budapest, Hungary. He received the M.D. degree from the University of Basel, Switzerland. He is a Professor of Medicine and Chief of the Pulmonary Division, University of Miami, School of Medicine, Miami, Florida. His research interests include mucociliary interaction, animal models of airway disease, and clinical aspects of asthma.

Methods in Bronchial Mucology,
edited by P. C. Braga and L. Allegra.
Raven Press, Ltd. © 1988.

4.3. IN VITRO METHODS

4.3.1. Culture of Tracheal Epithelial Cells

J. H. Widdicombe

Cardiovascular Research Institute, University of California–San Francisco, San Francisco, California 94143

Culture procedures
Results
Discussion
Appendix

As discussed in detail elsewhere (10), there are three basic approaches to culturing airway tissues. In organ culture, the original arrangement of tissues is maintained. In explant cultures, newly divided cells grow out from a piece of tissue. Cell cultures start from suspensions of individual disaggregated cells. Explant and organ cultures of airways have been successfully performed for many years (8). True cell cultures were first performed in the 1940s (16). However, the first uses of dispersed cells to initiate cultures of airway epithelium were not until the late 1970s (5,7). There are several advantages of dispersed isolated cells as a starting point for culture. For example, one can control the types of cell present. This may involve no more than excluding fibroblasts from the starting cell dispersion. In theory, however, it is possible to separate different cell types from one another and use suspensions of individual cell types to initiate cultures.

A major advantage of cell suspensions is that even seeding densities are obtained, resulting in complete confluency over the entire culture surface. The disadvantage of cell culture is that epithelial cells tend to dedifferentiate more than in explant or organ culture. However, for many studies of epithelial function, it is probably better to have a pure preparation of dedifferentiated epithelial cells than a mixture

291

of epithelial and other cell types. Also, studies with denuded tracheal grafts have shown that such dedifferentiation need not be permanent. In these studies, the epithelial lining of small tracheas is destroyed. The trachea is then seeded with dispersed cells obtained from primary cultures and implanted into immunosuppressed recipients (irradiated or nude mice). Under these conditions, the cells can regain a fine structure much the same as in the original tissue (9). Also, in some cases airway epithelial cells can be grown under more conventional culture conditions and retain normal structure and function (18).

In the last ten years, several groups have successfully cultured dispersions of airway epithelial cells. In some instances, these cultures have been passaged repeatedly to produce stable cell lines. The culture conditions vary greatly from laboratory to laboratory. Some form of growth support is generally needed to encourage cell growth. However, human nasal epithelial cells have been grown successfully on uncoated tissue culture plastic (19). Many investigators use serum, although hamster cells grow well in a serum-free, hormonally defined medium (18). These various approaches recently have been discussed in several comprehensive reviews (6,10,17).

Our methods for culturing tracheal epithelial cells are described in this chapter (1,13,14). These methods produce confluent cell sheets in which typical tight junctions confer a high electrical resistance and separate apical from basolateral cell membranes. The ion transport processes of these cultured cells resemble closely those of the original tissues. In particular, the Cl transport defect in cells grown from patients with cystic fibrosis is retained in culture (15).

CULTURE PROCEDURES

All our media are obtained from the Cell Culture Facility at the University of California–San Francisco, but they are available commercially (Microbiological Associates). We add the following antibiotics to all media: streptomycin (100 mg/liter), penicillin (10^5 U/liter), and gentamicin (50 or 100 mg/liter). The higher gentamicin concentration is used with human cells. Amphotericin B (2.5 mg/l) is present in the phosphate-buffered saline (PBS) and enzyme solution. In our early experiments, it was also present in the culture medium, although it is now generally omitted. No differences are observed between cells grown in the presence or absence of amphotericin B.

In our initial experiments on dogs, the tracheas were removed by sterile surgery after perfusion of the tracheal circulation to remove red blood cells. These steps are not necessary. We now remove tracheas as aseptically as possible and rinse them several times in PBS. We have found that tracheas can be left overnight at 4°C in PBS with no decline in viability of the final cell suspension.

The following procedures are performed in a sterile culture hood (Sterilgard) with instruments sterilized by autoclaving (Market Forge Sterilmatic). The trachea is split open by a longitudinal incision through the anterior surface and laid out, with the epithelium uppermost, in a dissecting tray. With a No. 11 scalpel blade, we make shallow longitudional cuts through the mucosa. These cuts are ≈5 mm apart and extend the full length of the trachea. The end of a mucosal strip so formed is clamped in a hemostat, and the entire length of strip is pulled off from the underlying tissue. The strips are placed in a small volume (≈2 ml) of enzyme solution and chopped into small pieces (≈4 mm^2 surface area). They are next placed in 50 ml of enzyme solution in a trypsinizing flask at room temperature. The enzyme solution consists of 120 mM NaCl, 20 mM NaHepes, 5 mM NaHCO$_3$, 1.2 mM NaH$_2$PO$_4$, 5.9 mM KCl, 5 mM dithiothreitol (DTT), 0.02% crude collagenase (type 1, Sigma Chemical Co.), 1% bovine serum albumin (Sigma), and 100 μg/ ml DNAase (Sigma). The DTT is important for preventing the formation of mucus globs, which tend to entrap cells. The DNAase and bovine serum albumin also help to prevent cell clumping.

At 90, 180, and 240 min after the start of enzymatic digestion, the collagenase solution is removed from the epithelial strips and replaced by fresh solution. The old solution is centrifuged for 10 min at 100 g, using a desktop centrifuge. After centrifugation, the supernatant is discarded and the cell pellet is resuspended in 2 to 5 ml of culture medium, a mixture of 50% Dulbecco's modified Eagle medium containing 1 g/liter glucose and 50% Ham's nutrient F12 medium, with 5% fetal calf serum (FCS) added. Cell counts and viability estimates on our three cell collections and on the pooled cells are made using trypan blue and a hemocytometer. On average, we obtain 1.5 × 10^8 cells of 95% viability. In our first experiments, the cells were preplated to remove fibroblasts (1). We now know this step to be unnecessary and omit it.

We have isolated dog tracheal cells essentially according to the method of Wu et al. (19). This involves incubating the tissue strips overnight in 0.1% protease (Sigma type XIV) in culture medium lacking serum. The next morning, agitation of the epithelial strips releases cells, and the protease is inhibited by addition of serum. Yields and viabilities with this method are the same as with collagenase digestion.

The isolated cells are suspended in an appropriate volume of culture medium and dispensed into culture dishes whose surfaces are coated with human placental collagen (Sigma type VI). A stock solution of human placental collagen is prepared by dissolving 50 mg of collagen in 100 ml of double distilled water containing 0.2% glacial acetic acid. The solution is then sterilized by passage through a 0.45 μm filter. We assumed that no collagen is lost during the filtration. The stock solution is diluted with double distilled water to produce collagen concentrations such that when added to the culture vessels there is 20 μg of collagen per cm^2 of surface area. The vessels are then incubated for 2 to 20 hr at room temperature before removing the collagen solution and allowing the vessels to dry. Prior to use, the collagen-coated flasks and dishes are rinsed with PBS and allowed to dry. We have tried a number of other growth supports (13), but human placental collagen produces the best attachment and growth (Fig. 1).

For most of our studies, we grow cells on filters. We obtain filters of 16 or 25

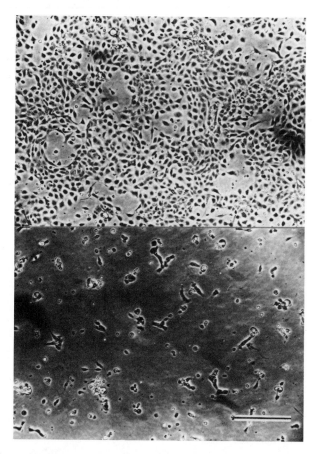

FIG. 1. Effects of human placental collagen on growth. Cells are from the same dog on day 4. Seeding density was 2.5×10^5 cells per cm^2. **Top:** Cells grown on a coating of human placental collagen. **Bottom:** Growth on uncoated tissue culture plastic. Scale bar = 200 μm. (From ref. 13.)

mm diameter from Nucleopore (polycarbonate, 0.8 μm pore size, 10 μm thick); the 25 mm filters are in stock, the 16 mm filters are custom made. They are sterilized by autoclaving (Market Forge Sterilmatic) at 121°C for 30 min. The 16 mm filters fit exactly in the bottom of wells in 24-well multiwell plates (Costar); no attachment is necessary. The 25 mm filters are attached to the bottom of wells in 6-well culture plates (Falcon) by touching the edge at four to six points with a hot soldering iron. Most recently, we have been growing cells in millicell inserts (Millipore). The electrical properties of such cell sheets are much the same as those grown on Nucleopore filters. For counting macroscopic cell features (e.g., domes), we grow cells on 60 mm dishes with grids of 2 × 2 mm (Corning).

Dishes and flasks are kept in an incubator (Forma Scientific) at 37°C in 6% CO_2/air. Media are changed at 24 hr and every 2 to 3 days thereafter. Because the filters are not transparent, assessment of monolayer formation is made by observing cell growth on wells lacking filters.

RESULTS

Dog tracheal cells are plated at 2.5×10^5 per cm^2, and about 15% attach. The cells divide approximately every 24 hr, and a confluent cell sheet forms after about 5 days. The cell sheet consists of several layers (Fig. 2), with typical tight junctions (Fig. 3) separating two distinct membranes. The membrane facing the overlying medium possesses microvilli and a pronounced glycocalyx; the membrane facing the growth support is relatively unspecialized. Pharmacological experiments reveal that the former corresponds to the apical membrane of the original epithelium, and the latter to the basolateral. Freeze-fracture studies reveal subtle changes in the basolateral membrane of the cultured cells. In the original tissue, this membrane has abundant square arrays, but gap junctions are small and infrequent. Cultured cells lack square arrays, but gap junctions are large and abundant (13).

The first evidence that cultures of cells from the dog's tracheal epithelium were actively transporting ions and water was provided by the appearance of domes. These structures are thought to be caused by active fluid absorption (4). The transported fluid accumulates under the epithelium, forcing the cell layer away from the culture surface. Domes continue to grow until the hydrostatic pressure within them ruptures the epithelium, and they subside. In our dog cells, domes appear on the first day after attainment of confluency. Their numbers reach a

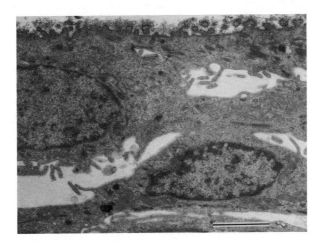

FIG. 2.   Low power electron micrograph of dog tracheal mucosa cells in culture. Note stubby microvilli and pronounced glycocalyx on apical membrane. Bar = 2 μm. [From Widdicombe (1986): *Clin. Chest Med.*, 7:299–305.]

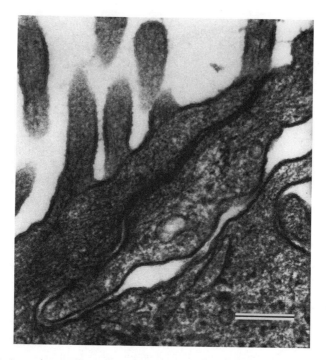

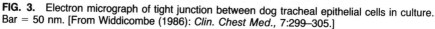

FIG. 3. Electron micrograph of tight junction between dog tracheal epithelial cells in culture. Bar = 50 nm. [From Widdicombe (1986): *Clin. Chest Med.*, 7:299–305.]

peak about a week later, and they disappear after another 2 weeks or so. The lifespans of individual domes range from 0.5 to 5 days. They average 300 μm in diameter and reach local densities of up to 175 per cm². A pair of small domes is illustrated in Fig. 4.

Cultured cell sheets mounted in Ussing chambers show much the same resistance as the original tissue (≈350 Ω·cm²). Short-circuit current (I_{sc}) and transepithelial p.d. are only one-fifth to one-tenth that of the original. However, despite this quantitative difference, the transport processes underlying the I_{sc} seem to be the same as in the original tissue. Thus, blockers of both chloride and sodium transport inhibit I_{sc} in cultured cell sheets with the expected directionality. Mucosal amiloride and serosal bumetanide or ouabain inhibit I_{sc}. Added to the opposite sides of the epithelium, these drugs are without effect.

Chloride secretion across dog tracheal epithelium is stimulated by a wide variety of substances: adrenergic agents, prostaglandins, leukotrienes, bradykinin, exogenous cyclic AMP (cAMP), vasoactive intestinal peptide, platelet-activating factor, the Ca ionophore A23187, and others. All these substances stimulate I_{sc} across cultured cell sheets (13). With certain substances (isoproterenol, bradykinin, PGE_2, dibutyryl cAMP), we have shown that the increase in I_{sc} is not seen in media

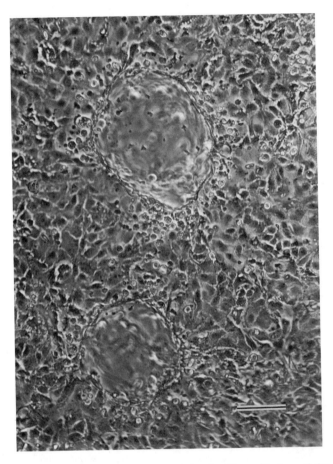

FIG. 4. Domes in cultured dog tracheal epithelial cells. The epithelium of the domes has been lifted above the focal plane of the rest of the cell sheet. Bar = 50 μm. [From Widdicombe (1986): *Clin. Chest Med.,* 7:299–305.]

where Cl has been replaced by the nontransported anions, gluconate or iodide (13).

In their responses to transport inhibitors and stimulators of Cl secretion, the cultured cells reveal that they have retained the transport properties of the original epithelium.

Our success at retaining differentiated transport function in dog cells led us to attempt similar experiments with humans (14). Cells are obtained after death. Isolation and culture procedures are identical to those used for the dog, except that shorter periods of enzymic digestion (≈ 2 hr) are usually sufficient. Even up to 20 hr after death, several million viable cells can be obtained per trachea. Tracheas obtained 5 to 10 hr after death yield approximately 10^8 cells. In the few cases where we have mounted pieces of the original trachea in Ussing chambers,

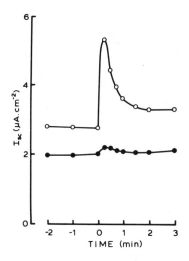

FIG. 5. Changes in I_{sc} induced by isoproterenol (10^{-5} M, serosal side) in normal human (open circles) and CF (closed circles) cells. Values are means of nine records from six sets of normal and eight records from four sets of cystic fibrosis cells.

we have found zero resistance and transepithelial p.d. However, the isolated cells will grow in culture to produce confluent cell sheets. In their resistance, p.d., and responses to stimulators and inhibitors of ion transport, these cell sheets closely resemble those of the dog (14).

The underlying defect in cystic fibrosis (CF) may be a reduced permeability of epithelia to chloride (3). Cystic fibrosis tracheal cells grow into cell sheets with baseline electrical properties very similar to those of sheets derived from control humans who do not have this disease (15). Chloride secretion can be induced across both normal and CF cell sheets by the Ca ionophore, A23187 (12). However, CF cells differ from normal cells in that increases in intracellular cAMP do not stimulate Cl secretion. Thus, although isoproterenol causes cAMP to rise by the same extent in CF and normal cells (12), it fails to stimulate I_{sc} across the CF cell sheets (Fig. 5). Microelectrode studies performed on our cells showed that the inability to secrete Cl was due to the absence of an apical membrane Cl conductance (15).

Patch-clamp studies (2,11) performed on tracheal cells cultured by our methods have confirmed more directly that cAMP is unable to open Cl channels in CF. The conducting part of the apical membrane Cl channels appears normal, however, and can be opened by Ca (2).

DISCUSSION

In a conventional Ussing chamber experiment, a dog trachea will yield at most seven tissues that will remain viable for about 10 hr. From the same trachea, our published methods will yield 40 or more cultured cell sheets that show constant

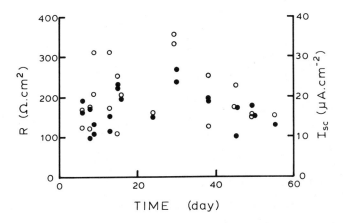

FIG. 6. Dependence of R (open circles) and I_{sc} (closed circles) on time after plating. Values are for individual cell sheets. All cell sheets came from the same dog. (From ref. 13.)

electrical properties for up to 2 months (Fig. 6). Recently, for biochemical purposes, we have been growing cells on smaller filters and can obtain up to 200 cell sheets from each dog. Miniaturization of our Ussing chambers has allowed us to use these smaller cell sheets in our studies on the electrical properties of the cells.

Our cells lack cilia and secretory granules. Therefore, they are useless for the study of certain aspects of the original cells' normal function. Despite this, they are proving useful in studies not only of electrical properties but also of prostaglandin metabolism, protein kinase activities, phosphorylation patterns, and glycocalyx production. In the hamster, it is possible to grow cells that in appearance are virtually indistinguishable from the native tissue (18). Such cells will prove useful in the study of several further functions.

I would like to emphasize the usefulness of cell culture in the study of human cells. For obvious reasons, it is very difficult to obtain appreciable amounts of human tissue of good viability. The tracheas that we have used were dead from the point of view of ion transport. However, one can collect the remaining living cells and culture them to produce tissues that retain the ion transport processes and other properties of the original tissue.

ACKNOWLEDGMENT

The original research described here was supported by NIH Program Project Grant HL-24136 and by grants from the Cystic Fibrosis Foundation, Cystic Fibrosis Research, Inc., and the Strobel Foundation of the American Lung Association of San Francisco.

REFERENCES

1. Coleman, D. L., Tuet, I. K., and Widdicombe, J. H. (1984): Electrical properties of dog tracheal epithelial cells grown in monolayer culture. *Am. J. Physiol.*, 246:C355–C359.
2. Frizzell, R. A., Rechkemmer, G., and Shoemaker, R. L. (1986): Altered regulation of airway epithelial cell chloride channels in cystic fibrosis. *Science*, 233:558–560.
3. Knowles, M. R., Stutts, M. J., Yankaskas, J. R., Gatzy, J. T., and Boucher, R. C. (1986): Abnormal respiratory epithelial ion transport in cystic fibrosis. *Clin. Chest Med.*, 7:285–297.
4. Lever, J. E. (1979): Regulation of dome formation in differentiated epithelial cell cultures. *J. Supramol. Struct.*, 12:259–272.
5. Marchok, A. C., Rhoton, J. C., Griesemer, R. A., and Nettesheim, P. (1977): Increased *in vitro* growth capacity of tracheal epithelium exposed *in vivo* to 7,12-dimethylbenz(a)anthracene. *Cancer Res.*, 37:1811–1821.
6. Nettesheim, P., and Barrett, J. C. (1984): Tracheal epithelial cell transformation: A model system for studies on neoplastic progression. *CRC Crit. Rev. Toxicol.*, 12:215–239.
7. Steele, V. E., Marchok, A. C., and Nettesheim, P. (1977): Transformation of tracheal epithelium exposed *in vitro* to *N*-methyl-*N'*-nitro-*N*-nitrosoguanidine (MNNG). *Int. J. Cancer*, 20:234–238.
8. Stoner, G. D., Katoh, Y., Foidart, J.-M., Myers, G. A., and Harris, C. C. (1980): Identification and culture of human bronchial epithelial cells. *Methods Cell Biol.*, 21A:15–35.
9. Terzhagi, M., Nettesheim, P., and Williams, M. L. (1978): Repopulation of denuded tracheal grafts with normal, preneoplastic, and neoplastic epithelial cell populations. *Cancer Res.*, 38:4546–4553.
10. Van Scott, M. R., Yankaskas, J. R., and Boucher, R. C. (1986): Culture of airway epithelial cells: Research techniques. *Exp. Lung Res.*, 11:75–94.
11. Welsh, M. J., and Liedtke, C. M. (1986): Chloride and potassium channels in cystic fibrosis airway epithelia. *Nature*, 322:467–470.
12. Widdicombe, J. H. (1986): Cystic fibrosis and β-adrenergic response of airway epithelial cell cultures. *Am. J. Physiol.*, 251:R818–R822.
13. Widdicombe, J. H., Coleman, D. L., Finkbeiner, W. E., and Friend, D. S. (1986): Primary cultures of the dog's tracheal epithelium: Fine structure, fluid and electrolyte transport. *Cell Tissue Res.*, 247:95–103.
14. Widdicombe, J. H., Coleman, D. L., Finkbeiner, W. E., and Tuet, I. K. (1985): Electrical properties of monolayers cultured from cells of human tracheal mucosa. *J. Appl. Physiol.*, 58:1729–1735.
15. Widdicombe, J. H., Welsh, M. J., and Finkbeiner, W. E. (1985): Cystic fibrosis decreases the apical membrane chloride permeability of monolayers cultured from cells of tracheal epithelium. *Proc. Natl. Acad. Sci. USA*, 82:6167–6171.
16. Willmer, E. N. (1965): Introduction. In: *Cells and Tissues in Culture. Methods, Biology and Physiology, Vol. 1*, edited by E. M. Willmer, pp. 1–17. Academic Press, New York.
17. Wu, R. (1986): *In vitro* differentiation of airway epithelial cells. In: *In Vitro Models of Respiratory Epithelium*, edited by J. Schiff. CRC Press, Boca Raton, FL.
18. Wu, R., Nolan, E., and Turner, C. (1985): Expression of tracheal differentiated functions in serum-free hormone-supplemented medium. *J. Cell Physiol.*, 125:167–181.
19. Wu, R., Yankaskas, J. R., Cheng, E., Knowles, M. R., and Boucher, R. C. (1985): Growth and differentiation of human nasal epithelial cells in culture: Serum-free, hormone-supplemented medium and proteoglycan synthesis. *Am. Rev. Respir. Dis.*, 132:311–320.

APPENDIX I: SOURCES OF EQUIPMENT AND SUPPLIES

Media

Microbiological Associates, Building 100, Biggs Ford Road, Walkersville, MD 21793

Chemicals

Collagenase: Type I (Cat. No. C-0130)
DNAase: Type III (Cat. No. D-4638)
Bovine albumin: Fraction V (Cat. No. A-9647)
Protease: Type XIV (Cat. No. P-5147)
Human placental collagen: Type VI (Cat. No. C-7521)
All from Sigma Chemical Company, P.O. Box 14508, St. Louis, MO 63178

Sterile Hood

Sterilgard, The Baker Company, Inc., Sanford, ME 04073

Autoclave

Sterilmatic, Market Forge Co., 35 Garvey Street, Everett, MA 02149

CO_2 Incubator

Forma Scientific, Division of Malinckrodt, Inc., Box 649, Marietta, OH 45750

Nucleopore Filters

Polycarbonate (25 mm, 0.8 μm pore, (stock No. 110609): Nucleopore, 7035 Commerce Circle, Pleasanton, CA 94120

Millicell Inserts

Millipore Corporation, Ashby Road, Bedford, MA 01730

Six-Well Culture Dishes

(Falcon 3046): Becton Dickinson Labware, 1950 Williams Drive, Oxnard, CA 93030

24-Well Culture Dishes

(Costar Cluster[24], stock No. 3424): Costar, 205 Broadway, Cambridge, MA 02139

60 mm Dishes (2 mm Grid)

Corning (stock No. 25011): Corning Glass Works, Corning, NY 14831

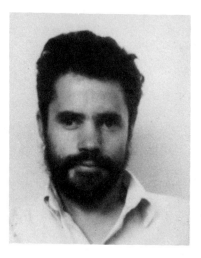

Jonathan Hilton Widdicombe was born in 1949 in London, England. He received the B.A. (Zoology) degree in 1971, Oxford, UK, and the Ph.D. in 1975, Oxford, UK. He is Associate Professor of Physiology and Senior Staff Member, Cardiovascular Research Institute, University of California, Medical School, San Francisco, California. Fields of interest include ion and water transport by airway epithelia and culture of airway epithelium.

Methods in Bronchial Mucology,
edited by P. C. Braga and L. Allegra.
Raven Press, Ltd. © 1988.

4.3.2. Methods for Studying Secretions from Airways

D. B. Borson, A. A. Gashi, and J. A. Nadel

Cardiovascular Research Institute, University of California–San Francisco, San Francisco, California 94143

In vivo methods
In vitro methods for studying intact tissues
Methods for studying secretion from specific cells
Appendix

The purpose of this chapter is to describe methods useful for studying secretory processes in airways. Understanding the roles of secretions in airway physiology is hampered by the high degrees of complexity in the systems responsible for different secretory products. Macromolecules, ions, and water are transported by different cells in the airways. Macromolecules that contribute to the properties of the mucus gel are synthesized and secreted by submucosal glands and by the surface epithelium. For mucociliary clearance to be normal, the physical properties of the gel must be held within narrow limits of viscosity and elasticity. Otherwise, the gel is unable to store energy imparted to it from the ciliary beating, and clearance is impaired. Furthermore, the thickness of the sol layer in which cilia beat must be closely regulated by the surface epithelial cells. If the sol layer is too thin, the mucus gel settles down onto the cilia, preventing them from beating effectively. If the sol layer is too deep, the cilia may not make contact with the gel layer, and thus the cilia will be prevented from propelling the gel.

This complexity results in many problems for studies *in vivo* because many mechanisms can stimulate secretion under different circumstances. For example, there are many reflex stimuli that result in secretion of mucus from submucosal glands in response to a variety of irritating stimuli, including sulfur dioxide, laryngeal irritation, pulmonary inflation (see ref. 34 for review), and chemical stimulation of bronchial C-fibers with capsaicin or bradykinin. These neural pathways involve both cholinergic (45) and adrenergic (20,24,36) mechanisms. Interaction between the different neural pathways in regulating secretion alters secretion (17). In addition, local mediators (e.g., metabolites of arachidonic acid and neuropeptides) may be released during inflammation of the airways. Mediators that cause secretion include the prostaglandins, leukotrienes (33,40), and peptides, including bradykinin (1) and the neuropeptides from sensory or motor nerves, substance P (SP) (1,13,16,22), and vasoactive intestinal peptide (VIP) (35).

Macromolecules are synthesized and released from the surface epithelial cell layer in response to a variety of extracellular proteinases from inflammatory cells and bacteria that commonly colonize airways (47). The materials released may contribute to the physical and chemical properties of the mucus blanket in the airway lumen. Thus, during physiological responses *in vivo,* multiple mechanisms may be active, making understanding of integrated responses difficult.

Therefore, *in vitro* methods were developed to overcome the shortcomings of *in vivo* conditions. The aims are to study the synthesis and release of macromolecular materials and ion transport phenomena using strategies that are specific for each component and each cell type. The strategies employed include measurement of fluid secretion directly, the release of radiolabeled macromolecules, the physical properties of the secretions, morphology and morphometry, and the release of cell-specific materials, such as lysozyme. Additional strategies include autoradiography, used for localization of specific materials to specific airway cells, determining which cells respond to specific stimuli, and for localizing autonomic receptors. Other strategies rely on immunological methods, using monoclonal antibodies to determine the localization of cell-specific materials, and enzyme-linked immunosubstrate assays (ELISA) are used to measure the release of cell-specific products.

IN VIVO METHODS

Some technical details of *in vitro* methods are described here because the same methods with modifications are also used for both *in vivo* and *in vitro* studies.

Fluid is the major component of secretions from submucosal glands. Because alterations in fluid secretion have important implications in mucociliary clearance and cough, methods have been developed to measure the volume of fluid secreted by individual glands. The two methods described are the hillocks and micropipette methods. The hillocks method is a visual method involving the measurement of mucus droplets as they appear on the tracheal surface. It is used primarily for screening studies in which assessment of changes in secretion from numerous glands simultaneously is desired. The method is relatively rapid to use but is only semiquantitative. Furthermore, it cannot be used accurately to study secretions from animals whose secretions are very thin (e.g., cats), but it is suitable for studying secretion in species whose mucus is more viscous (e.g., ferrets, dogs).

The micropipette method is more accurate for measuring the small volumes secreted by single glands. Additionally, by collecting the samples directly, the composition and properties of gland secretions can be studied. The major disadvantages of this method are that it is time consuming and cannot be used to study secretions in species whose mucus is thick and cannot be easily drawn into the narrow capillary tubes (e.g, dogs).

Because the macromolecules in mucus confer most of the viscoelastic properties to the secretions, several methods are used to study macromolecules. These include radiolabeling methods, measurement of specific secretory proteins (e.g., lysozyme), and immunological methods using monoclonal antibodies. These methods can be used for studies of secretion *in vivo* and *in vitro*.

Hillocks Method for Studying Fluid Secretion from Glands

The hillocks method is a semiquantitative procedure used to study fluid secretion from glands by observing the secretion droplets directly as they form over the gland ducts. By coating the airway surface before secretion with powdered tantalum or a similar dense powder, the visibility of the droplets is increased. An animal (e.g., dog) is anesthetized and artificially ventilated via an endotracheal tube introduced into the trachea at the thoracic outlet. Care must be taken to avoid damaging the recurrent laryngeal nerves, which are closely applied to the trachea. An incision is made in the anterior part of the proximal portion of the trachea remaining, and its edges are held apart with clamps. The surface of the trachea is dried by wiping it gently with tissue paper, and a thin layer of tantalum powder (mean mass diameter 0.5 μm, an inert metal) is then applied to the tracheal surface. After a 1- to 2-min baseline period, electrical stimulation of the superior or recurrent laryngeal nerves or injection of drugs into the tracheal circulation via the superior thyroid artery causes secretion to occur and hillocks to form.

There are several ways to express the amount of secretion. First, the number of hillocks formed reflects the number of glands activated. Some of the glands are active during the baseline secretion, but after electrical or pharmacological stimulation, the number of hillocks increases rapidly until most of the glands are secreting. The volume of a hillock can be estimated if it is small and round by measuring the diameter (d) using a videoimage shearing monitor. If we assume that the hillock has a hemispherical cross-section, its volume can be calculated as follows:

$$\text{Volume} = \frac{d^3\pi}{12}$$

The change in the secretory rate can be estimated by dividing the change in calculated volume by the time between measurements (e.g., 1 min). For thin secretions that do not form round hillocks, the area that the secretions cover can be measured by planimetry. If we assume that the thickness of the layer of secretions is approximately constant, changes in area reflect changes in volume (see Chap. 1.3.).

Micropipette Method for Studying Secretion from Glands

To measure accurately the volumes secreted by glands and to collect samples for analysis, the micropipette technique (45) is used. It is a modification of methods used to study the function of renal tubules. The micropipette and apparatus used for collecting secretions are shown in Fig. 1. Micropipettes are made from flint glass capillary tubes purchased commercially (Glass Company of America), have an internal diameter of 95 μm, and are bent at the tip to produce a 30 to 40 degree angle. To prevent damage to the epithelial surface, the tips are fire-polished. The micropipette is held in a larger, conical holding pipette with Eastman 910 adhesive, which is placed in a micropipette holder held by a fine excursion micromanipulator (modified David Kopf and Sensaur de Fonbrune). The micropipette is filled with Sudan black oil (Appendix I) and is placed over the gland duct opening of an anesthetized animal (e.g., cat), covering it completely. The trachea is illuminated by a cold fiberoptic light source aimed obliquely at the surface. The duct openings can be identified either by their characteristic funnel shape and their proximity to blood vessels or after staining the trachea with a 0.1% solution of neutral red dye. To ensure that no fluid from the surface epithelium contaminates the samples, the junction is covered with HEPES-equilibrated oil (Appendix I).

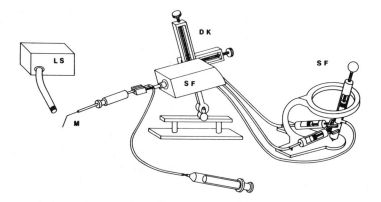

FIG. 1. Diagram of the micropipette apparatus used to collect samples from single submucosal glands. The micropipette (M) is held in a special holder, which in turn is held in a micromanipulator (SF), and placed over the opening of a gland duct (not shown). The screwdrive two-dimension manipulator (David Kopf; DK) is used to make coarse adjustments, and fine adjustments are made with a pneumatic-drive three-dimension micromanipulator (Sensaur de Fonbrune; SF). A 10-ml glass syringe attached to the pipette holder by a polyethylene tube (PE 200) is used to apply suction to the micropipette. Tissue is illuminated obliquely with light from a fiberoptic light source (LS). (From ref. 33a.)

To initiate flow into the oil-filled pipette, slight negative pressure is applied to the end of the pipette for a short time (1–5 sec) with a syringe attached, via tubing, to the pipette holder. After a timed collection period of 1 to 3 min, the pipette is raised transiently above the epithelium to allow a small quantity of paraffin oil to be aspirated. The pipette can be replaced over the duct for another collection. Using oil to separate the different samples, two or three collections can be made with one pipette (see Chap. 1.3.).

Because the collected samples are small (2–30 nl), special methods had to be developed to analyze them. The volume (V) is calculated from the radius (r) of the pipette and the length (l) of the fluid column, which is measured using a vernier micrometer and a stereomicroscope, and the volume is calculated according to the formula:

$$V = r^2 \pi l$$

A radioactive tracer can be used to calibrate the volume of the pipettes. A sample of water containing a known specific radioactivity is aspirated into the pipette. The length of this calibration sample is determined, and then the sample is diluted in 1.0 ml of water and its radioactivity is determined. The dilution of the radioactivity is equal to the dilution of the sample volume. From this, the volume of the calibration sample and the pipette's radius are calculated. Ion contents of the samples from glands are measured by atomic absorption spectroscopy, and the protein concentration is measured using a Lowry technique modified for nanoliter samples (46). Methods for studying viscoelastic properties of secretions are described elsewhere.

Measurement of Radiolabeled Macromolecules

Secretion of macromolecules has been studied by biochemical, cytochemical, immunological, and morphological methods. Many of the cells in the airway stain for carbohydrates with periodic acid-Schiff and alcian blue reagents (28). However, because it is impossible to quantify these methods, they are limited to use in morphological studies. Therefore, other methods have been developed to study neural and humoral mechanisms regulating secretion. Of these, the most widely applied are biochemical methods relying on radiolabeling. These methods have been valuable in studying neural and humoral regulation of tracheal secretion.

Using a method for measuring the release of $^{35}SO_4$-labeled macromolecules from cats *in vivo,* Gallagher et al. (20) found that electrical stimulation of the vagus nerves to the trachea causes secretion via muscarinic-cholinergic mechanisms. They also found that stimulation of the stellate ganglion causes secretion via β-adrenergic mechanisms. This method also was used to demonstrate vagal reflex responses to inhalation of irritant gases (38) and to laryngeal irritation (20) and to demonstrate that stimulating the vagi of geese causes secretion of radiolabeled mucins (37), indicating that in some species without glands, epithelial mucus secretion is under neural control.

Radiolabeling strategies rely on the fact that radioactive precursors of mucins are taken up by serous and mucus gland cells (20,21), by the surface epithelium (31,41,47), including goblet cells, and by ciliated cells and chondrocytes. However, in species with glands that have been studied, the surface epithelium does not usually secrete macromolecules in response to most secretagogues (11,19,31,41), indicating that in these species, the glands are the major sites of secretions of radiolabeled materials in response to autonomic agonists. Because mucus glycoproteins and proteoglycans contain a high percentage of serine and threonine (approximately 40%) (39), protein cores can be labeled using these amino acids. Galactose, *N*-acetylgalactosamine, *N*-acetylglucosamine, *N*-acetylneuraminic acid, and fucose comprise most of the carbohydrate residues (39), and precursors of these sugars [e.g., glucose (20), galactosamine (40)] can be used to label the carbohydrate portions of the molecules. A problem common to the use of each of these precursors is that they are incorporated into materials other than mucins. Many proteins contain serine and threonine, and the carbohydrate precursors (especially glucose) are used by cells for many purposes. Sulfate is present on many of the carbohydrate sidechains as the terminal residue (19), and because it is not metabolized, this tracer has advantages over the other precursors. However, none of the precursors is completely specific, and it is therefore necessary to determine which materials are labeled and what cell types are involved by using additional biochemical methods, including column chromatography, gel electrophoresis, and density gradient centrifugation. Discussion of these methods is outside the scope of this chapter.

Tissues can be incubated for short times (pulse labeling) or long times (steady-state labeling). Pulse labeling is useful for determining the transit times of the materials through the cells. Tissues are exposed to the radiolabel for short periods (e.g., 10–30 min), and then the label is replaced with unlabeled precursor. The specific radioactivity of the secretions increases with time to a maximum and then decreases. The time required to reach the maximum is the transit time, which also can be determined by measuring the disappearance of autoradiographic grains from over the structure. Steady-state labeling is used when all secretory pools must be labeled. This technique requires that the tissue be exposed to radiolabel for at least four times the transit time. In thick tissues (e.g., canine or human tracheal explants), the time required to reach steady-state may be quite long [up to 18 hr (8)], possibly because of long diffusion distances (up to 3 mm) in these tissues. During long *in vitro* incubations, cell function may change, possibly because of changes in receptor mechanisms secondary to denervation or loss of circulating mediators. To alleviate this difficulty, mucins can be labeled *in vivo* via the circulation. However, animals will remove or metabolize precursors, and the concentration of radiolabel in the blood will decrease, and as a consequence, tracheal secretion of radiolabeled materials decreases with time (20). Another alternative is to reduce the size of the tissue by dissection or cell isolation or to study animals with thin tracheas [e.g., ferrets (10), cats (35,36), or the posterior membrane of dogs (32)]. Using tissues less than 1 mm thick ensures that nutrients can diffuse into the core of the tissue (15) and thus maintain viability of cells in the interior of the tissue. Thus, the choice of method depends on the purpose of the study: to study the biochemistry of the secretions, a steady-state must be achieved. However, to study the regulation of secretory processes, steady-state labeling is not required; only enough mucin needs be labeled to allow one to measure changes in secretion. Failure to observe secretory responses does not necessarily mean that a secretory mechanism is not present because all of the secretory pools may not be labeled to steady-state during short labeling periods.

IN VITRO METHODS FOR STUDYING INTACT TISSUES

Many questions about the regulation of specific tissues or cells are difficult to answer using *in vivo* methods because of the presence of central nervous system reflexes or circulating mediators. Therefore, many of the methods described previously have been modified to study tissues *in vitro*. Secretion of fluid from submucosal glands can be measured using the micropipette or hillocks method, and secretion of mucins and proteoglycans from glands or the surface epithelium can be studied using radiolabeling methods. Viscosity and elasticity of glandular secretion can be studied with a microviscometer specially designed for the purpose.

Hillocks Method

The hillocks technique, modified for *in vitro* use, enables studies of secretion in the absence of the circulation or reflexes. A segment of trachea is incised along the posterior membrane and is mounted, luminal side up, in a plastic half-chamber 1 cm in diameter (Fig. 2). The edges of the tissue are held onto the chamber with a ring clamp. Tissue viability is maintained by circulating oxygenated Krebs-Henseleit solution on the submucosal side of the trachea (Appendix I).

After drying the trachea by gently wiping its luminal surface with tissue paper, a thin layer of the inert metal tantalum (mean mass diameter, 0.5 μm) is applied. Following a baseline period (1–2 min), secretion is evoked by electrical field stimulation or by drugs applied to the submucosal side of the tissue. After stimulation, the secretion droplets, or hillocks, can be seen easily through a dissecting microscope (Fig. 3), and the image can be recorded on a videotape recorder.

Electrical Stimulation of Nerves in vitro

To stimulate intramural nerves *in vitro,* short (0.5 msec or less) pulses of alternating electrical current are applied across the tissue via the pins that hold the tissue in the chamber (Fig. 2). The stimulator used should supply enough current to the tissue to achieve a supramaximal stimulus voltage (10–15 V). To show that secretory responses to electrical stimulation are mediated by nerves, a nerve conduction

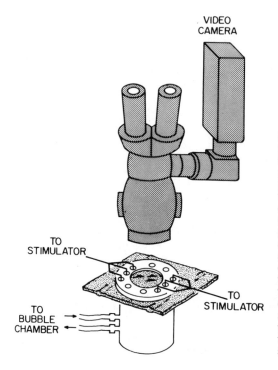

FIG. 2. Chamber and optical apparatus used for studies of fluid secretion from tracheal submucosal glands *in vitro.* A tracheal segment is impaled by pins and held, luminal side up, on top of a half-chamber using a ring clamp. The luminal surface of the segment is covered with a thin layer of powdered tantalum, viewed through a dissecting microscope, and the images are recorded on a videotape recorder and displayed on a videomonitor. Electrical field stimulation of the tissue is via six of the pins that are connected to a stimulator. Drugs are added to and removed from the solution bathing the submucosal side of the tissue via a bubbling chamber (not shown). (From ref. 12.)

blocker (e.g., tetrodotoxin) should be used. Tetrodotoxin prevents action-potential propagation by blocking voltage-dependent sodium channels in nerves (26), thereby abolishing electrically induced muscle contraction (25), the secretion of fluid (12) (Fig. 3) macromolecules (11), and the release of norepinephrine (14) from airways. To determine which neural mechanisms mediate secretion in response to electrical field stimulation, specific receptor antagonists are used.

Micropipette Method

Samples of secretions from single glands can be collected using the micropipette apparatus described. Tissues are mounted in a chamber such as the one described previously. It is then possible to study secretion in response to specific agonists in the absence of reflexes or the circulation.

Measurement of Physical Properties of Gland Secretions

The viscoelastic properties of the secretions from single glands can be studied by drawing the mucus through a microviscometer. The viscometer consists of a small capillary tube within a larger capillary tube (29) held on the stage of a

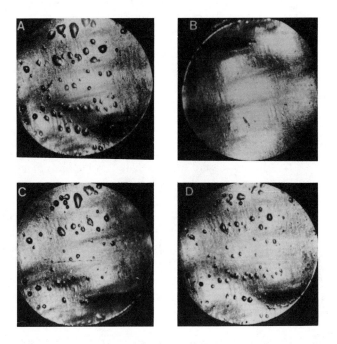

FIG. 3. Photographs of a segment of ferret trachea studied using the apparatus described above. **A:** Electrical field stimulation (intensity 10 V, pulse duration 0.5 msec, frequency 6 Hz for 1 min) caused the formation of hillocks seen in the tantalum layer. **B:** Electrical stimulation as in **A** but after incubating the tissue with the action potential blocker tetrodotoxin (10^{-7} M, 20 min). Tetrodotoxin prevented the secretory response to electrical field stimulation but not the responses to either the cholinergic agonist acetylcholine **(C)** or the α-adrenergic agonist phenylephrine **(D).** (From ref. 12.)

microscope ($\times 40$). The sample is transferred into the larger capillary and then pulled slowly through the smaller tube so that both menisci are in the large capillary, keeping the small capillary filled. Thus, the large surface forces ($>3,000$ dynes/ cm^2) at the menisci are equal and opposite and, therefore, can be ignored. To prevent desiccation, the ends of the sample are sealed with HEPES-equilibrated paraffin oil. The resistive property of a fluid to flow is the Newtonian viscosity (η) and is equal to the ratio of the shear stress (σ) to the rate of shear strain ($\dot{\gamma}$). The viscosity is calculated by measuring the flow rate through the small capillary in response to a constant pressure (ΔP). After steady flow is achieved, the linear displacement (l) is measured over a time period (t). The shear stress (σ) at the small capillary wall is calculated as follows:

$$\sigma = \frac{\Delta P \, r}{2 \, L}$$

where ΔP is the pressure gradient, and r is the radius of and L is the length of the smaller capillary tube. To calculate the rate of shear strain ($\dot{\gamma}$), the rate of displacement (l/t) and the radii of the larger (R) and smaller (r) capillaries are related according to the following formula:

$$\dot{\gamma} = \frac{1}{t}\frac{4R^2}{r^3}$$

The steady-state viscosity (η) is:

$$\eta = \frac{\sigma}{\dot{\gamma}} = \frac{\Delta P\, r^4\, t}{8\, R^2\, L \cdot l}$$

The resistive property of a solid to deformation is elasticity, and it is equal to the ratio of shear stress (σ) to the shear strain recovery (γ_r). To measure elasticity, the pressure difference (ΔP) that moves the fluid is released, and recoil distance (x) of the meniscus is measured at the capillary wall. During periods of high pressure, the meniscus is curved. After pressure is released, the centerline height of the meniscus (Δh) decreases. This change is used to correct the recoil distance. The shear strain recovery (γ_r) is therefore calculated according to the following formula:

$$\gamma_r = \frac{4\,R^2}{r^3}\left(x - \frac{\Delta h}{2}\right)$$

The elastic modulus (G) can be determined from the formula:

$$G = \frac{\sigma}{\gamma_r}$$

Because mucus is an elastic fluid, σ and $\dot{\gamma}$ are not independent, as they are for a Newtonian fluid. Therefore, measurement of viscosity is dependent on the shear rate at which it is measured and should be expressed as the apparent viscosity at a given shear rate (η). Similarly, the apparent elasticity must be expressed as the shear strain recovery obtained at a given shear stress. For studies of secretions from cats, we use shear rates of 0.3 and 1.0 sec^{-1} (29), which are estimated to correspond to the shear rates produced by cilia (18) (see Chap. 2.2.).

Measurement of Macromolecules from Glands and Epithelium

To measure macromolecular secretion from glands and epithelium *in vitro*, proteoglycans and glycoproteins can be labeled biochemically using the same radioactive precursors used to label macromolecules *in vivo*. By carefully regulating the composition of the medium in contact with the tissue, neurohumoral mechanisms of secretion can be studied. Using such a method, Borson et al. (10) demonstrated that stimulating nerves electrically *in vitro* causes secretion mediated by α- and β-adrenergic mechanisms and that nonadrenergic noncholinergic neural mechanisms also cause secretion, an effect possibly mediated by a neuropeptide, such as VIP

(35) or SP (1,13,22). *In vitro* methods have been used to study the roles of endogenous peptidases in regulating secretion induced by peptides. With these methods, Borson et al. have demonstrated a role of the peptidase, neutralendopeptidase (enkephalinase, E.C. 3.4.24.11), in regulating secretion induced by P (13). In addition to studying neural mechanisms, *in vitro* methods have been used to demonstrate that a variety of lipoxygenase (33) and cyclooxygenase (31,38) metabolites of arachidonic acid also cause secretion of macromolecules. Using another *in vitro* method, Varsano et al. (47) found that the epithelium produces macromolecules and releases them in response to proteinases.

Two main types of *in vitro* tracheal preparations have been used: segments of airway mounted in Ussing chambers separating the submucosal and the luminal solutions and explants incubated in flasks. The advantages of the first method are that the radiolabeled precursor can equilibrate with the submucosal side of the tissue for the duration of the experiment, during which time materials secreted into the lumen can be collected (9,32,36). The major disadvantage of this method is that secretion from glands cannot be studied in the absence of the epithelium because, without the epithelial diffusion barrier, the submucosal concentration of radiolabeled precursor does not remain constant. Furthermore, materials secreted toward each side could diffuse to the other side, and the advantage of separating the two sides is lost. The alternative method is to study secretion from explants cultured in flasks. This method is useful for studying secretions from glands and epithelium separately. The disadvantages of this method are (a) that secretions from submucosal and luminal sides of the trachea mix with each other and (b) that equilibration cannot be maintained during sampling.

Ussing Chambers

Segments of airway are mounted in plastic chambers (Fig. 4), and 5 ml of M199/Earles HCO_3 (Appendix I) equilibrated with 95% O_2–5% CO_2 at 38°C is added to each side. Then, 0.167 mCi of $^{35}SO_4$ is added to the submucosal side and is allowed to equilibrate with the tissue for the duration of the experiment. The luminal solution is collected every 15 min and replaced with fresh unlabeled medium. Samples are placed in cellulose dialysis tubing (e.g., Spectropore No. 2, 12,000–14,000 MW cutoff). The samples should be dialyzed against at least six changes of distilled water containing excess unlabeled SO_4 to remove ionically bound $^{35}SO_4$ and sodium azide (10 mg/liter) to prevent bacterial degradation (Appendix I). When the radioactivity in the dialysis water 3 hr after the last change is equal to the radioactivity of the water used for dialysis, the dialysis is complete. The radioactivity of the sample is then determined using a scintillation counter. An alternative to dialysis is chromatography on a desalting column (e.g., Sephadex G-50), but because many samples (>150) can be dialyzed simultaneously, it is easier to perform time course studies (Fig. 5). Most of the molecules remaining after dialysis or desalting are of very high molecular weight (>1,000,000) (11,

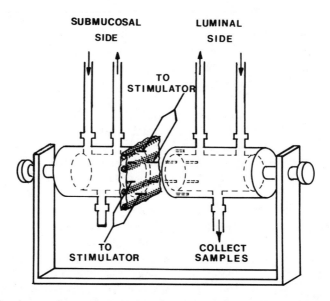

FIG. 4. Chamber used to study secretion of macromolecules from trachea. A segment of the trachea is impaled with pins and mounted between two half-chambers. Each side of the tissue is exposed to nutrient medium at body temperature and bubbled with 95% O_2–5% CO_2. For measurement of radiolabeled macromolecule secretion, $^{35}SO_4$ is added to the submucosal side and remains in contact with the tissue for the duration of the experiment. Samples collected from the luminal side are dialyzed, and the radioactivity in each is determined. Electrical fields are applied to tissue via the wires attached to pins that penetrate the tissue. (From ref. 11.)

20,40), suggesting that they are primarily mucins or proteoglycans. Further biochemical analyses can be performed on these samples, but discussion of them is beyond the scope of this chapter.

Secretion into the lumen increases rapidly after stimulation of nerves or after drugs are added to the submucosal side. For most stimuli, secretion returns to baseline within 30 min after the stimulus is removed (Fig. 5). The evoked response is the flux of bound $^{35}SO_4$ during the peak period minus the flux calculated for the period immediately before stimulation. The flux of bound $^{35}SO_4$ can be calculated from the counts per minute (cpm) in 50 μl of the hot-side medium, the cpm of the sample, the volumes of fluid on each side, the specific activity of the tracer in the medium, and the time interval (t) of sampling:

$$J_{SO_4} = \frac{(\text{cpm recovered/sample}) \times (\text{pmol cold } SO_4/5 \text{ ml on hot side})}{\text{sample interval (hr)} \times 0.5 \text{ cm}^2 \times \text{cpm in 5 ml of hot-side medium}}$$

The response can be expressed either as this value, as cpm secreted, or as the percent increase above the baseline. Using this method, repeated responses to stimulation can be obtained, allowing within-tissue experiments to be designed (see Chap. 4.4.1.).

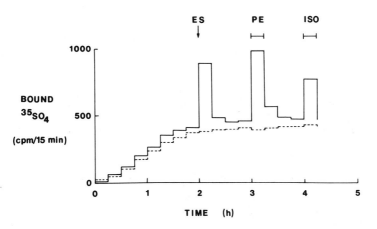

FIG. 5. Secretion of $^{34}SO_4$-labeled macromolecules from two tracheal segments from a ferret. In a control tissue (broken line), secretion increased rapidly for 1.5 hr after adding $^{35}SO_4$, but by 2 hr, release of bound sulfate reached relatively steady rates of secretion that were maintained over time. In another tissue (solid line), secretory responses were obtained by stimulating the tissue, first by electrical fields (ES) (intensity, 10 V, pulse duration, 0.5 msec biphasic, frequency 5 Hz for 5 min), then by phenylephrine (PE), and finally, by isoproterenol (ISO) (each drug, $10^{-5}M$, 15 min, added to the submucosal side). The flux of bound sulfate can be calculated, and changes in secretion are expressed as the absolute change or as functions of baseline secretion or previous responses in the tissue. (From ref. 33a.)

Secretion from Glands Versus Epithelium

When it is necessary to study secretion from glands or epithelium alone, the epithelium can be separated from the submucosa of dogs (48), cats (43), or ferrets (31) by exposing segments of airway to Ca^{2+}/Mg^{2+}-free medium for 15 min (Appendix I). After incubation, the epithelium can be removed as sheets using forceps. Cells isolated from this preparation have high viability (>90%) as determined by exclusion of vital dyes, such as tryphan blue or erythrosin B. Epithelial sheets and the gland-containing submucosa are incubated separately in a metabolic incubator (e.g., Dubnoff Incushaker) and exposed to 0.167 mCi of $^{34}SO_4$ for 2 to 4 hr. For longer incubation periods (e.g., 1–4 days), tissues must be cultured under sterile conditions in a tissue culture incubator. It is difficult to measure secretion accurately during the labeling period, so the tissues must then be washed in unlabeled medium. The medium is replaced every 15 min, and samples are treated as described. Baseline secretion decreases rapidly at first, but usually after 3 hr, secretion is approximately constant, and reproducible responses to stimuli can be obtained.

METHODS FOR STUDYING SECRETION FROM SPECIFIC CELLS

Cytochemical differences between cells have been described on the basis of the contents of acidic (alcian blue staining) and neutral (periodic acid-Schiff staining—PAS mucosubstances. The acidic mucosubstances can be further differentiated into those containing terminal neuraminic acid residues (i.e., that become PAS positive after neuraminidase) and those that do not (i.e., that remain alcian blue positive) (28). However, these methods are difficult to quantify. Therefore, other cell-specific techniques are required.

Although there are advantages in measuring the release of radiolabeled materials from mixed cell preparations, they all have the problem that no radiolabeled precursor yet identified selectively labels only one cell or macromolecular type. This problem led to the use of cell-specific methods, including morphology, morphometry, lysozyme immunocytochemistry and plate assay, autoradiography, and immunological methods using monoclonal antibodies. These methods are used to study the responsiveness of individual cell types to specific secretagogues. In ferrets, cholinergic and α-adrenergic agonists have potent effects on serous cells, causing both the release of lysozyme (44) and degranulation (7), whereas β-adrenergic agonists have less potent effects. In contrast, mucus cells are degranulated by β-adrenergic but not α-adrenergic agonists. Selectivity is reflected in the observation that α-adrenergic agonists cause large increases in fluid secretion from glands that are low in protein (46) and have low viscosity (29). Conversely, β-adrenergic agonists cause the secretion of less fluid that has more protein content (46) and higher viscosity (29).

Different strategies are used to study secretion from individual cell types. These include the measurement of cell-specific secretions (e.g., lysozyme) or *in situ* anatomic methods, including morphology, autoradiography, and immunocytochemistry.

Morphology and Morphometry

When activated, exocrine cells show morphological changes that distinguish them from resting cells. Characteristic changes include loss of secretory granules, convolution and expansion of the apical membranes, and vacuolization. Morphometric methods can be applied to distinguish between the effects of specific secretagogues on serous versus mucus cells (Fig. 6) (22). These methods can be used in conjunction with radiolabeling or immunological methods for measuring macromolecular secretion. A ferret or other experimental animal is anesthetized using a long-acting anesthetic (e.g., sodium pentobarbital, 45 mg/kg, i.p.), and a cannula is placed in the jugular vein for maintaining anesthesia. To ensure that the gland cells are filled with secretory granules, the animal is allowed to remain anesthetized for 3 hr. After this time, the trachea is removed and placed in Ham's F-12 medium and treated as described previously. At the end of the experiment, tissues are dissected into pieces 1 to 3 mm^2 × 1 mm thick and are fixed for electron microscopy at 4°C for 18 hr in 0.08 M cacodylate buffer containing 2.5% glutaraldehyde, 1% sucrose, and 5 mM $CaCl_2$ at pH 7.4. Pieces are then placed in a 4°C solution containing 1.5% OsO_4 in veronal acetate buffer, pH 7.4, for 4 additional hours.

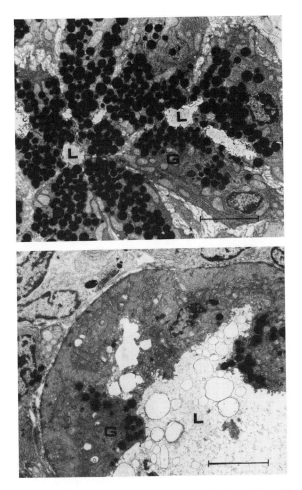

FIG. 6. Effect of substance P (SP) on submucosal glands of a ferret. **Top:** Electron micrograph of a ferret gland incubated for 3 hr in control medium, showing serous cells that contain granules (G) surrounding a narrow central lumen (L). **Bottom:** Electron micrograph of a different tissue from the same animal treated similarly, except for the addition of SP (10^{-5} M) for the last 30 min of incubation. Substance P causes a striking loss of serous cell granules (G), an increase in the area of the apical membrane, and enlarged lumens (L) that contain flocculent material and membrane fragments. Bar = 10 μm.

Tissues are dehydrated in ethanol, passed through propylene glycol, and embedded in Epon 812. Gland-containing blocks are trimmed to 1 × 1 mm, and sections for electron microscopy are obtained. Thin sections are collected on 200-mesh parlodion-coated copper grids, the sections are stained with 5% uranyl acetate and 0.4% lead citrate, and photographs are taken using an electron microscope (e.g., Zeiss EM-10). To ensure adequate sampling of structures in the glands, two blocks per animal per condition are sectioned, and the entire block faces are photographed and printed at ×5,800.

A coherent multipurpose lattice (parallel line length 0.5 cm) is laid over each micrograph to assess degranulation. Structures lying underneath one end of each line are considered "hits," which are recorded over granules, nongranular cytoplasm, nucleus, and gland lumen. The ratio of the number of points above granules to number of points above cytoplasm plus granules is equal to the volume density (V_v). Increases in the relative area of lumen to cellular elements in the gland profiles are proportional to losses in cytoplasm or granules. Changes in the number of points over cytoplasm reflect changes in cell size. Statistical differences between treated and untreated cells reflect the potency of the secretagogues in causing degranulation. Sufficient numbers of points must be counted to ensure that the standard error of the method is low. Therefore, morphometric methods are time consuming.

Lysozyme

An alternative to morphometric methods is to measure the presence and release of a cell-specific material. Although lysozyme is found in epithelial cells of human airways (27), in ferrets it is confined to serous cells of submucosal glands (44) (Fig. 7), indicating that lysozyme is a specific marker of serous cell activity in this species. Other materials are specific for other cell types.

Histochemical Localization of Lysozyme

Lysozyme is localized using the method of Sternberger (42). The embedding medium of the sections is removed, and the tissues remaining are treated for 30 min with normal goat serum (3%), followed by incubation for 48 hr at 4°C in a solution of phosphate-buffered saline (PBS) (Appendix I) containing 1% goat serum and rabbit antihuman lysozyme (1:2,500). Sections are then washed in PBS and treated sequentially with (a) normal goat serum (5 min), (b) goat antirabbit IgG (1:50, 30 min), (c) PBS (15 min), (d) 1% normal goat serum (15 min), and (e) peroxidase-antiperoxidase (1:60, 30 min). Finally, the sections are washed with 0.05 M Tris-HCl (pH 7.4) and incubated in 0.05% 3,3'-diaminobenzidine tetrahydrochloride (DAB) and 0.002% hydrogen peroxide. During the reaction, sections are examined under a light microscope to determine when sufficient time has elapsed for the reaction product to develop with minimal background staining. The optimal time is approximately 10 min. Sections are then washed with distilled water, counterstained with methyl green, dehydrated in graded alcohols, and cleared with xylene.

To control for endogenous peroxidase activity, sections are processed as described, except that normal rabbit serum replaces the rabbit antihuman lysozyme.

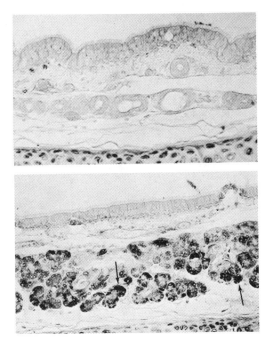

FIG. 7. Changes in immunocyto-chemical localization of lysozyme in serous cells of a ferret tracheal gland in response to stimulation. **Top:** Tissue stimulated with bethanechol (10^{-5} M, 30 min), a muscarinic agonist, and stained using rabbit antiserum raised against human lysozyme (1:2,500), demonstrating the depletion of lysozyme immunoreactivity from the glands. **Bottom:** Control tissue treated the same as the tissue above except for omission of the secretagogue, showing that immunoreactivity for lysozyme is localized to serous cells (arrows) in glands. ×300. (From ref. 44.)

To determine the specificity of the antilysozyme antibody, sections are pretreated with antihuman lysozyme preabsorbed with 0.1 μg/ml of purified human lysozyme.

Radial-Diffusion Assay for Lysozyme

To measure the secretion of lysozyme into the incubation medium, a radial-diffusion plate assay is used (44). Thirty milligrams of *Micrococcus lysodeikticus* is suspended in 1% melted agarose in 0.05 M Tris-HCl (pH 7.0) (Appendix I). Twenty milliliters of this medium is poured into each of several Petri dishes (10 × 10 cm) and allowed to set. Wells, 3 mm in diameter, are made in the plates and filled with 3 μl of either reference standards or the unknown sample. The plates are incubated at 37°C for 20 hr, after which zones of lysis appear. A standard curve is obtained by measuring radii of the lytic zones for the standards and plotting the radius against the logarithm of the concentration. To determine the concentration in unknown samples, the diameters of their zones of lysis are compared to those of the standards.

Autoradiography

Another important strategy for studying specific cells is autoradiography. Autoradiography is useful for localizing the cellular sites of uptake, synthesis, storage, and release of any macromolecules that can be radiolabeled. Additionally, autoradiography is a sensitive technique used to localize cell surface receptors in tissues, including those on tracheal submucosal glands and airway smooth muscle. Both methods rely on the incorporation of radiolabeled tracers into sections of tissues on slides, covering the slide with photographic emulsion, and allowing radioactive decay to expose the silver in the emulsion, producing a dense grain over the site of the tracer. The tissue sections are counterstained to allow identification of the labeled structures. The major advantage of these methods is that the sites of incorporation, storage, release, and binding can be determined anatomically. When used in conjunction with other methods, autoradiography can be a powerful tool in the study of cellular mechanisms of secretion.

Effects of Secretagogues on Specific Cells

Autoradiography can be used with scintillation spectrometry to determine the sites of uptake and release of radiolabeled materials from submucosal glands. Using this method, it is possible to observe the migration of labeled materials through cells and to determine the effects of secretagogues on release of radiolabeled macromolecules from specific cell types (23) (Fig. 8).

Preparation of tissues

To perform autoradiographic studies, tissues from animals are studied. Experimental animals (e.g., ferrets) are anesthetized with sodium pentobarbital, and a cannula is placed in the jugular vein for delivery of additional anesthetic. The animals remain anesthetized for 3 hr and then the trachea is removed and placed in Ham's F-12 medium at 37°C and equilibrated with 95% O_2–5% CO_2. After a 30-min period, tissues are transferred into F-12 medium containing 1 mCi of $Na_2 \cdot {}^{35}SO_4$, and, after an additional 20 min (pulse period), the tissues are blotted on filter paper to remove excess label and transferred into unlabeled medium for different periods of time (chase period). In addition to ${}^{35}SO_4$, ${}^3H$-glucosamine, ${}^3H$-serine, ${}^3H$-threonine, or other radiolabeled precursors can be used. The tissues are fixed for 18 hr with conventional fixatives (e.g., 2.5% glutaraldehyde, 0.08 M cacodylate buffer, 1% sucrose, and 5 mM $CaCl_2$). Tissues are then postfixed in 1.5% OsO_4 in 30 mM veronal acetate buffer, pH 7.4, for 24 hr. Segments are dehydrated in ethanol, passed through propylene oxide, and embedded in Epon 812. Sections 0.5 μm in thickness are cut, placed on acteone-cleaned glass slides, and dipped in photographic emulsion (e.g., Kodak NTB-2) mixed with distilled water (1:1). All sections from the same experiment are treated at the same time to prevent differences between slides caused by decay of the radiolabel during the intervening periods. Two weeks after coating the sections with emulsion, slides are developed in D-19 for 3 min at 17°C, stopped in distilled water (1 min), and fixed (e.g., Kodak Rapidfix without hardener) for 3 additional min. The slides

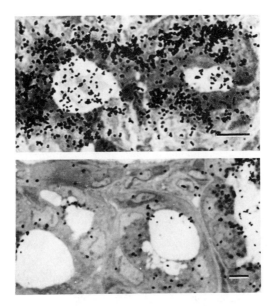

FIG. 8. Demonstration of the secretory effect of a cholinergic agonist using autoradiography. Tracheal segments from a ferret were incubated with 1 mCi of $^{35}SO_4$ for 1 hr and then washed out every 30 min for 3.5 hr. **Top:** Control tissue showing autoradiographic grains over gland cells. **Bottom:** Another tissue treated as the control except for the addition of the cholinergic agonist bethanechol (10^{-5} M, 30 min), showing the loss of autoradiographic grains over the glands and loss of granules from mucus cells. Bar = 10 μm.

are rinsed in distilled water, fixed with formalin, stained with toluidine blue, and viewed under an oil immersion lens, and photographs are made at ×1,000 (Fig. 8).

To quantify autoradiographic grains over glands, regional tissue areas are determined using a digitizer. Silver grains are counted manually and in sufficient quantity to ensure that the coefficient of variation is less than 0.05%. Grain counts are normalized to exposure time and specific activity of the tracer. Nonspecific grain density is determined by counting the grains/unit area of tracheal lumen. This nonspecific density is subtracted from the densities of grains over the epithelium, submucosal glands, and cartilage, yielding values for specific grain densities. To determine the grain density within clusters of grains, the area of each cluster is measured using a digitizer, and these areas are divided by the average area per grain. This method underestimates the densities of clusters containing superimposed grains, but because superimposed grains occur primarily in unstimulated tissues, the errors favor minimizing differences between unstimulated and stimulated tissues. Thus, if differences are observed, they are probably not due to errors in the method. Average grain densities are computed for one block of tissue per condition for each animal. Differences in grain densities can be compared using standard statistical methods (e.g., analysis of variance, *t*-tests) (Fig. 8).

Localization of Cell Surface Receptors

Physiological and pharmacological studies of airways have indicated that secretory phenomena can be elicited by activating muscarinic receptors (34). However, the identity of the specific tissues and cells that mediate these responses may not be apparent from physiological studies alone. Therefore, methods were developed to use anatomical methods for localizing receptors that rely on radioligand binding. The strategy used to localize receptors to specific cells is to bind a radiolabeled analog of a neurotransmitter to the cells, fix the tissue, cut sections, overlay the sections with photographic emulsion, and after an appropriate period, develop the slides. Using this technique, several investigators in our group (2,3,5) demonstrated the presence of cholinergic and adrenergic receptors on airway glands and smooth muscle cells. Because tissues are prepared similarly for localization of all types of autonomic receptors, the methods common to all are described first.

Tissue preparation

Tissues are treated *in vitro* as described, except that tissues are exposed to the radioactively labeled receptor ligand in the absence or presence of a specific, unlabeled receptor antagonist. After exposure to the ligand, the tissues are fixed in either 10% paraformaldehyde in 1.5 M cacodylate buffer, pH 7.4, or 1% acrolein, 2.3% glutaraldehyde in 0.1 M cacodylate buffer, and 5 mM $CaCl_2$, pH 7.4. After fixation for 18 hr at 4°C, tissues are dehydrated in methanol, passed through propylene oxide or α-terpinol, and vacuum imbedded in araldite, glycolmethacrylate, or paraffin. Sections of araldite- or glycolmethacrylate-imbedded tissues 2 or 2.5 μm thick or paraffin sections 10 μm thick are mounted on glass slides and dipped in emulsion (Kodak NTB-2) diluted 1:1 in distilled water. Slides are dried and stored in lightproof boxes at 4°C for 1 to 8 months before development.

Development of autoradiographs

Autoradiographs are developed at 4°C first in D-19 for 3 min, rinsed in water for 1 min, and then in Kodak Rapidfix without hardner. To determine which structures underlie autoradiographic grains, araldite or glycolmethacrylate sections are lightly stained with toluidine or methylene blue, and paraffin sections are stained with cresyl violet. Slides are finally dehydrated in ethanol, cleared in xylene, and mounted under coverslips.

Analysis of autoradiographic data

Because autonomic receptors are located on cell surfaces, grain densities must be calculated on the basis of cell membrane surface area. To determine cell membrane surface area (MSA), the cell boundaries on low power electron micrographs (×3,600) are traced, and the cell area (CA) and perimeter (P) are calculated using a computer (e.g., Hewlett-Packard model 9815A) interfaced with the digitizer. The volume (V) of gland tissue in the section is equal to the total gland area times the section thickness. Because the ratio of perimeter to cell surface area is equal to the ratio of section area to section volume, the surface area of cell membrane is:

$$MSA = V \times P/CA$$

Receptor density (RD) can be calculated for each cell type from the number of specific grains (grains displaced by specific antagonist, G), the number of radioactive decays (D) required to produce one grain, the number of decays (C) per day per Ci tracer, the exposure time (t), Avogadro's number (6.025×10^{20} molecules/mmol, A), and the specific activity of the ligand (S):

$$RD = (GD/t) \times A/(S\,C)$$

Localization of muscarinic receptors

Muscarinic receptors can be localized to tissues using light autoradiography (Fig. 9), but localization to cellular or subcellular sites can be determined only using electron microscopy. To label muscarinic receptors, we use ^{3}H-propylbenzilyl-choline mustard (^{3}H-PrBCM) at a specific activity of either 15 or 42 Ci/mmol. This ligand, when activated, will bind irreversibly to muscarinic receptors, allowing the tissue to be fixed for morphological preservation without losing the tracer. A concentrated stock solution (2.4×10^{-5}M) of tracer is diluted before use to a working concentration of 10^{-6}M. This solution is kept slightly alkaline (pH 7.6) at room temperature to allow cyclization and activation of the aziridinium ion in the ligand. To label muscarinic receptors, tissues are exposed to labeled PrBCM (5×10^{-9}M) for 80 min at 30°C in the absence or presence of atropine, a muscarinic receptor antagonist (10^{-4}M), and then washed in Krebs-Henseleit solution for 45 min to remove unbound tracer. Two fixatives can be used. The first consists of 10% paraformaldehyde in 1.5 M cacodylate buffer, pH 7.4. The second consists of 1% acrolein and 2.3% glutaraldehyde in 0.1 M cacodylate buffer, with 4 mM $CaCl_2$, pH 7.4. Samples are kept in these fixatives for approximately 18 hr (4°C), after which time they are dehydrated in methanols, passed through propylene oxide or α-terpineol, and vacuum embedded in araldite, glycolmethacrylate, or paraffin. Araldite sections (2 μm) are cut using a Porter-Blum Mt-2B ultramicrotome. Glycolmethacrylate sections (2.5 μm) are cut using a JB-4 microtome, and paraffin sections (10 μm) are cut using a rotary microtome. Sections are treated as described previously.

Measurement of autoradiographic silver grains over muscarinic receptors in the glands, muscle, and epithelium is performed using methods already described. For the muscle and epithelium, most grain counts are made directly from microscope slides, using an ocular grid with a ×100 objective. The final magnification at which grain counts are made is ×1000. The number of grains counted should exceed the number required to give a coefficient of variation of 0.05 or less.

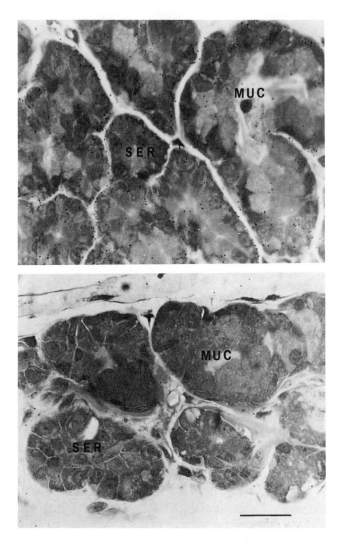

FIG. 9. Autoradiographic localization of muscarinic receptors in ferret tracheal glands. **Top:** Tissue exposed to the muscarinic ligand, ³H-Pr-BCM. Note the autoradiographic grains over basolateral membranes. **Bottom:** Tissue pretreated with atropine (10^{-4} M) and then ³H-Pr-BCM, demonstrating nonspecific binding of the ligand. Bar = 25 μm. MUC, mucus cells; SER, serous cells. (From ref. 5.)

To examine regional differences within the muscle, photographic prints ($\times 2,000$) are made of the entire thickness of the muscle. Because of the parallel orientation of the cells, it is possible to lay a transparent grid over each photograph that divides the muscle into 5 μm zones, starting from the adventitial surface. The smooth muscle caveolar membranes are excluded in making these measurements. The number of grains in each zone is divided by the area of the zone to give regional grain densities. Because muscarinic receptors occur on cell surfaces, we calculate the area of cell surface contained in each unit area of a tissue section, using methods previously described. To ensure sufficient accuracy, average values should be obtained from measurements made on at least 20 cells of each type (serous, mucus, smooth muscle, and epithelium).

Localization of adrenergic receptors

To localize adrenergic receptors, a somewhat different strategy is necessary (Fig. 10). The adrenergic receptor ligands used to not bind irreversibly, as do the muscarinic ligands, so the tissue cannot be fixed using conventional histological methods, and sections from frozen tissues must be studied. The α-adrenergic receptor ligand used is ^{3}H-prazosin, an α-adrenergic antagonist. The β-adrenergic receptor

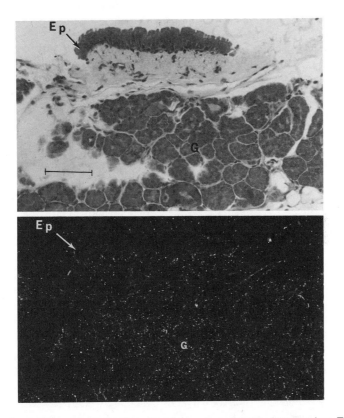

FIG. 10. Autoradiographic localization of β-adrenergic receptors in ferret trachea. **Top:** Bright-field photomicrograph of a segment of ferret trachea exposed to the β-adrenergic ligand, ^{3}H-dihydroalprenolol (^{3}H-DHA) and stained with cresyl violet, showing the locations of the epithelium (Ep) and submucosal glands (G). **Bottom:** Darkfield photomicrograph of the same section of trachea showing bright dots representing silver grains over the ligand binding sites. Bar = 100 μm. (Photomicrograph courtesy of C. B. Basbaum.)

ligand used is ^{3}H-dihydroalprenolol (DHA), a β-adrenergic antagonist. The trachea is cleared of loose connective tissue and cut into lengths approximately 5 mm long, which are rapidly frozen in freon 22 cooled by liquid nitrogen, and the rings are mounted on cryostat chucks using OCT embedding fluid (Lab Tek Products, Naperville, IL). Cryostat sections either 8 μm thick (for autoradiography) or 16 μm thick (for scintillation counting) are cut at −11°C and thaw-mounted onto gelatinized glass microscope slides. These slides are stored overnight at −20°C and then used in the binding reaction.

Radioligand binding was performed by incubation of the slide-mounted tracheal sections with the appropriate radioligand ([^{3}H]DHA or [^{3}H]PZ), using conditions that provided optimal specific (receptor) binding as previously determined in binding reactions to sections of ferret lung (2,3). Because binding of these ligands is reversible, each radioligand was used at a concentration that approximated its dissociation constant (K_D) determined in lung sections. Sections from the same animal are incubated with each radioligand on the same day. For labeling of β-adrenoceptors, [^{3}H]DHA (specific activity 101 Ci/mmol, New England Nuclear) is added to Tris-HCl buffer (pH 7.4) at a concentration of 1.0 nM, and sections are incubated for 20 min. For labeling $α_1$-adrenoceptors, [^{3}H]PZ (specific activity 20.2 Ci/mmol, New England Nuclear) is added at a concentration of 0.5 nM, and sections are incubated for 20 min. Nonspecific binding is determined by incubating adjacent sections with an excess of unlabeled antagonist. For [^{3}H]DHA binding, 1 μM L-propranolol was used, and for [^{3}H]PZ binding, 10 μM phentolamine was used. Under these conditions, [^{3}H]DHA labeled $β_1$- and $β_2$-receptors, and [^{3}H]PZ selectively labeled $α_1$-receptors. After incubation, sections are washed in ice-cold Tris-HCl buffer for 10 min. For scintillation counting, 16 μm sections are studied (five tracheal sections/slide), and after washing, the sections are wiped from the slide into scintillation vials using glass fiber filters (Whatman GF/C) and incubated overnight at 55°C in tissue solubilizer (0.5 ml Protosol, New England Nuclear). Radioactivity in the tissue sections is measured by liquid scintillation spectrometry. Scintillation counting showed that specific binding accounted for >70% of total counts bound for each radioligand (3). For autoradiography, 8 μm sections are washed as described and dried rapidly in a stream of cold air to prevent diffusion of the radioligand. The slides are then stored overnight in a desiccator.

Autoradiography is performed by placing the sections in contact with glass coverslips that previously had been coated in emulsion (Kodak NTB2). Coverslips are fixed at one end with cyanoacrylate adhesive and held in apposition to the section using binder clips. The emulsion is then exposed at 4°C, and test slides are developed at monthly intervals. In our studies, the optimal exposure time for [^{3}H]DHA was 2 months and for [^{3}H]PZ 4 months. The emulsion is developed after separation of one end of the coverslip from the slide by a polypropylene tube spacer, and the section is stained with 2% cresyl violet or alcian blue and periodic acid-Schiff (AB/PAS). After mounting, the sections are observed with a Zeiss microscope suitable for both brightfield and darkfield illumination. Grain counts over glands, airway epithelium, and muscle are made, using a calibrated eyepiece and a ×40 or ×100 objective lens. Specific autoradiographic grain densities are computed by counting grains/1,000 μm^2 over each major cell type and subtracting nonspecific grain counts after correcting both for background counts. Estimates of receptor density are then obtained.

Immunological Methods Using Monoclonal Antibodies

Monoclonal antibodies can be made that recognize specific antigenic determinants unique to single secretion products or cell types (6). Thus, these methods offer unique opportunities to study a variety of cell-specific materials. The major advantages of this method are derived from the fact that single antigenic determinants can be measured, conferring a high degree of specificity for single products. Furthermore, morphological methods can localize the sites of production of specific materials (Fig. 11).

The strategy involves immunization of mice with materials secreted from tracheal explants *in vitro* in response to stimulation by autonomic drugs. Hybridomas are produced by fusion of the mouse spleen cells with cells of a nonsecreting myeloma line such as SP2/0. Hybridoma supernatants are screened by immunofluorescence, using goat anti-mouse IgG-fluorescein isothiocyanate on frozen sections of trachea (6). Those cells producing antibodies with affinity for secretory materials from a single cell type (i.e., serous, mucus, goblet) are subcloned, expanded, and injected into mice for production of ascites fluid. The antibodies can be used to localize antigens by immunocytochemistry (Fig. 11) and to measure release of antigens in enzyme immunoassays (ELISA). Additionally, antibodies can be used in immunoaffinity chromatography, a technique used to purify and subsequently characterize

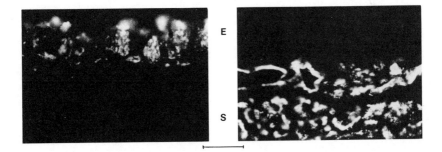

FIG. 11. Use of monoclonal antibodies to demonstrate cell specificity of secretion products. Antibodies were prepared against lyophilized secretions from sheep trachea stimulated by the combination of bethanechol, phenylephrine, and isoproterenol (each drug, 10^{-5} M, 24 hr). Sections were first exposed to monoclonal antibodies and then to goat antimouse IgG-fluorescein isothiocyanate. **Left:** Section stained with monoclonal antibodies directed against an antigen present in epithelial cells (E) but not in submucosal glands (S). **Right:** Adjacent section stained with a monoclonal antibody directed against an antigen present in submucosal glands but not in epithelial cells. Bar = 30 μm.

the specific secretion products. However, discussion of these methods is outside the scope of this chapter.

Preparation of Immunogen

Because the tracheas of sheep produce large quantities of secretory macromolecules, sheep are anesthetized using sodium pentobarbital (40 mg/kg), the extrathoracic region of tracheas are removed and rinsed (4 times) in 500 ml sterile PBS, and loose connective tissue is removed by sterile dissection. Tracheas are cut into segments that will fit compactly into beakers containing 100 ml of fluid; they are equilibrated for 30 min in Ham's F-12 nutrient medium, maintained at 37°C, and bubbled with 95% O_2–5% CO_2 in a Dubnoff metabolic shaker. The pieces are then transferred to a second beaker containing 100 ml of the same medium and the autonomomimetic agonists carbamyl-β-methylcholine Cl (muscarinic, Sigma), L-phenylephrine HCl (α-adrenergic, Sigma), and isoproterenol HCl (β-adrenergic, Sigma) (10^{-5} M), and gentamicin (1 U/ml). Pieces are removed from the solution each day after 24 hr, and the solution is dialyzed at 4°C (Spectropor tubing, MW cutoff, $\approx$13,000 dalton) against 25 volumes of PBS for 2 hr and concentrated overnight by centrifugal evaporation (Speed Vac). The protein content of the desiccated material is assayed by the method of Lowry (30), and the remainder is stored at −80°C prior to use.

Immunization and Preparation of Clones

Balb/C mice are injected intraperitoneally with 100 μg of the desiccated secretions dissolved in 100 μl sterile PBS emulsified with 100 μl Freund's complete adjuvant. The mice are boosted 3 weeks later with an i.p. injection, and 5 weeks later with an i.v. injection of the immunogen.

Three days after the i.v. injection, spleens are removed under sterile conditions from immunized mice and homogenized between slides of frosted glass. The homogenates are filtered, suspended in PBS, and fused with azaguanine-resistant SP2/0 myeloma cells using polyethylene glycol. The pellet containing fused cells is resuspended and plated into 96-well plates containing thymocyte feeder cells, DME H21, 20% fetal calf serum, and hypoxanthine, aminopterin, and thymidine.

Immunofluorescence

Tissue sections used for screening hybridoma supernatants are obtained by fixing pieces of trachea, intestine, and salivary gland in 0.1 M PO_4 buffer containing 4% paraformaldehyde, pH 7.4 (2 hr, 4°C). Sections are then cryoprotected by 18-hr incubation in 30% sucrose in 0.1 M PO_4 buffer, pH 7.4, and frozen in embedding molds containing OCT compound (Miles). Sections 5 μm thick are made and melted onto gelatinized glass slides. Slides are rinsed briefly in PBS to remove the OCT. Hybridoma supernatants are diluted 1:1 with PBS containing 2% normal goat serum (NGS) and 0.6% triton. The diluted supernatants are applied to the sections for 2 hr at room temperature, after which time sections are rinsed in PBS containing 1% NGS and 0.3% triton. They are then incubated with goat antimouse IgG-fluorescein isothiocyanate (FITC 1:40, Cappel) for 30 min at room temperature. Next, they are rinsed in PBS and covered with glycerin:PBS, 3:1, and glass coverslips. Slides are viewed in a Zeiss fluorescence microscope.

Enzyme-linked Immunosubstrate Assay (ELISA)

To quantify the secretion of tracheal antigens, ELISAs are performed on plates activated with 0.1% glutaraldehyde in 0.1 M $Na_2 \cdot CO_3$ buffer (pH 9.0) for 1 hr at room temperature (4). Plates are rinsed in distilled water and incubated in L-polylysine (20 μg/ml) in 0.05 M $Na_2 \cdot CO_3$ buffer for 18 hr at 4°C and washed four times with buffer. Antigenic material is collected using methods described earlier and diluted in buffer containing 1% glutaraldehyde. Fifty μl of each antigen solution is added to each well and dried overnight at 40°C. Nonspecific binding is reduced by addition (1 hr) of a blocking solution consisting of 1% bovine serum albumin (BSA, Sigma type V) and 0.05% Tween 20 in 0.01 M PBS. Plates are incubated with hybridoma supernates (1:10–1:100 dilution, 2 hr, room temperature) and are washed four times with blocking solution; then the second antibody is added (sheep antimouse IgG (FAB′)₂ conjugated to a β-galactosidase (Bethesda Research Labs, 2 hr). Plates are rinsed with PBS containing 1.5 mM $MgCl_2$, 0.05% NaN_3, and 2 mM 2-mercaptoethanol before adding substrate (1.0 mg/ml dinitrophenyl β-D-galactoside in PBS containing 1.5 mM $MgCl_2$) for 30 min at room temperature). The reaction is stopped by adding 100 μl of 0.5 M $Na_2 \cdot CO_3$ (pH 11.5), and plates are read at 405 nm in a Titertek Multiscan (Flow Labs, McClean, VA). The amount of antigen in the unknown wells is determined by comparing the intensity of staining with the intensity of staining of standard amounts of antigen.

REFERENCES

1. Baker, A. P., Hillegass, L. M., Holden, D. A., and Smith, W. J. (1977): Effect of kallidin, substance P, and other basic polypeptides on the production of respiratory macromolecules. *Am. Rev. Respir. Dis.*, 115:811–817.
2. Barnes, P. J., Basbaum, C. B., Nadel, J. A., and Roberts, J. M. (1982): Localization of beta-adrenoreceptors in mammalian lung by light microscopic autoradiography. *Nature*, 299:444–447.
3. Barnes, P. J., Basbaum, C. B., Nadel, J. A., and Roberts, J. M. (1983): Pulmonary alpha-adrenoceptors: Autoradiographic localization using [³H] prazosin. *Eur. J. Pharmacol.*, 88:57–62.
4. Basbaum, C. B., Chow, A., Macher, B. A., Finkbeiner, W. E., Vessiere, D., and Forsberg, L. S. (1986): Tracheal carbohydrate antigens identified by monoclonal antibodies. *Arch. Biochem. Biophys.*, 249:363–373.
5. Basbaum, C. B., Grillo, M. A., and Widdicombe, J. H. (1984): Muscarinic receptors: Evidence for a nonuniform distribution in tracheal smooth muscle and exocrine glands. *J. Neurosci.*, 4:508–520.
6. Basbaum, C. B., Mann, J., Chow, A., and Finkbeiner, W. E. (1984): Monoclonal antibodies as

probes for unique antigens in secretory cells of mixed exocrine organs. *Proc. Natl. Acad. Sci. USA,* 81:4419–4423.

7. Basbaum, C. B., Ueki, I., Brezina, L., and Nadel, J. A. (1981): Tracheal submucosal gland serous cells stimulated *in vitro* with adrenergic and cholinergic agonists: A morphometric study. *Cell Tissue Res.,* 220:481–498.

8. Boat, T. F. (1982): Quantitation of mucous glycoprotein secretion by airways epithelium. *Chest,* 81:29S–31S.

9. Borson, D. B. (1982): *Neural regulation of secretion from tracheal submucosal glands.* Ph.D. Dissertation. University of California, San Francisco.

10. Borson, D. B., Charlin, M., Gold, B. D., and Nadel, J. A. (1982): Nonadrenergic noncholinergic nerves mediate secretion of macromolecules by tracheal glands of ferrets. *Fed. Proc.,* 41:1754.

11. Borson, D. B., Charlin, M., Gold, B. D., and Nadel, J. A. (1984): Neural regulation of $^{35}SO_4$-macromolecule secretion from tracheal glands of ferrets. *J. Appl. Physiol.,* 57:457–466.

12. Borson, D. B., Chinn, R. A., Davis, B., and Nadel, J. A. (1980): Adrenergic and cholinergic nerves mediate fluid secretion from tracheal glands of ferrets. *J. Appl. Physiol.,* 49:1027–1031.

13. Borson, D. B., Corrales, R., Varsano, S., et al. (1987): Enkephalinase inhibitors potentiate substance P-induced secretion of $^{35}SO_4$-macromolecules from ferret trachea. *Exp. Lung Res.,* 12:21–36.

14. Borson, D. B., and Nadel, J. A. (1981): Cholinergic nerves inhibit adrenergic neurotransmission to tracheal submucosal glands of ferrets. *Fed. Proc.,* 40:254.

15. Cascarano, J., and Zweifach, B. W. (1961): Physical and metabolic factors in diffusion of solutes into tissue slices. *Am. J. Physiol.,* 200:1285–1292.

16. Coles, S. J., Bhaskar, K. R., O'Sullivan, D. D., Neill, K. H., and Reid, L. M. (1984): Airway mucus: Composition and regulation of its secretion by neuropeptides *in vitro.* In: *Mucus and Mucosa. CIBA Foundation Symposium 109,* edited by J. Nugent and M. O'Connor, pp. 40–60. Pitman Publishing Co., London.

17. Davis, B., Borson, D. B., and Graf, P. D. (1985): Effect of interaction of sympathetic and parasympathetic nerves on tracheal gland secretion in dogs. *Fed. Proc.,* 44:642.

18. Dulfano, M. J., Adler, K., and Philippoff, W. (1971): Sputum viscoelasticity in chronic bronchitis. *Am. Rev. Respir. Dis.,* 104:88–98.

19. Ellis, D. B., and Stahl, G. H. (1973): Biosynthesis of respiratory-tract mucins. Incorporation of radioactive precursors into glycoproteins by canine tracheal explants *in vitro. Biochem. J.,* 136:837–844.

20. Gallagher, J. T., Kent, P. W., Passatore, M., Phipps, R. J., and Richardson, P. S. (1975): The composition of tracheal mucus and the nervous control of its secretion in the cat. *Proc. R. Soc. Lond.* [*Biol.*], 192:49–76.

21. Gashi, A. A., Benaron, L., and Basbaum, C. B. (1982): Uptake, transport, and release of ^{35}sulfate in secretory cells of the trachea: autoradiographic studies in cat, ferret, and rabbit. *Fed. Proc.,* 41:666.

22. Gashi, A. A., Borson, D. B., Finkbeiner, W. E., Nadel, J. A., and Basbaum, C. B. (1986): Neuropeptides degranulate serous cells of ferret tracheal glands. *Am. J. Physiol.,* 251(*Cell Physiol.,* 20):C223–C229.

23. Gashi, A. A., Nadel, J. A., and Basbaum, C. B. (1987): Autoradiographic studies of the distribution of ^{35}sulfate label in ferret trachea: effects of stimulation. *Exp. Lung Res.,* 12:83–86.

24. German, V. F., Ueki, I. F., and Nadel, J. A. (1980): Micropipette measurement of airway submucosal gland secretion: laryngeal reflex. *Am. Rev. Respir. Dis.,* 122:413–416.

25. Gershon, M. (1967): Effects of tetrodotoxin on innervated smooth muscle preparations. *Br. J. Pharmac. Chemother.,* 29:257–279.

26. Katz, B., and Miledi, R. (1966): The production of end-plate potentials in muscles paralyzed by tetrodotoxin. *J. Physiol.,* 185:5–6P.

27. Konstan, M. W., Chen, P. W., Sherman, J. M., Thomassen, M. J., Wood, R. E., and Boat, T. F. (1981): Human lung lysozyme: Sources and properties. *Am. Rev. Respir. Dis.,* 123:120–124.

28. Lamb, D., and Reid, L. (1969): Histochemical types of acidic glycoprotein produced by mucous cells of the tracheobronchial glands in man. *J. Pathol.,* 98:213–229.

29. Leikauf, G. D., Ueki, I. F., and Nadel, J. A. (1984): Autonomic regulation of viscoelasticity of cat tracheal gland secretions. *J. Appl. Physiol.,* 56:426–430.

30. Lowry, O. H., Rosebrough, N. J., Farr, A. L., and Randall, R. J. (1951): Protein measurement with the folin phenol reagent. *J. Biol. Chem.,* 193:265–275.

31. Mackay, A. D., Borson, D. B., Jensen, E. M., and Nadel, J. A. (1983): Endogenous and exogenous inflammatory mediators cause secretion of $^{35}SO_4$-labeled macromolecules from ferret trachea. *Physiologist,* 26:A35.

32. Marin, M. G., Estep, J. A., and Zorn, J. P. (1982): Effect of calcium on sulfated mucous glycoprotein secretion in dog trachea. *J. Appl. Physiol.*, 52:198–205.

33. Marom, Z., Shelhamer, J. H., and Kaliner, M. (1981): Effects of arachidonic acid, monohydroxyei-cosatetraenoic acid and prostaglandins on the release of mucous glycoproteins from human airways *in vitro*. *J. Clin. Invest.*, 67:1695–1702.

33a. Nadel, J. A., Borson, D. B., Basbaum, C. B., and Widdicombe, J. H. (1984): Techniques for studying airway mucus, secretion, ion transport, and water movement. In: *Techniques in Respiratory Physiology*, Part 1, edited by A. B. Otis, pp. 1–35. Elsevier Scientific Publishers Ireland Ltd., County Clare, Ireland.

34. Nadel, J. A., Widdicombe, J. H., and Peatfield, A. C. (1985): Regulation of airway secretions, ion transport, and water movement. In: *Handbook of Physiology. The Respiratory System*, edited by A. P. Fishman and A. B. Fisher, pp. 419–445. The American Physiological Society, Bethesda, MD.

35. Peatfield, A. C., Barnes, P. J., Bratcher, C., Nadel, J. A., and Davis, B. (1983): Vasoactive intestinal peptide stimulates tracheal submucosal gland secretion in ferret. *Am. Rev. Respir. Dis.*, 128:89–93.

36. Phipps, R. J., Nadel, J. A., and Davis, B. (1980): Effect of alpha-adrenergic stimulation on mucus secretion and ion transport in cat trachea *in vitro*. *Am. Rev. Respir. Dis.*, 121:359–365.

37. Phipps, R. J., Richardson, P. S., Corfield, A., et al. (1977): A physiological, biochemical and histological study of goose tracheal mucin and its secretion. *Philos. Trans. R. Soc. Lond.*, 279:513–540.

38. Richardson, P. S., Phipps, R. J., Balfre, K., and Hall, R. L. (1978): The roles of mediators, irritants and allergens in causing mucin secretion from the trachea. In: *Respiratory Tract Mucus*, edited by CIBA Foundation Symposium 54 (new series), pp. 111–131. Elsevier/Excerpta Medica/North-Holland, Amsterdam.

39. Roussel, P., Degard, P., Lamblin, G., Laine, A., and Lafitte, J. J. (1978): Biochemical definition of human tracheobronchial mucus. *Lung*, 154:241–260.

40. Shelhamer, J. H., Marom, Z., and Kaliner, M. (1980): Immunologic and neuropharmacologic stimulation of mucous glycoprotein release from human airways *in vitro*. *J. Clin. Invest.*, 66:1400–1408.

41. Sherman, J. M., Cheng, P. W., Tandler, B., and Boat, T. F. (1981): Mucous glycoproteins from cat tracheal goblet cells and mucous glands separated with EDTA. *Am. Rev. Respir. Dis.*, 124:476–479.

42. Sternberger, L. A. (1974): *Immunocytochemistry*, pp. 129–172. Prentice-Hall, Englewood Cliffs, NJ.

43. Tandler, B., Sherman, J., and Boat, T. F. (1981): EDTA-mediated separation of cat tracheal lining epithelium. *Am. Rev. Respir. Dis.*, 124:469–475.

44. Tom-Moy, M., Basbaum, C. B., and Nadel, J. A. (1983): Localization and release of lysozyme from ferret trachea: Effects of adrenergic and cholinergic drugs. *Cell Tissue Res.*, 228:549–562.

45. Ueki, I., German, V. F., and Nadel, J. (1980) Micropipette measurement of airway submucosal gland secretion: autonomic effects. *Am. Rev. Respir. Dis.*, 121:351–357.

46. Ueki, I., and Nadel, J. A. (1981): Differences in total protein concentration in submucosal gland fluid: Alpha-adrenergic vs. cholinergic. *Fed. Proc.*, 40:622.

47. Varsano, S., Basbaum, C. B., Forsberg, L. S., Borson, D. B., Caughey, G. H., and Nadel, J. A. (1987): Dog tracheal cells in culture synthesize sulfated macromolecular glycoconjugates and release them from the cell surface upon exposure to extracellular proteinases. *Exp. Lung. Res.*, 13:157–184.

48. Widdicombe, J. H., Basbaum, C. B., and Highland, E. (1981): Ion contents and other properties of isolated cells from dog tracheal epithelium. *Am. J. Physiol.*, 241:C184–C192.

APPENDIX I. SOLUTIONS USED TO STUDY SECRETION FROM THE AIRWAYS

Sudan Black Oil

This oil and HEPES-equilibrated oil (next item) require prior preparation. Both require water-equilibrated oil, which is made by adding 5.0 ml of water to 250 ml of paraffin oil and storing for 1 week in a jar. To make the dye, 1.0 g Sudan black dye (Sigma) is dissolved in 5.0 ml chloroform and then added to 100 ml of water-equilibrated oil and mixed. Store the solution in an open jar (≈ 1 week) to allow chloroform to dissipate.

HEPES-equilibrated Oil

250 ml H$_2$0
5.958 g Na HEPES buffer (*N*-2-hydroxyethylpiperazine *N'*-2-ethanesulfonic acid, Sigma)
0.526 g NaHCO$_3$ (Sigma)

Add 250 ml water-equilibrated paraffin oil and bubble with 95% O$_2$–5% CO$_2$ for ½ hr. Check pH.

Krebs-Henseleit Solution (1 liter)

Substance	*Weight* (*g/liter*)
NaCl	6.82
KCl	0.418
CaCl$_2$·2H$_2$O	0.279
MgSO$_4$·7H$_2$O	0.296
NaHCO$_3$	2.10
NaH$_2$PO$_4$·H$_2$O	0.179
Glucose	1.008

Dissolve NaCl, KCl, and MgSO$_4$ together. Dissolve CaCl$_2$ separately and add. Dissolve NaH$_2$PO$_4$ separately and add. Dissolve and add glucose and NaHCO$_3$. Equilibrate with 95% O$_2$–5% CO$_2$ at 37°C, and adjust pH to 7.4.

Medium 199 Earles HCO$_3$

This multipurpose medium contains all essential fatty acids, amino acids, sugars, nucleotides, and vitamins and is buffered with bicarbonate. This can be purchased commercially (e.g., Gibco Inc., Santa Clara, CA). Add 100 U/ml each of penicillin and streptomycin, equilibrate with 95% O$_2$–5% CO$_2$ at the temperature to be used, and adjust the pH to 7.4.

Ca^{2+}/Mg^{2+}-free Krebs-Henseleit Solution (1 liter)

Substance	*Weight* (*g/liter*)
NaCl	6.85
KCl	0.44n

NaHCO$_3$	2.09
NaH$_2$PO$_4$	0.166
Glucose	1.062

For these media, stock solutions of glucose, NaHCO$_3$, and the salt mixtures can be made at 10 × the above concentrations, stored in the refrigerator, and mixed and diluted to achieve the proper working concentrations. The working solution should be equilibrated at 37°C with 95% O$_2$–5% CO$_2$ by bubbling with humidified gas (30 min) before use and the pH adjusted to 7.4.

Ham's F-12 Medium

Similar to Medium 199 but slightly less complex. Purchase commercially (Gibco). Add 100 U/ml each of penicillin and streptomycin, equilibrate with 95% O$_2$–5% CO$_2$ at the temperature to be used, and adjust the pH to 7.4.

Dialysis Medium (4 liters)

4 liters distilled water
40 mg NaN$_3$
5 g Na$_2$SO$_4$

0.05 M Phosphate-Buffered Saline (PBS) (1 liter)

Substance	Weight
Na$_2$HPO$_4$·7H$_2$O	11.17 g
NaH$_2$PO$_4$·H$_2$O	1.15 g
NaCl	9.0 g
H$_2$O	1.0 liter

Adjust pH to 7.4 if necessary.

Suspension of *Micrococcus lysodeikticus* for Lysozyme Assay

Add 30 mg *Micrococcus lysodeikticus* to 1 g agarose dissolved in 100 ml of 0.05 M Tris-HCl, pH 7.0. Warm until agarose melts, then pour 20 ml into assay plates (10 cm × 10 cm) and allow to cool.

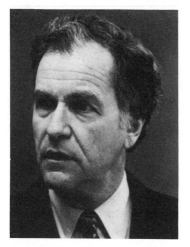

Jay A. Nadel was born in Philadelphia, Pennsylvania, in 1929. He received the M.D. degree from Jefferson Medical College. He is currently Professor of Medicine, Physiology and Radiology, Chief of the section of Pulmonary Diseases, UCSF. His main interest is in pulmonary physiology and cell biology.

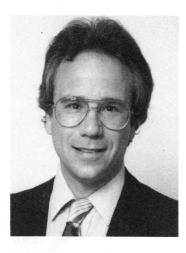

Daniel B. Borson was born in Berkeley, California, in 1946. He received the M.A. degree from the University of California, Riverside, and the Ph.D from the University of California, San Francisco, where he is currently Adjunct Lecturer in Physiology. His main interests are the regulation of airways and the roles of peptides and proteinases in regulation.

Methods in Bronchial Mucology,
edited by P. C. Braga and L. Allegra.
Raven Press, Ltd. © 1988.

4.4. ELECTROPHYSIOLOGICAL METHODS

4.4.1. Electrical Methods for Studying Ion and Fluid Transport Across Airway Epithelia

J. H. Widdicombe

Cardiovascular Research Institute, University of California–San Francisco, San Francisco, California 94143

Methods
    Ussing's short-circuit current technique
    Electrical measurement of volume flows
Results
Discussion
Appendix

Airway epithelia possess transepithelial ion transport processes that may help to regulate the fluid content of airway secretions. Chloride secretion promotes fluid movement from blood to airway lumen. Active absorption of sodium favors fluid movement in the opposite direction. The balance between these two processes can be altered by a number of agents that stimulate chloride secretion (11). The importance of ion transport for normal mucociliary clearance is suggested by the finding that airway epithelia in patients with cystic fibrosis are unable to secrete chloride (18). This defect may cause the characteristically sticky and tenacious mucus secretions, which are the major cause of death in this disease.

METHODS

Ussing's Short-Circuit Current Technique

Diffusional ion movements across a membrane obey Ussing's flux ratio equation (15):

$$J_{12}/J_{21} = (a_1/a_2) \cdot e^{(EF/RT)}$$

Where J_{12} and J_{21} are the two unidirectional fluxes of a particular ion, a_1 and a_2 are its activities on either side of the membrane, E is the potential difference in volts across the membrane, R is the universal gas constant (8.314 joules $\cdot$ mol^{-1} $\cdot$ Å^{-1}), F is Faraday's constant ($96,500$ coulombs $\cdot$ Eq^{-1}), and T is the temperature in Å.

If $a_1 = a_2$ and $E = 0$, then for diffusional movement, $J_{12} = J_{21}$. If under these conditions, J_{12} does not equal J_{21}, factors other than diffusion must be involved in the movement of the ion. These factors could include primary active transport where the flux of an ion is driven by the energy released from a chemical reaction, or the ion flux could be linked to the movement of another chemical present (e.g., solvent drag). The second possibility can be eliminated by ensuring that the activities of all substances present (including water) are the same on either side of the membrane. In other words, if a membrane is bathed with media of identical ionic compositions and there is no potential difference and no osmotic or hydrostatic pressure gradients across the tissue, the only force that can bring about net movement of an ion across the membrane is the tissue's own metabolism. This is the principle of Ussing's short-circuit current technique.

Active transport of ions by epithelia can be essentially electroneutral, as in the case of Na and Cl absorption by the gallbladder. Alternatively, transport can be electrogenic in the sense that it generates a transepithelial potential difference (p.d.), e.g., Na absorption by frog skin or Cl secretion by dog tracheal epithelium. Any transepithelial p.d. generated by the active transport process will cause net diffusional ion movements through shunt or leak pathways within the tissue. Thus, current will cycle within the tissue through the active and shunt pathways. If both sides of the tissue are now connected by a wire of infinitely low resistance, the current normally flowing in the tissue shunt will be drawn off, and the current in the wire will be equal to the sum of the currents generated by all the active tranport processes of the tissue.

This is essentially the experiment performed on frog skin by Ussing and Zerahn (16). They mounted a sheet of skin between plastic half chambers such that it separated serosal and mucosal bathing solutions of identical ionic composition. Oxygenation and stirring of the solutions were achieved with gas-lift oxygenators. The transepithelial p.d. was measured with agar bridges connected via calomel half cells to a high impedance electrometer. Agar bridges at the backs of the half-chambers were connected to an external circuit used to bring the p.d. across the epithelium to zero. In practice the external circuit used by Ussing and Zerahn was not a wire of infinitely low resistance but rather a circuit containing a variable current source. The current flowing through the external circuit was adjusted to maintain the transepithelial p.d. at zero. This current is known as the short-circuit current (I_{sc}) and is equal to the sum of all the active transport processes operating across the tissue.

Electrical continuity between the media bathing the frog skin and the external current-passing circuit was made by Ag/AgCl wires. Thus, when the frog skin moves an Na ion from outside to in, the Cl^- left behind is taken up at the anode by the reaction:

$$Cl^- + Ag \rightarrow AgCl \downarrow + e^-$$

The electron generated flows through the external circuit to neutralize the actively transferred Na^+ by liberating a Cl^- ion at the cathode according to the reaction:

$$AgCl + e^- \rightarrow Ag + Cl^-$$

Details of our own Ussing chamber setup are shown in Fig. 1. Our Ussing chambers are cylindrical, with a variety of internal diameters giving exposed tissue areas of from 0.5 to 2 cm^2. The walls are 4 mm thick, and six pins are spaced evenly in the wall at the open end of one cylinder, projecting 3 mm parallel to the cylinder's main axis. The pins fit into corresponding holes in the wall of the open end of the other cylinder. For mounting, tissues are laid out with the cell side uppermost on a block of paraffin wax. The pins on the half-chamber are then pushed through the tissue, which is then picked up together with the half-chamber. The two half-chambers are clamped together, with the tissue in the middle separating the volumes of the two half-chambers. The surfaces of the half-chambers in contact with the epithelial sheet are coated with high vacuum silicone grease (Dow Corning) in order to prevent edge damage (7). Two holes in the tops of each half-chamber serve to connect them with a gas-lift perfusion apparatus (MRA Inc., Clearwater, FL) which is water-jacketed at 37°C and contains 10 to 20 ml of physiological saline. Single holes in the bottoms of the chambers are connected to three-way stopcocks that are used for draining or filling. The sides of the chambers contain holes for the p.d.-sensing and current-passing bridges. The p.d. bridges (PE 205 tubing containing 150 mM NaCl in 3% agar) are positioned ≈2 mm from the tissue. It is important to position these bridges close to the tissue in order to minimize the resistance of the solution lying between the tissue and the bridges. The value of this solution resistance must be known before the transepithelial p.d. can be clamped to zero. The current needed to bring the transepithelial p.d. to zero, the short-circuit current (I_{sc}), is related to the current needed to bring the p.d. across the agar bridges to zero (I'_{sc}) by the formula (13):

$$I_{sc}/I'_{sc} = (R_T + R_s)/R_T$$

R_T is the tissue resistance, and R_s is the solution resistance. Obviously, the smaller the value of R_s, the less is the difference between I_{sc} and I'_{sc}, and the less is the error in the estimate of I_{sc}. One can buy voltage clamps (Department of Bioengineer-

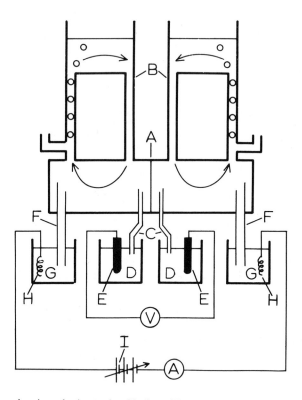

FIG. 1. Ussing chamber. A sheet of epithelium (A) separates media (B) bathing the two faces of the tissue. Fluid is circulated (arrows) by gas-lift oxygenators. Agar bridges (C) are connected to pots of saturated KCl (D) containing calomel half-cells (E), which are connected to a high impedance voltmeter (V) for recording transepithelial potential difference (p.d.). Agar bridges at the backs of the chambers (F), connect to pots of normal saline (G), which are connected via Ag/AgCl wires (H) to a variable current source (I). Current flowing in this external circuit is monitored with an ammeter Ⓐ.

ing, University of Iowa) that will automatically compensate for solution resistance. The p.d. bridges are connected via calomel cells to a high impedance electrometer. Routinely, we match the half-cells so that the imbalance is <0.5 mV. However, our voltage clamp allows us to dial out any imbalance between the half-cells. The current-passing bridges (PE 320 tubing containing 150 mM NaCl in 3% agar) are positioned 1.5 cm from the tissue. The exact distance is not critical. However, for uniform voltage clamping, the current-passing bridges need to be sufficiently far away to ensure similar current densities across all parts of the tissue. A variety of tricks can be used to prevent leaks at the points of insertion of the agar bridges. Making agar bridges with eppendorf pipette tips on their ends and then pushing the tapered tip firmly into the hole in the lucite forms an effective seal. Coating the tips of the bridges with a layer of paraffin wax also works. A coating of petroleum jelly is somewhat less effective. The tips of the bridges should be cut at 45 degrees, with the cut surface facing the tissue.

We have cultured tracheal cells on porous filters and mounted the confluent cell sheets in Ussing chambers (18). With cultured cells, care must be taken in mounting the cell sheet to avoid displacing the cells from the filter. First, we disconnect the gas-lift oxygenators. Fluid is then introduced from 20 ml syringes via three-way stoptaps at the bottom of the apparatus. When filling the perfusion apparatus, the level on the mucosal side is always kept ≈ 1 cm above that of the serosal side. This serves to press the cells against the filter. Even quite small pressure gradients in the opposite direction can push the cells off the filter. Overly vigorous circulation of fluid also can remove the cells. Therefore, before connecting the oxygenators, we always record the p.d. and the resistance of the monolayer (as given by the change of p.d. in response to a current pulse of 100 μA). Solutions can be changed by pumping fluid into the bottom of the chambers with a peristaltic pump while simultaneously removing fluid from the tops of the reservoirs with a vacuum line. In this way, changes in hydrostatic pressure are avoided.

Once properly mounted, the tissues (whether native or cultured) are short-circuited, and a continuous record of I_{sc} is obtained on a chart recorder. Resistance can be determined by disconnecting the current-passing circuit and recording the open-circuit p.d. Resistance is then given by the ratio of p.d. to I_{sc}. If the voltage clamp has a pulse generator, a better way of recording resistance is to pass current pulses at regular intervals in order to shift the p.d. from zero to some other known value. From the size of the current and voltage pulses, the tissue resistance can be determined. Current pulses should be of small magnitude and short duration (≈ 100 msec) to avoid artifacts due to tissue polarization (14).

To determine what active transport processes are responsible for the I_{sc}, one can employ both direct and indirect approaches. Indirect approaches include the use of specific transport blockers and ion substitution experiments. For instance, abolition of the I_{sc} on replacement of Cl by gluconate would suggest that active Cl transport was the only active transport process present. Likewise, inhibition of I_{sc} by mucosal amiloride (which blocks apical membrane Na channels) would suggest the presence of active Na absorption.

Direct determination of the transport processes responsible for the I_{sc} can be made using radioactive tracers. Ideally, both unidirectional fluxes of a particular ion should be performed on the same tissue using different isotopes of the same ion. This can be done for sodium using ^{24}Na and ^{22}Na. In practice, however, the two unidirectional fluxes for a particular ion are measured on a pair of tissues that are closely matched in terms of their short-circuit currents and electrical conductances. Unidirectional fluxes of several ions can be determined simultaneously taking advantage of differences in half-life and type of radiation between isotopes. We routinely determine Na and Cl fluxes on the same sheets of airway epithelia. Boucher et al. (3) simultaneously determine the fluxes of ^{22}Na, ^{42}K, and ^{36}Cl. It is very important that differences in the passive fluxes between the two members of the tissue pair do not obscure the flux due to the active transport process. In pairing tissues, one should bear in mind the following two relations: (a) the sum of the diffusional ion fluxes across a short-circuited tissue (i.e., with zero transepithelial p.d.) in μEq$\cdot$cm$^{-2}\cdot$hr^{-1} is almost identical to the conductance in mS$\cdot$cm^{-2}

(8), and (b) an I_{sc} of 26.8 $\mu A \cdot cm^{-2}$ is equivalent to a net ion flux of 1 $\mu Eq \cdot cm^{-2} \cdot hr^{-1}$. Most of the passive ion fluxes will be carried by Na and Cl. Therefore, a mismatch in conductances of 1 mS $\cdot cm^{-2}$ between the members of a pair could obscure active Na and Cl fluxes in the order of 15 to 20 $\mu A \cdot cm^{-2}$.

Fluxes are calculated according to the formula:

$$J(\mu Eq \cdot cm^{-2} \cdot hr^{-1}) = \frac{(cpm\ B - fcpm\ A) \times [ion] \times V}{cpm/ml\ (hot\ side) \times A \times t}$$

A and B refer to two successive 1 ml samples from the cold side; f is a factor correcting for dilution of the radioactivity when the 1 ml sample is replaced by 1 ml of fresh Krebs-Henseleit solution (for a 15 ml reservoir, f will be $\frac{14}{15}$; [ion] is the concentration of the ion in mM; V is the reservoir volume in ml; A is the surface area in cm^2; t is the time interval between samples in hours.

Electrical Measurement of Volume Flows

Our apparatus for measuring volume flows across airway epithelia was modified from that described by Wiedner (19). It involves the measurement of the distance between a fluid meniscus and the tip of a capacitance probe (Mechanical Technology Inc.). It is illustrated schematically in Fig. 2, and the principles of its use are described in the legend. A detailed diagram of the apparatus has been published elsewhere (17).

RESULTS

Melon was the first to apply Ussing's short-circuit current technique to airway epithelia (10). He found that the I_{sc} across rabbit tracheal epithelium and several different nasal epithelia could be accounted for largely by active absorption of Na. Since then, ion transport has been studied across a wide variety of airway epithelia. The results described briefly below are reviewed in detail elsewhere (1,2,11).

There is considerable variation among short-circuited airway epithelia in the relative magnitudes of active Cl secretion and active Na absorption. The tracheal epithelium of the fetal sheep shows only Cl secretion. The cow trachea, like the dog's has both active Na absorption and Cl secretion. Many airway epithelia *in vitro* show only Na absorption. In some cases (e.g., cat and ferret tracheal epithelium), Cl secretion can be induced by mediators. Other epithelia cannot be induced to secrete Cl by physiological means. These latter epithelia, however, can be induced to secrete Cl by amiloride, due to hyperpolarization of the apical membrane and an increase in the driving force for Cl exit. Thus, the various membrane proteins needed for Cl secretion are all present, and it seems possible that under certain conditions most airway epithelia show active secretion of Cl *in vivo*.

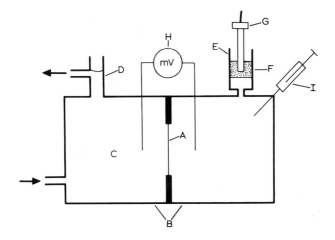

FIG. 2. Apparatus for measurement of transepithelial fluid flow. A sheet of epithelium (A) is mounted between Lucite half-chambers (B). Warm, oxygenated physiological saline is circulated continuously across the mucosal face of the tissue (C). A tube (D) on the mucosal side allows one to apply a small hydrostatic pressure to press the tissue against a wire screen, thereby preventing bulging or flapping. The fluid on the serosal side of the tissue is introduced into a tube (E), and layered with paraffin oil (F). A capacitance probe (G) in the paraffin oil senses the distance between the probe tip and the meniscus of the serosal salt solution. Tissue viability is assessed from the transepithelial potential difference, which is measured with Ag/AgCl wires and a voltmeter (H). Calibration is performed by injecting fluid into the closed serosal chamber with a Hamilton syringe (I). Fluid movements across the tissue are registered as changes in the capacitance sensed by the probe.

Active Na absorption across airway epithelia is insensitive to mediators. However, a large number of compounds have been shown to stimulate Cl secretion: β-adrenergic agents, prostaglandins E_1, D_2, and $F_{2\alpha}$, leukotrienes C_4 and D_4, bradykinin, vasoactive intestinal peptide, platelet-activating factor, substance P and related peptides, major basic protein, acetylcholine, and histamine. The last two compounds have relatively minor actions on active Cl secretion; their major effects on ion movements seem to be secondary to stimulation of gland secretions. Somatostatin, neurotensin, leukotrienes A_4 and B_4, HETEs and α-adrenergic agents are essentially without effect on Cl secretion.

We have performed Ussing chamber studies on primary cultures of tracheal cells (18). Dog tracheal cells in culture behaved in a qualitatively identical fashion to the original tissue. For instance, stimulators of Cl secretion across the original tissue increased I_{sc} across cultured dog cells, and these increases in I_{sc} were virtually abolished in Cl-free (gluconate) medium. Primary cultures of human tracheal cells resembled those cultured from dog trachea. Figure 3 shows increases in I_{sc} across human cells in response to several mediators. However, in tracheal cells cultured from patients with cystic fibrosis, the response to agents expected to raise intracellular cAMP levels was greatly reduced.

Fluid transport across epithelia is secondary to the generation of osmotic gradients by active transepithelial solute transport (5). Chloride secretion across airway epithelia will make the lumen electrically negative to the serosa and cause net movement

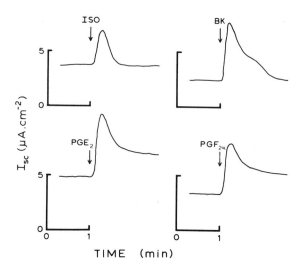

FIG. 3. Changes in short-circuit current across cultures of normal human trachea induced by endogenous mediators. ISO, 10^{-5} M isoproterenol on serosal side, BK, 10^{-6} M bradykinin on serosal side, and prostaglandins (10^{-6} M) were added to both the serosal and mucosal baths. [From Widdicombe et al. (1985): *J. Appl. Physiol.*, 58:1729–1735.]

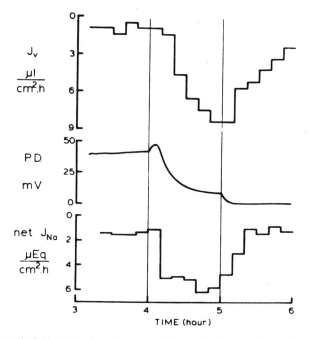

FIG. 4. Changes in fluid volume flow (J_v) and net Na flux (J_{Na}) induced by adding amphotericin B (3×10^{-5} M) to luminal bath at 4 hr and adding ouabain (10^{-2} M) to luminal bath at 5 hr. Middle panel shows record of transepithelial potential difference obtained from tissue in volume-flow apparatus. (From ref. 12.)

of Na toward the lumen down the favorable electrical gradient. The resulting transfer of salt from blood to lumen should cause water flow toward the lumen by osmosis. Similar reasoning shows that active absorption of Na should tend to promote fluid movement from lumen to blood. *In vivo,* the volume and direction of fluid flow presumably depend on the relative magnitudes of Cl secretion and Na absorption. These processes may, therefore, contribute to the regulation of the depth of the periciliary sol layer and the degree of hydration of the mucus blanket.

To test these ideas, we measured fluid movement across open-circuited tissues (i.e., with no current flowing in the external short circuit) using the apparatus shown in Fig. 2. We found that stimulation of active Cl secretion led to fluid secretion (17), whereas stimulation of active Na absorption led to fluid absorption (12). Stimulation of salt and fluid absorption following stimulation of active Na absorption by amphotericin B is illustrated in Fig. 4, which also shows that inhibition of active Na transport with ouabain abolishes the effects of amphotericin B.

DISCUSSION

Ussing chambers are easy to operate and provide important initial information about the types of ion transport present in any particular sheet of epithelium. Because I_{sc} can be recorded continuously on a pen recorder, it is easy to screen drugs for their effects on ion transport. For screening purposes, it is possible to run several Ussing chambers simultaneously. Flux studies are also easy to perform; isotope is added to one side of the tissue and timed samples are withdrawn from the other, cold side. Such flux studies can be used to study transport of organic solutes, such as glucose, proteins, and mucins, as well as ions.

Ussing chambers treat the tissue as a black box and provide only indirect information about the types of ion transport present and their mechanisms. To study mechanisms in detail, the components of the black box must be separated from one another using further techniques, such as intracellular microelectrodes, membrane vesicles, and patch-clamping.

Our method for measuring fluid flows is highly sensitive but is difficult to operate, and one can run only one tissue at a time. It is also expensive to set up.

Fluid flow across airway epithelia has been measured by other means. Durand et al. (6) mounted bovine tracheal epithelium in a modified Ussing chamber and connected the closed serosal chamber to a horizontal glass tube. They measured volume flow by using a photocell to record the movement of the meniscus along the tube. Loughlin et al. (9) introduced physiological saline into the lumen of a ferret trachea *in vitro* and then sandwiched the saline between layers of mineral oil. They measured fluid movement as changes in the inulin content of the luminal fluid. If one assumes that fluid transported by airway epithelia is isotonic NaCl solution, one can estimate fluid movements from the size of the net Na and Cl fluxes across open-circuited tissues (2,4).

REFERENCES

1. Al-Bazzaz, F. J. (1986): Regulation of salt and water transport across airway mucosa. *Clin. Chest Med., 7:*259–272.
2. Boucher, R. C., Narvarte, J., Cotton, C., et al. (1982): Sodium absorption in mammalian airways. In: *Fluid and Electrolyte Abnormalities in Exocrine Glands in Cystic Fibrosis,* edited by P. M. Quinton, J. R. Martinez, and U. Hopfer, pp. 271–287. San Francisco Press, San Francisco, CA.
3. Boucher, R. C., Stutts, M. F., and Gatzy, J. T. (1981): Regional differences in bioelectric properties and ion flow in excised canine airways. *J. Appl. Physiol., 51:*706–714.
4. Corrales, R. J., Coleman, D. L., Jacoby, D. B., et al. (1986): Ion transport across cat and ferret tracheal epithelia. *J. Appl. Physiol., 61:*1065–1070.
5. Diamond, J. M. (1979): Osmotic water flow in leaky epithelia. *J. Membr. Biol., 51:*195–216.
6. Durand, J., Durand-Arczynska, W., and Haab, P. (1981): Volume flow, hydraulic conductivity and electrical properties across bovine tracheal epithelium *in vitro:* Effect of histamine. *Pflugers Arch., 392:*40–45.
7. Helman, S. I., and Miller, D. A. (1971): *In vitro* techniques for avoiding edge damage in studies of frog skin. *Science,* 173:146–148.
8. Linderholm, H. (1952): Active transport of ions through frog skin with special reference to the action of certain diuretics. A study of the relation between electrical properties, the flux of labelled ions, and respiration. *Acta Physiol. Scand.,* 27 (Suppl. 97): 10–35.
9. Loughlin, G. M., Gerencser, G. A., Crowder, M. A., Boyd, R. L., and Mangos, J. A. (1982): Fluid fluxes in the ferret trachea. *Experientia,* 38:1451–1452.
10. Melon, J. (1968): Activite secretoire de la muquese nasale. *Acta Otorhinolaryngol. Belg.,* 22:11–244.
11. Nadel, J. A., Widdicombe, J. H., and Peatfield, A. C. (1985): Regulation of airway secretions, ion transport and water movement. In: *Handbook of Physiology, Section 3: The Respiratory System, Vol. I. Circulation and Nonrespiratory Functions,* edited by A. P. Fishman and A. B. Fisher, pp. 419–445. American Physiological Society, Bethesda, MD.
12. Nathanson, I. T., Widdicombe, J. H., and Nadel, J. A. (1983): Effect of amphotericin B on ion and fluid movement across dog tracheal epithelium. *J. Appl. Physiol., 55:*1257–1261.
13. Rehm, W. S. (1975): Ion transport and short-circuit technique. *Curr. Top. Memb. Transp., 7:*217–271.
14. Rehm, W. S., Shoemaker, R. L., Sanders, S. S., Tarvin, J. T., Wright, J. A., and Friday, E. A. (1973): Conductance of epithelial tissues with particular reference to the frog's cornea and gastric mucosa. *Exp. Eye Res.,* 15:532–552.
15. Ussing, H. H. (1949): The distinction by means of tracers between active transport and diffusion. The transfer of iodide across the isolated frog skin. *Acta Physiol. Scand.,* 19:43–56.
16. Ussing, H. H., and Zerahn, K. (1951): Active transport of sodium as the source of electric current in the short-circuited isolated frog skin. *Acta Physiol. Scand.,* 23:110–127.
17. Welsh, M. J., Widdicombe, J. H., and Nadel, J. A. (1980): Fluid transport across the canine tracheal epithelium. *J. Appl. Physiol., 49:*905–909.
18. Widdicombe, J. H. (1986): Ion transport by tracheal epithelial cells in culture. *Clin. Chest Med., 7:*299–305.
19. Wiedner, G. (1976): Method to detect volume flows in the nanoliter range. *Rev. Sci. Instru.,* 47:775–776.

ACKNOWLEDGMENTS

Supported by NIH Program Project Grants HL-06285 and HL-24136 and by grants from the Cystic Fibrosis Research Foundation, Cystic Fibrosis Research Inc., and the Strobel Foundation of the American Lung Association of San Francisco.

APPENDIX I. SOURCES OF EQUIPMENT AND SUPPLIES

Silicone Grease

Dow Corning high vacuum grease: Fisher Scientific Company, 52 Faden Road, Springfield, NJ 07081

Gas-Lift Perfusion Chambers

Catalogue No. M93: MRA Corporation, 1058 Cephas Road, Clearwater, FL 33515

Calomel Half-Cells

Radiometer Copenhagen No. K401: The London Company, 811 Sharon Drive, Cleveland, OH 44145

Catalogue No. 13–639–56: Fisher Scientific Company, 52 Faden Road, Springfield, NJ 07081

Voltage Clamp

Model 742C Dual Voltage Clamp: Department of Bioengineering, The University of Iowa, Iowa City, IA 52242

Model DVC-1000 Dual Voltage Clamp: World Precision Instruments, 60 Fitch Street, P.O. Box 3110, New Haven, CT 06515

Capacitance Probe

Accumeasure System 1000: Mechanical Technology, Inc., 968 Albany-Shaker Rd., Latham, NY 12110

5. Clinical Methods of Analysis

Methods in Bronchial Mucology,
edited by P. C. Braga and L. Allegra.
Raven Press, Ltd. © 1988.

5.1. MUCUS TRANSPORT AND CLEARANCE MEASUREMENT

5.1.1. Roentgenographic Technique

A. Wanner

Division of Pulmonary Disease, University of Miami,
Miami Beach, Florida 33101

Technical details and procedure
Results
Discussion

Nonabsorbable materials introduced into the lower airways are deposited on the mucosa and subsequently cleared by mucociliary transport. If the material is radiodense, its clearance from the airways can be followed externally. This principle forms the basis of several techniques that use markers that are sufficiently radiodense and have a high enough mass for satisfactory radiographic detection. For human use, the radiopaque markers additionally have to be inert, and one must use a method of introduction into the lower airways that is safe and readily acceptable by volunteers and patients. Insufflation of tantalum powder (1) and bronchoscopic placement of Teflon particles rendered radiodense (2) meet these requirement. A discussion of the latter technique in human subjects is the purpose of this chapter.

TECHNICAL DETAILS AND PROCEDURE

The subjects are seated upright in a dental chair (Fig. 1) or lie supine on an examining table. The nasal passages and the posterior pharynx are sprayed with a 4% lidocaine solution for topical anesthesia. A fiberoptic bronchoscope is passed through either the nose or the mouth, and its distal tip is positioned above the

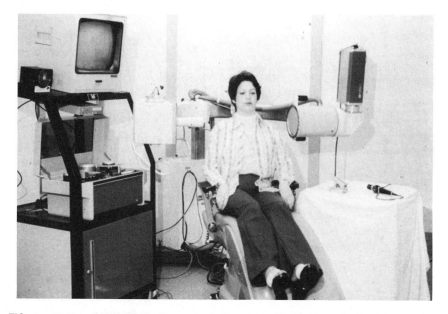

FIG. 1. Measurement of tracheal mucus velocity using radiographic method in sitting position. Note bronchoscope, Teflon punch, and fluoroscopy unit with videotape and monitor.

glottis. At the end of a normal inspiration, several radiopaque disks (Teflon mixed with 50% by volume of bismuth trioxide powder) 1.0 mm in diameter are blown onto the tracheal mucosa through the inner channel of the fiberoptic bronchoscope by means of a punch connected to an air source (3). The movement of the deposited disk in the cervical trachea is visualized with a television monitor connected to a portable image intensifier unit and recorded on videotape while time from a digital clock is displayed (Fig. 2). The distance traveled is measured with a ruler, and the linear velocity of each disk is computed by dividing the distance traveled by the elapsed time. Tracheal mucus velocity is expressed in units of millimeters per minute. Calibration of the image size is obtained by placing a grid adjacent to the trachea during the filming. An average of 15 disks is deposited per filming run, and all visible disks are included in the statistical analysis. Each filming run lasts 2 to 4 min. The individual velocities of all analyzed disks are averaged and are expressed as a single value for any given run. Disks with caudad movement are considered as having no motion.

RESULTS

Normal Subjects

Values of tracheal mucus velocity for normal subjects are available from three studies that were carried out in the same laboratory using the radiographic Teflon

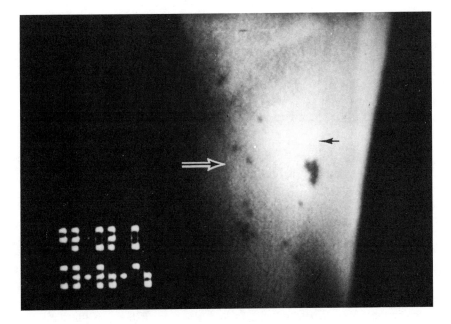

FIG. 2. Photographic copy (lateral view) of videotape showing radiopaque disks in the proximal trachea. Arrows mark anterior (right) and posterior (left) wall of the trachea. Time is displayed in lower left corner.

disk technique as described (2,4,5). Mean tracheal mucus velocity in 27 normal nonsmokers between the ages of 21 and 30 years was 11.5 mm/min (range 6.0–19.4 mm/min). The standard deviation was 2.7, hence the coefficient of variation was 23%; 48% of the subjects had a mucus velocity between 10 and 12 mm/min. This indicates a wide intersubject variability of mucus transport in the healthy trachea. The reasons for this variability are not clear. The upper airway anesthesia with lidocaine solution is unlikely to induce changes in mucus transport (Chap. 4.2.2.). The measurement itself may introduce an inconsistent artifact in that different people exhibit differential mucosal responses to the intubation of the upper airway with the fiberoptic bronchoscope or other stimuli associated with the procedure. True interindividual differences in baseline mucus transport rates are, however, more likely, since a considerable variability in mucociliary clearance among normal subjects has been reported for other, less invasive methods, such as radioaerosol clearance. Camner et al. (6,7) have suggested a genetic determination of mucociliary clearance in human subjects. They reported highly comparable clearance patterns in monozygotic twins and least similarity among normal unrelated nonsmokers.

Friedman et al. (2) also examined the effect of gravity on Teflon particle transport in the trachea of normal subjects. In five subjects, the authors found a mean (SD) mucus velocity of 11.5 mm/min (4.7) in the sitting position and 11.7 mm/min (3.9) in the supine position (p = NS). Thus, gravity appears not to reduce the cephalad motion of particles as heavy as Teflon disks (0.6 mg) in young normals. In contrast, young smokers with chronic bronchitis may be influenced by gravity, probably due to excessive secretions (8). In this case, the weight of the secretions rather than the weight of the Teflon disk appears to be responsible for the slower cephalad transport rate in the sitting position than in the supine position.

Induced or Spontaneous Changes in Transport

The radiopaque Teflon disk technique has been used in several clinical studies involving patients with airway disease and in normal subjects exposed acutely to inhalants or pharmacological agents (4,8–11). The results of those investigations have shown that this method is capable of demonstrating abnormalities of mucociliary transport in patients with chronic bronchitis and asthma and of detecting minimal airway effects of inhaled materials in normal subjects.

Cigarette smoke and cigarette smoke-induced chronic bronchitis seem to impair tracheal mucus clearance independently (8). In that study, tracheal mucus velocity of healthy young current smokers was lower than that of age-matched nonsmokers, and in healthy young ex-smokers higher than in healthy young current smokers but lower than in age-matched nonsmokers (Fig. 3). Patients with simple and obstructive chronic bronchitis had markedly decreased tracheal mucus velocity as compared to age-matched lifetime nonsmokers. In selected smokers, tracheal mucus velocity was measured before and within 10 minutes after smoking one cigarette, and there was no consistent change in this parameter.

Abnormal tracheal mucus transport also has been observed in patients with asthma. In one study, tracheal mucus velocity and respiratory mechanics were measured in asymptomatic asthmatic patients with ragweed hypersensitivity before

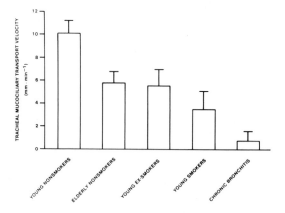

FIG. 3. Independent effects of age, cigarette smoking, and chronic bronchitis (in elderly ex-smokers) on mean tracheal mucus velocity (SE reflected by bracket) in different populations.

and after inhalation of specific antigen and with or without cromolyn sodium pretreatment (5). The airway response to bronchial provocation was monitored by measurements of forced expiratory volume in 1 second (FEV_1) and specific airway conductance. Tracheal mucus velocity was significantly less (6.3 $\pm$ 2.3 mm/min, mean $\pm$ SD) in the six asymptomatic asthmatic patients than in seven normal subjects (11.6 $\pm$ 3.6 mm/min). In the asthmatic patients, mean tracheal mucus velocity diminished to 72% of baseline immediately after bronchial provocation when specific airway conductance was decreased to 65% of baseline or less, with a further decrease in tracheal mucus velocity to 47% of baseline after 1 hr, at which time respiratory mechanics had returned to baseline values. Pretreatment with cromolyn sodium prevented the decrease in tracheal mucus velocity after bronchial provocation. This suggests that in asymptomatic patients with allergic asthma, baseline tracheal mucus velocity is impaired, inhalation of specific antigen causes a marked decrease in tracheal mucus velocity independent of the degree of bronchospasm, and the decrease in tracheal mucus velocity may be related to the release of chemical mediators.

In another study, the effect of an anticholinergic bronchodilator aerosol (ipratropium bromide) on tracheal mucociliary transport was assessed in 14 patients with mild asthma (11). Tracheal mucus velocity and the FEV_1 were measured before and serially for 120 min after inhalation of either 40 µg ipratropium bromide or placebo in a double-blind crossover design. Baseline mean $\pm$ SE tracheal mucus velocity and FEV_1 were comparable before the two treatments (4.4 mm/min $\pm$ 1.1 and 4.9 mm/min $\pm$ 0.9). Neither ipratropium bromide nor placebo had a significant effect on mean tracheal mucus velocity throughout the 120-min observation period. Mean FEV_1 was slightly higher after ipratropium bromide than after placebo ($p < 0.05$) (Fig. 4). These results suggest that, at the dosage used, inhaled ipratropium bromide reduced airflow obstruction without an appreciable effect on mucociliary transport in the central airways, where the drug concentration is highest.

In contrast, inhalation of an apparently safe cosmetic aerosol produced an appreciable decrease of tracheal mucus transport in normals (4). The acute effects of a commercially available aerosol hair spray preparation and a freon propellant on various pulmonary function tests and tracheal mucociliary transport were studied in 12 normal nonsmokers who were not habitual hair spray users. In 7 subjects exposed to hair spray by directing the aerosol to the hair for 20 sec, no significant changes occurred in any of the various pulmonary function parameters, whereas mean tracheal mucus velocity decreased by 57% ($p < 0.001$) 1 hr after exposure. This effect was transient and could not be demonstrated after 3 hr. No significant changes in tracheal mucus velocity or pulmonary function tests were observed in the 5 control subjects exposed to the freon propellant alone. These observations suggest that acute exposure to aerosol hair spray produces a transient impairment of a pulmonary defense mechanism and that measurement of mucociliary transport is a more sensitive indicator of this type of airway irritation than conventional pulmonary function tests.

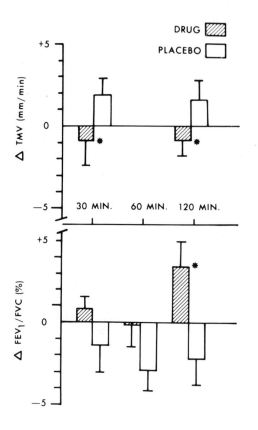

FIG. 4. Mean (SE in bracket) changes in tracheal mucus velocity (TMV) and FEV$_1$/FVC in 14 patients with mild asthma, before and after inhalation of 40 µg ipratropium bromide or placebo (freon propellant). Asterisks indicate significant difference between drug and placebo.

DISCUSSION

The radioactive microsphere bolus technique (12), the tantalum powder technique (1), and the radiographic Teflon marker technique (2) all have the advantage of measuring mucus transport in an anatomically defined airway. In addition, the radioaerosol bolus and Teflon disk measurements can be repeated at short time intervals, thereby allowing the detection of transient changes in mucus transport. Of the three methods, inhalation of a radioactive bolus is the least and insufflation of tantalum powder the most invasive. No single technique can be said to be superior to the others, and the choice of methodology for a clinical study should be based on the questions to be answered and the availability of equipment.

REFERENCES

1. Gamsu, G., Weintraub, R. M., and Nadel, J. A. (1973): Clearance of tantalum from airways of different caliber in man evaluated by a roentgenographic method. *Am. Rev. Respir. Dis.*, 107:214–224.

2. Friedman, M., Stott, F. D., Poole, D. O., et al. (1977): A new roentgenographic method for estimating mucous velocity in airways. *Am. Rev. Respir. Dis.,* 115:67–72.
3. Sackner, M. A., Rosen, M. J., and Wanner, A. (1973): Estimation of tracheal mucous velocity by bronchofiberscopy. *J. Appl. Physiol.,* 23:495–499.
4. Friedman, M., Dougherty, R., Nelson, S. R., White, R. P., Sackner, M. A., and Wanner, A. (1977): Acute effects of an aerosol hair spray on tracheal mucociliary transport. *Am. Rev. Respir. Dis.,* 116:281–286.
5. Mezey, R. J., Cohn, M. A., Fernandez, R. J., Januszkiewicz, A. J., and Wanner, A. (1978): Mucociliary transport in allergic patients with antigen-induced bronchospasm. *Am. Rev. Respir. Dis.,* 118:677–684.
6. Camner, P., Philipson, K., and Friberg, L. (1972): Tracheobronchial clearance in twins. *Arch. Environ. Health,* 24:82.
7. Camner, P., Mossberg, B., and Afzelius, B. A. (1975): Evidence for congenitally nonfunctioning cilia in the tracheobronchial tract in two subjects. *Am. Rev. Respir. Dis.,* 112:807–809.
8. Goodman, R. M., Yergin, B. M., Landa, J. F., Golinvaux, M. H., and Sackner, M. A. (1978): Relationship of smoking history and pulmonary function tests to tracheal mucous velocity in nonsmokers, young smokers, ex-smokers, and patients with chronic bronchitis. *Am. Rev. Respir. Dis.,* 117:205–214.
9. Goodman, R. M., Yergin, B. M., and Sackner, M. A. (1978): Effects of S-carboxymethylcysteine on tracheal mucus velocity. *Chest,* 74:615–618.
10. Ahmed, T., Greenblatt, D. W., Birch, S., Marchette, B., and Wanner, A. (1981): Abnormal mucociliary transport in allergic patients with antigen-induced bronchospasm: Role of slow reacting substance of anaphylaxis. *Am. Rev. Respir. Dis.,* 124:110–114.
11. Bell, J. A., Bluestein, B. M., Danta, I., and Wanner, A. (1984): Effect of inhaled ipratropium bromide on tracheal mucociliary transport in bronchial asthma. *Mt. Sinai J. Med.,* 51:215–217.
12. Yeates, D. B., Aspin, N., Levinson, H., Jones, M. T., and Bryan, A. C. (1975): Mucociliary tracheal transport rates in man. *J. Appl. Physiol.,* 39:487–495.

Methods in Bronchial Mucology,
edited by P. C. Braga and L. Allegra.
Raven Press, Ltd. © 1988.

5.1.2. Radioaerosol Technique

D. B. Yeates

*Section of Environmental and Occupational Medicine, Department of Medicine,
University of Illinois at Chicago, Chicago, Illinois, 60612*

Technical details and procedure
Results
Discussion

A noninvasive technique for measuring tracheal mucus velocity (TMV) by radioaerosol techniques was developed to assess the mucociliary transport system without mechanical, chemical, or pharmacological perturbation. When a person inhales via the mouth an aerosol of relatively large particle size with a high inspiratory flow rate, aerosol particles impact on the bifurcations of the larger pulmonary airways to form relatively high local concentrations of deposited radiotagged particles. These local concentrations of particles are transported by mucociliary activity along the airways and up the trachea. The positions of these boluses of activity in the trachea are measured as a function of time using either a gamma camera or a scintillation detection system. This radioaerosol technique was first described by Yeates et al. in 1975 (19) and has since undergone progressive development along with its use as an assay to measure the effects of drugs, disease, and pollutants on mucociliary transport.

TECHNICAL DETAILS AND PROCEDURE

Both aqueous and dry radioaerosols have been generated for deposition in the airways of the human lung. Aqueous aerosols have been generated either from denatured albumin microspheres tagged with technetium-99m (20) or a radiotagged iron oxide sol (10). Such sols, aerosolized by ultrasonic nebulizers, are delivered as an aqueous aerosol (11,13,17–19). To produce a dry, radiotagged iron oxide aerosol, a spinning disk aerosol generator (Fig. 1) was used (2–5,7–9). The spinning disk aerosol generator is advantageous because the particle size of the aerosols may be regulated by either varying the percentage of colloid in the aqueous sol or by adjusting the speed of the disk.

Initially, local aerosol deposition on the bifurcations of the large airways was obtained by inhaling at 1 liter/sec a small volume of aerosol inserted toward the end of a tidal breath using a pulsed aerosol deposition system (13). However in later studies (Fig. 2), 9 μm mass medial aerodynamic diameter (MMAD) iron oxide aerosols produced with the spinning disk aerosol generator were inhaled throughout the inspiration with a 1.4 liter tidal breath inhaled at a flow rate of 1 liter/sec (2,5). This latter technique has the advantage of not requiring a pulsed aerosol deposition system with a fast response time.

Measurements of the positions of these local concentrations of deposited particles (boluses) were made initially by imaging the trachea with the subject seated facing a gamma camera (13). Serial scintiphotos of the profiles of the activity in the trachea were generated during 30 sec to 5 min intervals depending on the velocity of the transported bolus. The peak in each sequential longitudinal profile of the trachea was divided into two portions of equal area, and its position was noted. The slope of the least-squares fit of peak position as a function of time was

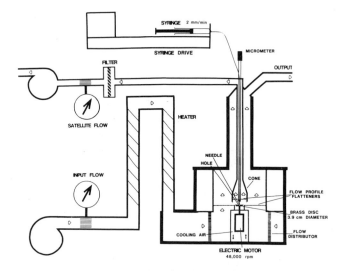

FIG. 1. Schematic drawing of a spinning disk aerosol generator. The radiotagged colloid is fed at 1 to 2 ml/min into the center of a brass disk 3.9 cm in diameter that is rotated by a three-phase electric motor (TRW Globe Motors, Dayton Ohio, model 75A-1645). at 800 Hz. Satellite particles are small and are entrained within the air that flows through the inner cone, whereas inertial forces carry the larger primary particles into the main airstream and up the tower, where they are dried by the warm air and then delivered to the subject.

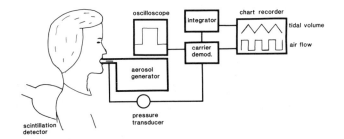

FIG. 2. Aerosol delivery system. The subject inhales the radiotagged aerosol by following a tracing of a predetermined breathing pattern on an oscilloscope. The flow of the aerosol is measured with a pneumotacograph (Validyne MP45) connected to a carrier demodulator (Validyne CD 19) and displayed on a long persistence oscilloscope. In this case, the inspiration should be at 1 liter/sec for 1.4 sec. The flow signal is integrated to give volume (Validyne FV 156). Both the flow and volume signals are transferred to a chart recorder. A scintillation detector placed at the midline of the chest is used to ensure that enough radioactivity is deposited to obtain good data and not so much that people are subjected to any unwarranted increased risk.

taken to be the TMV. Such analysis has also been computerized (1). TMVs have been measured also when the subjects were seated with their back to the gamma camera (3). However, additional radiation shielding and scattering by the backbone and possibly the increased distance from the trachea during imaging makes tracheal mucociliary transport rates more difficult to obtain when the subject is thus positioned.

Boluses of activity being transported in the trachea have been detected using a scanning scintillation detector fitted with a parallel slit collimator (19). With the patient in the supine position, the probe scanned back and forth along the trachea at a rate of 19 cm/min, and the activity was measured with a ratemeter connected to a chart recorder. The TMV was calculated from these serial activity profiles of the trachea. Using this technique, the activity in the whole trachea is monitored consecutively rather than continuously. It is desirable, however, to obtain a continuous record of activity throughout the trachea, using as little radioactivity as practical. To accomplish this, multidetector probes were designed that fit snugly against the neck and can be used with the subject in either the sitting or supine position.

The use of a multidetector probe to measure TMVs is illustrated in Fig. 3. The subject is seated with the head immobilized with both head and chin supports. The multidetector probe is placed against the neck between the cricoid cartilage and the collar bones. The photopeaks in each detector are discriminated for by the appropriate analyzers, and the output pulses are integrated using ratemeters with time constants adjustable between 10 and 50 sec. Each of the six ratemeters is connected to one channel of a Y-T chart recorder, which is operated between 2 and 10 cm/min. Chart recordings of a bolus of activity moving up the trachea are shown in Fig. 4. The position, in time, of each peak due to a local concentration of activity being transported up the trachea is determined by dividing each peak into portions of equal area. As the distance between each detector is known, the TMV is determined from the slope of the line of least-squares fit.

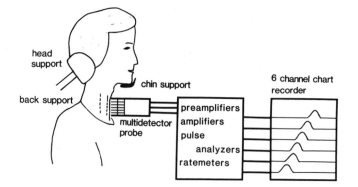

FIG. 3. Measurement of TMVs using a multidetector probe.

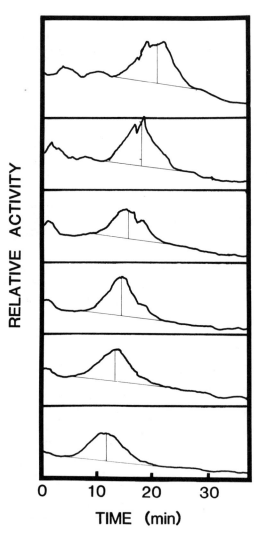

FIG. 4. A local concentration of activity is shown moving in time from the lowest detector sequentially to the highest detector. The construction lines demonstrating how the position of each peak is located are shown. In this example, the chart speed was 3 mm/min.

Two multidetector probes have been used to measure TMVs, each having six scintillation phosphors. One probe used six aligned sodium iodide (Tl) crystals, each 1 cm high, 2.7 cm deep, and 4 cm wide, and separated by 1.2 mm thick lead-antimony plates. The probe was suspended anterior to the subject over the midline of the trachea. It was used in a whole-body counting chamber that reduced background radiation (7–9,17,18). Each detector was connected to its own amplifier, single channel analyzer, ratemeter, and channel of a six-channel Y-T chart recorder. Based on the experience with this probe, a second multidetector probe was designed for improved performance and to be used in a clinical setting in conjunction with a gamma camera or scintillation probe system (16). This probe uses a combination of conventional collimation and active collimation using a phoswich design to provide high resolution, high sensitivity, and a low background. Its curved scintillation crystals are thinner and wider. These features allow closer positioning to the trachea with less distortion caused by subject movement. The design, operation and related circuitry have been described in detail (16). This multidetector phoswich probe is the detector of choice for measuring TMVs using radioaerosol techniques.

RESULTS

Results of studies using the radioaerosol technique to measure TMV are described so that the future experimenter may become familiar with both the characteristics of this technique and the physiological data that can be obtained by its use.

Mean TMVs and their standard deviations for healthy volunteers are shown in Table 1. The mean TMVs measured with radioaerosol techniques are generally lower than those measured by other methods (14). It is likely that the more invasive methods stimulate mucociliary transport (14). There are larger differences in TMVs between subjects than within subjects; thus when the effects of active agents are being studied, it is desirable to use each subject as his or her own control. Although TMVs vary within a single study, each local concentration of particles is transported

TABLE 1. *Mean tracheal mucociliary transport rates in healthy humans*

Mean TMV ± SD	No. of subjects	Age	Reference
4.7 ± 3.1	42	28	13
4.4 ± 1.3	7	26	11
5.5 ± 2.4	6	~24	3
4.3 ± 1.9	10	28	8
5.1 ± 2.9	22	31	17
6.7 ± 3.0	12	21–38	5
6.7 ± 4.1	13	22–30	2

at its own constant velocity (13). Thus, it is best to make as many measurements as possible. In one study using the phoswich multidetector probe, as many as 10 ± 4 TMVs were measured in each subject (2).

As the aerosol is deposited in local concentrations on the bifurcations of the large airways, there is a delay period between the deposition of the aerosol and the appearance of boluses in the trachea. This has been defined as the large airway transit time. Interestingly, in studies using smaller diameter aerosols, this large airway transit time [52 ± 24 min using a 4.2 μm MMAD aerosol (17)] was longer than when larger aerosols were used [15 ± 14 min using a 9.4 μm diameter particle (2)]. This is due to the difference in deposition pattern of large compared to small diameter aerosols. Larger particles impact on larger bifurcations than the small particles, thereby reducing the distance to be traveled between the sites of deposition and their subsequent detection in the trachea.

Air velocities in the trachea during cough may be between 20 m/sec and 200 m/sec resulting in high shear forces on the mucus lining. In healthy people who presumably have scant mucus, the local concentrations of deposited radiotagged particles are little affected by coughing (11,13). However, when excess mucus is in the trachea, as in people with cystic fibrosis, cough is effective in its removal (11,19).

Using the radioaerosol technique to measure TMVs in the tracheae of people with cystic fibrosis, it has been shown that patients could be divided into three groups on the basis of their tracheal mucociliary transport rates: (a) those who had normal mucociliary transport rates, (b) those who demonstrated some normal mucociliary transport rates but also had mucus in the trachea that was not transported, and (c) those in whom no positive transport of mucus in the trachea could be detected (19). Such observations are consistent with the variability of presentation of the disease and suggest that abnormal mucociliary transport is not a general defect in persons with cystic fibrosis. Mucus transport in the trachea differs in many people with cystic fibrosis compared to healthy people in that it is noticeably affected by the force of gravity, supporting the concept that postural drainage may be beneficial to these patients (11).

The trachea (with the exception of a few measurements in the major bronchi) is the only airway in which mucus velocity has been measured; therefore, transport velocities in all the other airways have been calculated based on these measurements (6,12,15).

Acute respiratory tract infections can also affect mucus transport in the trachea. Two days after an influenza infection, mucus transport becomes impaired and the clearance of mucus is accomplished by coughing (4). However, tracheal mucus transport appeared normal 2 days after a rhinovirus infection (4).

The trachea provides a more accessible airway in which the components of the mucociliary transport can be studied. Agents that alter mucus transport in the trachea can be anticipated to result in the same directional change in the intrapulmonary airways. However, changes in mucus transport in the trachea induced by active agents do not necessarily reflect the response of the lung. When 20 mg of orciprenaline was administered orally, tracheal transport increased and lung muco-ciliary clearance did not (18). Conversely, other studies demonstrate changes in mucus transport in the intrapulmonary airways but not in the trachea. Inhaled sulfuric acid aerosols at low concentrations increased lung mucociliary clearance and at higher levels decreased lung mucociliary clearance (8). However, no signifi-cant changes in TMVs were observed in the range of doses tested (7–9).

In the healthy unchallenged lung, mucociliary transport rates in the trachea are correlated with those in the major bronchi (3) and with clearance of particles deposited in the bronchial airways (17). However, this close coordination of muco-ciliary transport in the extrapulmonary and intrapulmonary airways can be perturbed by drugs (18) and inhaled pollutants (8). Such temporal variations in mucociliary transport can be accommodated in healthy subjects but may contribute to the pathogenesis or exacerbation of disease in lungs that are compromised.

DISCUSSION

Fundamental to the successful application of the radioaerosol technique for mea-suring TMVs is the necessity to inhale via the mouth a relatively large aerosol (4 μm to 10 μm MMAD) at a relatively high inspiratory flow rate (approximately 1 liter/sec). At slow rates of inhalation, local concentrations of particles will not be of sufficient magnitude to discriminate detectable boluses. The intensity of such boluses decreases with decreasing particle size and takes longer to transverse from the site of deposition to the trachea.

It takes longer to conduct TMV measurements with radioaerosols than with the fiberoptic bronchoscopic methods, since there is a delay between the deposition of the aerosol and its detection in the trachea. In addition, each bolus of activity is followed for about 2 inches compared with the generally much shorter distances in the fiberoptic bronchoscopic methods. Since this technique only detects local concentrations that are being transported up the trachea, it would seem that these measured rates would likely represent the faster mucociliary streaming and that the overall effective mean transport rate of mucus may indeed be lower (if there are some undetected areas of mucus stasis) than the mean of the measured values.

The radioaerosol technique has been shown to consistently measure TMVs that are responsive to drugs that predictably increase or decrease mucus transport. In other techniques where the baseline TMVs have been measured at about 20 mm/min, further stimulation by adrenergic agents was not observed.

The amount of radioactivity deposited in the lungs is only a few microcuries when low background counters are used and tens of microcuries when the multidetec-tor probe is used in conjunction with a gamma camera. This latter activity is required to obtain statistically significant counts on the camera rather than to be limited by the multidetector probe. Of the aerosol deposited in the lungs, each bolus has been estimated to contain 1% of the total activity deposited in the lungs. Thus, it is unlikely that there is any effect on TMV due to radiation.

The radioaerosol technique for measuring tracheal mucus velocity is now well established and has been used to study the physiology of healthy airways and how they are perturbed by drugs, disease, and inhaled pollutants.

REFERENCES

1. Bassett, P. G., Wong, J. W., and Aspin, N. (1979): An interactive computer system for studying human mucociliary clearance. *Comput. Biol. Med.*, 9:97–105.
2. Cotromanes, E., Gerrity, T. R., Garrard, C. S., et al. (1985): The effect of low serum theophylline levels on aerosol penetration and mucociliary transport. *Chest*, 88:194–200.
3. Foster, W. M., Langenback, E., and Bergofsky, E. H. (1980): Measurements of tracheal and bronchial mucus velocities in man. *J. Appl. Physiol.*, 48:965–971.
4. Garrard, C. S., Levandowski, R. A. Gerrity, T. R., Yeates, D. B., and Klein, E. (1985): The effects of acute respiratory tract infection on tracheal mucous velocity. *Arch. Environ. Health.*, 40(6):322–325.
5. Gerrity, T. R., Cotromanes, E., Garrard, C. S., Yeates, D. B., and Lourenco, R. V. (1983): The effect of aspirin on human lung mucociliary clearance. *N. Engl. J. Med.*, 308:139–141.
6. Gerrity, T. R., Garrard, C. S., and Yeates, D. B. (1982): A mathematical model of particle retention in the airspaces of the human lung. *Br. J. Ind. Med.*, 40:121–130.
7. Leikauf, G. D., Spektor, D. M., Albert, R. E., and Lippmann, M. (1984): Dose-dependent effects of submicrometer sulfuric acid aerosol on particle clearance from ciliated human lung airways. *Am. Ind. Hyg. Assoc. J.*, 45:285–292.
8. Leikauf, G., Yeates, D. B., Wales, K. A., Albert, R. E., and Lippmann, M. (1981): Effects of sulfuric acid aerosol on respiratory mechanics and mucociliary particle clearance in healthy non-smoking adults. *Am. Ind. Hyg. Assoc. J.*, 42(4):273–282.
9. Spektor, D. M., Leikauf, G. D., Albert, R. E., and Lippmann, M. (1985): Effects of submicrometer sulfuric acid aerosols on mucociliary transport and respiratory mechanics in asymptomatic asthmatics. *Environ. Res.*, 37:174–191.
10. Wales, K. A., Petrow, H. G., and Yeates, D. B. (1980): Production of Tc-99m-labelled iron oxide aerosols for human lung deposition and clearance studies. *Int. J. Appl. Radiat. Isotopes*, 31:689–694.
11. Wong, J. W., Keens, T. G., Wannamaker, E. M., et al. (1977): Effects of gravity on tracheal mucus transport in normal subjects and in patients with cystic fibrosis. *Pediatrics*, 60:146–152.
12. Yeates, D. B., and Aspin, N. (1978): A mathematical description of the airways of the human lungs. *Respir. Physiol.*, 32:91–103.
13. Yeates, D. B., Aspin, N., Levison, H., Jones, M. T., and Bryan, A. C. (1975): Mucociliary tracheal transport rates in man. *J. Appl. Physiol.*, 39(3):487–495.
14. Yeates, D. B., Gerrity, T. R., and Garrard, C. S. (1982): Particle deposition and clearance in the bronchial tree. *Ann. Bioeng.*, 9:577–592.
15. Yeates, D. B., Gerrity, T. R., and Garrard, C. S. (1982): Characteristics of tracheobronchial deposition and clearance in man. In: *Inhaled Particles V. Ann. Occup. Hyg.*, 26(1–4):245–257.
16. Yeates, D. B., and Mayhugh, M. (1984): A phoswich multidetector probe for measuring tracheal mucus velocity. *Clin. Phys. Physiol. Meas.*, 5(4):313–320.
17. Yeates, D. B., Pitt, B. R., Spektor, D. M., Karron, G. A., and Albert, R. E. (1981): Coordination of mucociliary transport in the human trachea and intrapulmonary airways. *J. Appl. Physiol.*, 51(51):1057–1064.
18. Yeates, D. B., Spektor, D. M., and Pitt, B. R. (1986): Effect of orally administered orciprenaline on tracheobronchial mucociliary clearance. *Eur. J. Respir. Dis.*, 69:100–108.
19. Yeates, D. B., Sturgess, J. M., Kahn, S. R., Levison, H., and Aspin, N. (1976): Mucociliary transport in the trachea of patients with cystic fibrosis. *Arch. Dis. Child.*, 51(1):28–33.
20. Yeates, D. B., Warbick, A., and Aspin, N. (1974): Production of Tc-99m-labelled albumin microspheres for lung clearance studies and inhalation scanning. *Int. J. Appl. Radiat. Isotopes*, 25:578–580.

ACKNOWLEDGMENT

This work was supported by the Medical Service of the Veterans Administration and the National Institutes of Health grant, HL 33461.

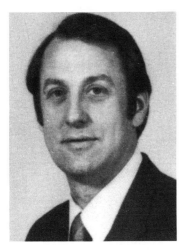

Donovan Byron Yeates was born in 1943, Perth, Western Australia. He received the Associate Applied Physics degree, the M.Sc., and Ph.D. in 1967, 1969, and 1975 from the Perth Technical College, the University of Surrey, UK, and the University of Toronto, Canada, respectively. He is Director, Occupational Health and Safety Center, Research Associate Professor, Department of Medicine at the University of Illinois at Chicago, and Research Physiologist, Veterans Administration, West Side Medical Center. His interests include mucociliary transport, aerosol deposition and clearance, pathogenesis of asthma and chronic bronchitis, and lung defense mechanisms.

Methods in Bronchial Mucology,
edited by P. C. Braga and L. Allegra.
Raven Press, Ltd. © 1988.

5.1.3. Radioaerosols for the Study of Lung Function

D. Pavia

Department of Thoracic Medicine, The Royal Free Hospital, Hampstead, London, United Kingdom

Aerosols
Mechanisms for aerosol deposition
Factors affecting aerosol deposition
Generation of aerosols
Radioaerosols as tracers for lung function studies
Lung ventilation and permeability studies
Lung mucociliary clearance

Radioaerosols have several applications in the study of lung function (4,5,13). At present, the three main applications are (a) ventilation imaging as part of the ventilation/perfusion comparison for the diagnosis of pulmonary embolism or simply for ventilation imaging used for assessing lung function or regional distribution of lung function, (b) measurement of lung permeability, and (c) assessment of mucus clearance either by mucociliary transport or by cough. In performing such measurements in humans successfully, a good understanding is required of the type of aerosol that needs to be used, the appropriate radionuclide with which to label the aerosol, the apparatus for generating the aerosol, the mechanisms involved in the deposition of aerosols, and the various factors that will affect the amount and site of deposition of inhaled aerosols in the human lung.

AEROSOLS

The definition of an aerosol is any system of solid particles or droplets sufficiently small in diameter to maintain some stability as a suspension in air (11). Since the properties of an aerosol are determined to a large extent by the interaction between the air and particles, these particles must be, on the one hand, large enough not to diffuse like gas molecules and, on the other hand, small enough to remain airborne for some period of time. Aerosols cover a wide range of sizes, from tobacco smoke (particles much smaller than 1 μm in diameter) to foundry dusts and pollens (approximately 100 μm in diameter).

Monodisperse aerosols comprise particles of approximately the same size. Since, in practice, perfectly monodisperse aerosols do not exist, an aerosol is said to be monodisperse if the coefficient of variation (standard deviation expressed as a percentage of the mean size) of the spectrum of particle sizes is less than 20%. Most naturally occurring aerosols are heterodisperse. Such aerosols have a much wider spread of sizes, and the distribution is often skewed toward particles of a small size. Under such conditions, it is often more useful to consider the mass distribution of the aerosol because the volume of an aerosol particle and, hence, its mass are proportional to the cube of its radius. For example, a particle with a radius of 10 μm would have a mass of 1,000 particles (of the same density) with a 1 μm radius.

It is possible for two particles with different physical diameters to behave aerodynamically in the same way. In order to overcome the difficulty of particles of different density, the term ''aerodynamic diameter'' (d_a) is used, which is defined as the physical diameter of the particle (d) multiplied by the square root of the density (ρ) of the particle:

$$d_a = d\rho^{1/2}$$

Effectively, the aerodynamic diameter of a particle is equal to the equivalent diameter of a unit density particle that has the same settling velocity in still air as the particle in question.

The mass distribution of heterodisperse aerosols is best characterized by the mass median aerodynamic diameter (MMAD), such that half the mass of the distribution is contained in particles larger than this size, and by its geometric standard deviation (GSD), which is equivalent to the ratio of the 84.1% size to the 50% size (or 50% size to the 15.9% size) in the cumulative mass distribution. (The values of 84.1% and 15.9% represent the mean ± SD of the gaussian distribution, and ratios must be calculated because the horizontal axis displaying size in μm is plotted on a logarithmic scale.) Aerosols with a GSD less than 1.22 are termed ''monodisperse.''

MECHANISMS FOR AEROSOL DEPOSITION

The three main mechanisms for aerosol deposition in the human lungs are inertial impaction, gravitational sedimentation, and Brownian diffusion (1,9).

Inertial Impaction

This is the most important mechanism for deposition in the respiratory tract for particles with diameters greater than 1 μm. If the inhaled particles are heavy or are travelling at high velocities (i.e., high inspiratory flow rates) they may not be able to follow the airstream when it changes direction within the respiratory tract, for instance, in the upper airways (pharynx/larynx) or at bifurcations; this gives rise to the particles impacting on the airway walls.

Aerosol deposition due to impaction takes place predominantly in the central airways, where the overall cross-sectional area of any one airway generation is small. Deposition of aerosol in the airways by impaction increases with (a) increases in aerodynamic diameter, (b) obstruction of the airways, and (c) increase in flow rates.

Gravitational Sedimentation

A particle allowed to settle under gravity accelerates until it reaches a steady terminal velocity, at which time the gravitational force is balanced by the resistance of the air through which it falls. A 6 μm unit density particle has a settling velocity of 0.11 cm sec^{-1}, whereas a 2 μm unit density particle has a settling velocity of 0.013 cm sec^{-1}. Deposition of inhaled aerosols into the human lung by gravitational sedimentation is favored in the more distal airways where the airway diameters are smaller, and thus the particles have a smaller distance to travel before depositing for any given time during breath holding or during the course of steady breathing, provided the frequency of breathing is low.

Brownian Diffusion

Particles smaller than 0.5 μm when entering the airways of the lungs are displaced by random bombardment of gas molecules and thus collide (hence depositing) with the airway walls. The Brownian displacement for large particles, e.g, 1 μm, is only 13 μm sec^{-1}; thus aerosol deposition by this mechanism even at such small particle size is still only a small percentage of the total deposition for particles of this size. Deposition of particles due to Brownian diffusion is of importance for particles less than about 0.5 μm in diameter.

FACTORS AFFECTING AEROSOL DEPOSITION

There are three main factors that affect the site of deposition of inhaled particles into the human lungs; (a) the physical properties of the aerosol, (b) the mode of inhalation of the aerosol, and (c) the patency of the airways (1,13,14).

Physical Properties of Aerosols

The main properties of aerosols that affect their site of deposition in the lungs are (a) particle size, (b) density of the particles, (c) hygroscopicity, and (d) electric charge. In general, the larger the diameter of the particles, the greater is the probability of their deposition nearer to the mouth due to impaction. For any given particle size, increasing the density of the material from which the aerosol is made results in an increase in its aerodynamic diameter. An aerosol made from a hygroscopic substance will absorb water from the nasal/oropharyngeal region on its way to the lungs and will thus increase in size and deposit nearer to the mouth than intended. The effects of electric charge carried by the particles on deposition are not yet well defined. However, the effect of electric charge on deposition is believed to result mainly from the formation of image charges in the airway walls rather than from electrostatic interaction between particles. Evidence indicates that quite high charges are needed on particles in the respirable range (i.e., 1–10 μm in diameter) to give comparable deposition to that arising from inertial and gravitational forces. The electrical charges on freshly produced aerosols can be reduced through the use of a charge neutralizing system, e.g., an ionizing radiation source.

Mode of Inhalation of Aerosol

The mode of inhalation can have profound effects on the site of deposition within the lungs of inhaled aerosols. All other things being equal, the bigger the breath taken, the more particles will be carried to the peripheral airways and be deposited there. Inspiratory flow rate is also of paramount importance; the higher the flow rate, the more particles will deposit in the central airways due to turbulence (impaction). If a breath-holding pause is introduced after inspiration of an aerosol, enhancement of deposition of aerosols at their furthest point of entry into the lungs will result. For instance, a 5 μm unit density particle has a settling velocity of approximately 0.07 cm sec^{-1}. Therefore, during a 3-sec breath-holding pause, all particles in airways less than 2 mm in diameter ($3 \times 0.07 = 0.21$ cm) will have deposited by gravitational sedimentation. Aerosol deposition during steady breathing is also increased at very low breathing frequencies because the mean residence time of the airborne particles in the airways is correspondingly raised. Paradoxically, total lung deposition is also increased at very high breathing frequencies as a result of inertial impaction of the fast moving particles. Furthermore, the lung volume at the commencement of an aerosol inhalation will govern its site of deposition within the lungs. An aerosol inhaled as a bolus at a given lung volume will be deposited in a different manner to aerosol inhaled throughout the breath. Particles inhaled during the first half of a deep inhalation may be deposited relatively diffusely throughout the lung, whereas aerosol given as a bolus nearer the end of the breath will result in a proximal deposition within the airways. A bolus of aerosol inhaled at low volume may be distributed preferentially in the upper lobes.

Airway Patency

The architecture of the airways of the subject inhaling an aerosol is very important in determining the site of deposition of the inhaled particles (3). In healthy subjects, there is a large intersubject variability in deposition that is probably a reflection of the random anatomical differences in airway dimensions (e.g., length and diameter of airways, angles at bifurcations of the airways). In patients with airway obstruction (due to bronchoconstriction or presence of excess mucus), aerosol penetration to the peripheral airways is decreased (6).

GENERATION OF AEROSOLS

Perhaps the cheapest and easiest way of generating heterodisperse aerosols is through the use of jet nebulizers (12,19). Compressed gas is fed into the nebulizer containing the material to be aerosolized. Large particles are entrapped by baffles within the nebulizer and returned to the reservoir; smaller particles leave the reservoir and are available for inhalation or for modification to smaller and more uniform-sized particles. The aerosol output rate and particle size for any one liquid are dependent on the type of nebulizer used and on its operating conditions, in particular, on the flow rate of the air through the device. Ultrasonic nebulizers are widely used for the generation of heterodisperse aerosols. In such a device, the energy required to atomize the liquid is produced by a piezoelectric crystal, vibrating at a frequency in the range of 1 to 2 mHz. The vibrations are transmitted through a coupling liquid to the nebulizer solution, and a fountain of droplets is formed in the reservoir, with the smaller droplets carried away by the inhalation stream. The mean particle size of aerosol produced by an ultrasonic nebulizer is generally inversely proportional to the operating frequency.

For the generation of monodisperse aerosols, the spinning top generator has so far been the instrument of choice. A spray of uniform droplets is generated when liquid is fed onto the center of a rapidly rotating disk that can be driven by either compressed air or an electric motor. In order to produce particles small enough for inhalation, disk speeds in excess of 10^4 rpm are necessary. The faster the disk speed, the smaller is the particle size of the aerosol generated. There are other devices for generating monodisperse aerosols, such as condensation and vibrating orifice generators, although to date these devices have not been used as extensively as the spinning top generator.

RADIOAEROSOLS AS TRACERS FOR LUNG FUNCTION STUDIES

When assessing lung ventilation or permeability, the aim is to deposit the tracer-inhaled radioaerosol predominantly or, if possible, exclusively in the alveolated regions of the lungs (2). Clearance of deposited, insoluble material from these nonciliated regions of the lungs is extremely slow, with a biological half-life in the order of 3 to 4 months. Depositing insoluble radioaerosols labeled with radionuclides in the alveoli for lung ventilation studies could result in unacceptably high absorbed radiation doses in patients, depending on the physical half-life ($T_{1/2}$) of the radionuclide used (17). Aerosols made from soluble or biodegradable substances are thus favored for such investigations. Gluconate, diethylenetriamine pentaacetic acid (DTPA), and albumin microspheres have been used for ventilation imaging, and DTPA has been used also for lung permeability studies. The versatile radionuclide ^{99m}Tc, with a physical $T_{1/2}$ of 6 hr and emitting gamma rays with an energy (E_γ) of 140 keV, is the most commonly used radionuclide for labeling such aerosols. ^{113m}In, with a $T_{1/2}$ of 1.7 hr and E_γ of 393 keV, and ^{111}Im, with a $T_{1/2}$ of 2.8 days and E_γ of 171 and 245 keV, have also been used, although these radionuclides have rather high gamma ray energies for appropriate detection with a gamma camera.

For lung mucociliary clearance studies, it is important that the aerosols used be insoluble in the lung fluids and that the radiolabel be tagged firmly onto the particles. Aerosols for the study of mucociliary clearance have been made from polystyrene, Teflon, iron oxide, Lucite, carbon, and resin. A small group of investigators use biodegradable aerosols of human albumin and erythrocytes. Once again, the radionuclide of choice for labeling such aerosols has been ^{99m}Tc. If observation periods longer than 2 days are needed, other radionuclides, such as ^{111}In ($T_{1/2}$ of 2.8 days, E_γ of 171 and 245 keV) and ^{198}Au ($T_{1/2}$ of 2.7 days, E_γ of 412 keV) need to be given consideration despite somewhat high gamma ray energies.

LUNG VENTILATION AND PERMEABILITY STUDIES

When performing lung ventilation studies using radioaerosols, the aim is to produce very fine particles with properties similar to a gas, so that they can mimic the information obtained when using radioactive xenon or krypton gases for such assessment (7,8,20). The particles must deposit in the alveolated regions of the lungs in much the same way as when using radioaerosols for assessing alveolar permeability. Alveolar permeability is a measure of the rate of transference of the labeled, soluble aerosol from the lungs into the bloodstream and is expressed as the half-time in minutes, i.e., the time it takes for half the deposited particles to get into the bloodstream (10).

For routine diagnostic procedures, the easy use of jet nebulizers to generate heterodisperse aerosols outweighs the more expensive and somewhat esoteric use of generators producing monodisperse aerosols. The wide range of particle size produced by jet nebulizers can be narrowed by permitting the bigger particles to settle out in a reservoir or by causing the larger particles to impact on obstacles or baffles placed in the output path of the nebulizer. (The appropriate particle size for such studies is less than 2 μm in diameter.) Both of these methods are in current use commercially. The Pulmoscint uses a helix for particle size modification, the SynteVent uses baffles, and the VentiCIS uses a filter. The percentage efficiency with several nebulizer systems, when expressed as actual lung deposition as a percentage of the activity initially present in the nebulizer, has been reported to be less than 2%. Much higher efficiencies have been claimed for inhalation from a settling bag. Systems using nebulizers with obstacles or baffles placed in their output path have advantages in relation to radiation shielding, since they are more compact.

A possible future development may be the use of extremely small particles (<0.1 μm in diameter), called "pseudogas." Theoretically, such small particles would behave almost like a gas, with deposition being determined by gaslike diffusion rather than by impaction and sedimentation.

When administering radioaerosols, due care must be taken in generating the appropriate-sized aerosol for the investigation and in the mode of inhalation and degree of healthiness of the patients' lungs. Simple pulmonary function tests, such as measure of the patient's peak expiratory flow rate using a peak flowmeter, should indicate whether the subject has airway obstruction. In patients with airway obstruction, even greater care must be taken in the mode of inhalation of the radioaerosol to avoid hot spots, i.e., impaction of radioaerosol on the conducting airways. The presence of hot spots could complicate the interpretation of the data. Such patients might be advised to inhale either tidally or preferably more slowly, taking full inspirations and if possible breath-holding at the end of each inspiration. Inhalation through a mouthpiece and exhalation via a filter must be the route of choice as opposed to the use of a face mask, in order to avoid possible radioactive contamination of the patient's face, of the environment, and of the monitoring system, e.g., the gamma camera.

LUNG MUCOCILIARY CLEARANCE

The conducting airways (trachea to terminal bronchioles) are lined with ciliated epithelium. The cilia beating in a watery, periciliary layer propel the overlying lung secretions, containing trapped insoluble material and locally produced biological debris, cephalad. The efficiency of this nonspecific host defense mechanism of the lungs can be altered by disease, pollutants, physiological factors, and pharmacological intervention (15).

The efficiency of the mucociliary escalator can be assessed by monitoring the removal of inhaled, deposited insoluble radioaerosols from the ciliated airways of the lungs (16,18). Some investigators prefer to measure the rate of flow of mucus in anatomically well-defined airways, such as the trachea and main bronchi. Others prefer to sample the efficiency of the mucociliary escalator from the proximal ciliated airways, from predominantly distal ciliated airways, and from all the ciliated airways of the lungs. Depending on which method one wishes to use, due attention must be paid to the particle size of the monodisperse aerosol and the mode of inhalation.

For the measurement of mucus velocity in the trachea or main bronchi using the radioaerosol bolus technique, the subject must inspire the radioaerosol from near total lung capacity with a high flow rate. The aerosol will then deposit mainly in local boli in the large airways.

In order to measure mucociliary clearance from predominantly central airways, perhaps it is necessary over the first four to six airway generations for the subject to inhale relatively large particles (MMAD greater than 5 μm) with a high inspiratory flow rate (>60 liters min^{-1}), with the radioaerosol being available throughout the inspiration maneuver.

A predominantly distal deposition of radioaerosol can be achieved with small particles (MMAD 1–3 μm) and with a large breath taken at a low inspiratory flow rate (<20 liters min^{-1}), followed by a relatively large breath-holding pause (e.g., 5–10 sec).

For a more uniform pattern of deposition in the airways, an aerosol with an MMAD in the range of 3 to 6 μm needs to be generated and inhaled from approximately functional residual capacity with an inspiratory flow rate of less than 30 liters min^{-1}. The size of the breaths taken may be equivalent to those in tidal breathing (0.5 liters). At the end of inspiration, an adequate breath-holding pause (e.g., 2–3 sec) will tend to enhance deposition of aerosol at its farthest point of entry into the lungs.

REFERENCES

1. Agnew, J. E. (1984): Physical properties and mechanisms of deposition of aerosols. In: *Aerosols and the Lung: Clinical and Experimental Aspects,* edited by S. W. Clarke and D. Pavia, pp. 49–70. Butterworths, London.
2. Agnew, J. E., Francis, R. A., Pavia, D., and Clarke, W. S. (1982): ^{99m}Tc-DTPA aerosol ventilation imaging: Theoretical and practical assessment. In: *Nuclear Medicine and Biology,* edited by C. Raynaud, pp. 2018–2021. Pergamon Press, Paris.
3. Chopra, S. K., Taplin, G. V., Tashkin, D. P., Trevor, E., and Elam, D. (1979): Imaging sites of airway obstruction and measuring functional responses to bronchodilator treatment in asthma. *Thorax,* 34:493–500.
4. Clarke, S. W., and Pavia, D. (eds.). (1984): *Aerosols and the Lung: Clinical and Experimental Aspects.* Butterworths, London.
5. Dolovich, M. B., Coates, G., Hargreave, F., and Newhouse, M. T. (1985): Aerosols in diagnosis: Ventilation, airway penetrance, airway reactivity, epithelial permeability and mucociliary transport. In: *Aerosols in Medicine: Principles, Diagnosis, and Therapy,* edited by F. Morén, M. T. Newhouse, and M. B. Dolovich, pp. 225–260. Elsevier, Amsterdam.
6. Dolovich, M. B., Sanchis, J., Rossman, C., and Newhouse, M. T. (1976): Aerosol penetrance: A sensitive index of peripheral airways obstruction. *J. Appl. Physiol.,* 40:468–471.
7. Fazio, F., Wollmer, P., Lavender, J. P., and Barr, M. M. (1982): Clinical ventilation imaging with In-113m aerosol: A comparison with Kr-81m. *J. Nucl. Med.,* 23:306–314.

8. Francis, R. A., Agnew, J. E., Sutton, P. P., Pavia, D., and Clarke, S. W. (1981): Ventilation imaging with easily prepared ^{99m}Tc aerosols. *Nucl. Med. Commun.,* 2:203–208.
9. Heyder, J. (1981): Mechanisms of aerosol particle deposition. *Chest,* 80 (Suppl):820–823.
10. Jones, J. G., Minty, B. D., and Royston, D. (1982): The physiology of leaky lungs. *Br. J. Anaesth.,* 54:705–721.
11. Morrow, P. E. (1981): An evaluation of the physical properties of monodisperse and heterodisperse aerosols used in the assessment of bronchial function. *Chest,* 80 (Suppl.):809–813.
12. Newman, S. P. (1984): Production of radioaerosols. In: *Aerosols and the Lung: Clinical and Experimental Aspects,* edited by S. W. Clarke and D. Pavia, pp. 71–91. Butterworths, London.
13. Newman, S. P., Agnew, J. E., Pavia, D., and Clarke, S. W. (1982): Inhaled aerosols: Lung deposition and clinical applications. *Clin. Phys. Physiol. Meas.,* 3:1–20.
14. Newman, S. P., and Pavia, D. (1985): Aerosol deposition in man. In: *Aerosols in Medicine: Principles, Diagnosis, and Therapy,* edited by F. Morén, M. T. Newhouse, and M. B. Dolovich, pp. 193–218. Elsevier, Amsterdam.
15. Pavia, D., Bateman, J. R. M., and Clarke, S. W. (1980): Deposition and clearance of inhaled particles. *Bull. Eur. Physiopathol. Respir.,* 16:157–177.
16. Pavia, D., Bateman, J. R. M., Sheahan, N. F., Agnew, J. E., Newman, S. P., and Clarke, S. W. (1980): Techniques for measuring lung mucociliary clearance. *Eur. J. Respir. Dis.,* 61 (Suppl. 110):157–177.
17. Philipson, K. (1981): Radioisotope labelling of aerosols for the study of lung function. *Chest,* 80 (Suppl.):818–820.
18. Sutton, P. P. (1984): Chest physiotherapy and cough. In: *Aerosols and the Lung: Clinical and Experimental Aspects,* edited by S. W. Clarke and D. Pavia, pp. 156–169. Butterworths, London.
19. Swift, D. L. (1985): Aerosol characterization and generation. In: *Aerosols in Medicine: Principles, Diagnosis, and Therapy,* edited by F. Morén, M. T. Newhouse, and M. B. Dolovich, pp. 53–76. Elsevier, Amsterdam.
20. Taplin, G. V., and Chopra, S. K. (1978): Inhalation lung imaging with radioactive aerosols and gases. *Prog. Nucl. Med.,* 5:119–143.

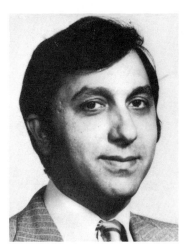

Demetri Pavia was born in Alexandria, Egypt, in 1944. He received the M.Sc. from the University of Surrey in 1969 and the Ph.D. in 1974 from London University. He is Principal Scientific Officer and Hon. Senior Lecturer in the Department of Thoracic Medicine in the Royal Free Hospital and School of Medicine, London. Fields of interests are measurement of tracheobronchial clearance in man, the generation, administration, and deposition of therapeutic aerosols, and regional depositions of inhaled industrial aerosols.

Methods in Bronchial Mucology,
edited by P. C. Braga and L. Allegra.
Raven Press, Ltd. © 1988.

5.1.4. Bronchial Clearance Measurement with Radioaerosols in Humans

H. Matthys

Robert Koch Klinik, Medizinische Universitasklinik, Freiburg, West Germany

---

Aerosols and their characteristics
Inhalation device
Airway geometry
Clinical importance of mc and tc

Bronchial clearance includes mucociliary transport and cough clearance. Both are influenced by gravity, the rheology of the mucus, and especially by the shear rate, which is a function of the lower serous layer and the local airflow. The measurement of mucociliary (mc) and tussive (tc) clearance in humans should be noninvasive and easily reproducible without additional drug therapy (e.g., local anesthesia) on untrained subjects. Therefore, the radioaerosol technique is the most widely used method to obtain an efficiency index of mc and tc.

AEROSOLS AND THEIR CHARACTERISTICS

Various types of aerosols are used to measure mc and tc. The particles may be either liquid (but insoluble) or solid, and they may be either approximately all of the same size (monodisperse) or of a wide variety of sizes (heterodisperse) (Fig. 1). The particles can be characterized according to their shape, surface area, chemical

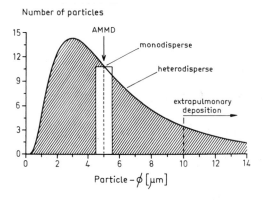

Number of particles

FIG. 1. Heterodisperse aerosol with nongaussian distribution of the particle size. AMMD = aerodynamic mass median diameter of the aerosol. Particles with a diameter of more than 10 μm are practically all deposited outside the lung. Particles with an AMMD of 5 ± 0.5 μm are called "monodisperse" particles.

composition, density, radioactivity, dissolution rate, electrical charge, and so on. Size is best described for heterodisperse aerosols by aerodynamic mass median diameter (AMMD). Particles with an AMMD of more than 10 μm do not allow any significant pulmonary deposition. Heterodisperse diagnostic aerosols should have an AMMD of 5 ± 3 μm. This means 50% of the volume or mass distribution is larger and 50% is smaller than the median-sized particles. A particle spectrum with a geometric standard deviation below 1.22 is by definition called "monodisperse" (27).

Particle Size

The particle size should be as monodisperse as possible so that under standardized breathing maneuvers and constant airway patency there is a reproducible deposition pattern. The most widely used radioactive tracer is [99m]Tc. There is general agreement that only monodisperse aerosols with a mean AMMD between 3 and 8 μm should be used in order to achieve a more-or-less peripheral bronchial deposition. In our laboratory, we use radioactive tagged erythrocytes with a special device to avoid the formation of doublets and triplets. Monodisperse particles for mc and tc clearance measurements are commercially available (^{99m}Tc-microspheres) or can be produced by special disk nebulizers.

Labeled Erythrocyte Method

We use an aerosol of ^{99m}Tc-labeled erythrocytes because they are essentially monodisperse, cost-free and easy to load with high levels of activity (36). Only a very few inexpensive ingredients are needed: some blood of the patient or from the blood bank (type O), normal saline solution, radioactive ^{99m}Tc-pertechnate from a molybdean-generator, and a solution of 25% glutaraldehyde, as used for electron microscopy.

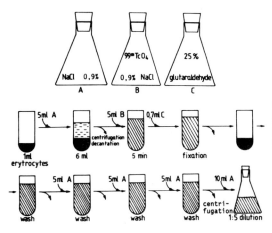

FIG. 2. Preparation and labeling of human erythrocytes with ^{99m}Tc for the measurement of mucociliary and tussive clearance in man.

Ten milliliters of blood is washed three times in 0.9% NaCl and centrifuged at 5,000 rpm for 5 min. As indicated in Fig. 2, 1 to 3 ml of centrifuged erythrocytes is first suspended in 5 ml physiological normal saline solution A. Then ^{99m}Tc solution B, with the same osmolarity as solution A, is added. During an incubation time of 5 min with 60 mCi ^{99m}Tc O_4 at room temperature, 60% of the ^{99m}Tc O_4 will be weakly bound to the hemoglobin. After this, the erythrocytes are fixed with 2 ml 25% glutaraldehyde. In this way, the ^{99m}Tc is enclosed in the erythrocytes. After an incubation period of 10 min at 60°C, the erythrocytes are washed four times with 0.9% NaCl and again centrifuged at 5,000 rpm for 2 min, then rediluted with solution A by a factor of 1:5 after measurement of radioactivity in the supernatant (which should be below 1%). At this point, the monodisperse particles are ready to be inhaled. Nevertheless, it is possible that some erythrocytes are still clumped together. Therefore, a device is needed to eliminate doublets and triplets.

INHALATION DEVICE

Our device for aerosol application for diagnostic and therapeutic purposes is shown in Fig. 3A. It allows one to define a narrow particle spectrum. The simple combination of a helix (Fig. 3B) with a rubber balloon (Fig. 3C), fed by a conventional nebulizer (Fa.Pari, Starnberg, FRG), allows one to obtain a high mist concentration and to eliminate doublets and triplets.

In 30 secs, the collapsed balloon is filled by the aerosol, which previously has passed the helix (coil). The tap is opened, and the patient is able to inhale the aerosol. A valve system separates the inhaled and exhaled aerosol. The stenosis serves the purpose of limiting inspiratory flow at 250 ml/sec. The filter on the expiratory side prevents contamination of the environment by the radioactive tracer.

Figure 3B shows how the centrifugal force acts as a selective mechanism for the particle spectrum that escapes from the helix. The deviation distance from

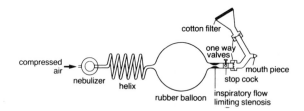

FIG. 3.A. Inhalation device (Fa. Pari, Starnberg, FRG) for monodisperse particle deposition in the lung to measure mucociliary and tussive clearance.

the mean radius of the helix (s) is a function of the velocity (V) of the airstream times the particle diameter (d) squared; n is the number of turns (8), ρ is the density of the particle (1 g/cm^3); η is the Newtonian viscosity of the carrier gas air (1.8 10^{-4} g/cm).

When the diameter of the circular helix lumen (D) is 8 mm, only particles with diameters smaller than 6.7 μm can escape the helix for a given particle velocity of 120 cm/sec within the coil. Choosing different diameters (D) and numbers of turns (n) of the helix allows one to determine at constant air velocity different maximal sizes of particles. The balloon, shown in Fig. 3C, allows:

1. Storage of the aerosol for the slow inspiratory vital capacity maneuver
2. Additional selection of smaller particles by gravity settlement
3. Prevention of aerosol evaporation

The balloon keeps the aerosol under ATPS-conditions, and as a time-related function, the concentration of bigger particles is reduced. Figure 3C shows the velocity of the particle (v), due to gravity settlement (g), which is a function of the particle radius alone for water droplets in the air. The broken line shows the selective power of our balloon with a content of 5 liters and an inflated height of 150

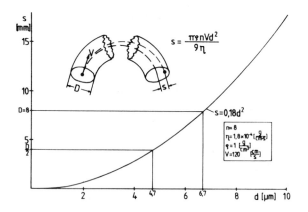

FIG. 3.B. Stokes law for selection of defined particle spectra. (d) Particle diameter; (D) helix lumen diameter; (V) particle velocity; (ρ) particle density; (n) number of turns of the helix.

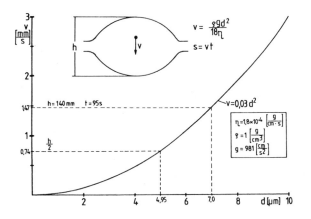

FIG. 3.C. Storage of radioactive particles to be inhaled. (η) Newtonian viscosity of gas inside the balloon; (g) gravitational constant; (ρ) density of the particle (water); (d) diameter of the particles; (s) sedimentation distance; (t) time allowed for gravity settlement; (v) velocity of sedimentation of the particles.

mm. After a duration of 95 sec gravity settlement, we have no particles bigger than 4.95 µm in our balloon. This device also helps to select smaller particles. Therefore, our inhaled erythrocytes have an AMMD of 6 ± 1 µm with a volume of about 100 µm³.

Deposition

To measure mc and tc, we prefer a relatively central deposition pattern because it allows us to shorten the observation period. Cough and mucociliary clearance is more efficient in the central bronchi and the trachea (downstream segment) than in the peripheral bronchi without cartilage support. In the peripheral airways, mc is slower and also more difficult to assess because the particles can move to and from the gamma camera without detectable longitudinal transport.

Penetration Index

Changing airway patency and different breathing maneuvers can influence the deposition pattern of monodisperse aerosols in the bronchial tree. The deeper the penetration and deposition of the particles, the longer the traveling distance to eliminate the particles.

The more peripheral the particles are deposited, the slower is the local mucociliary and tussive transport. Therefore, it is important to have the same initial starting point for comparative measurements. This means that mc and tc measurements need mapping of the initial deposition using either a rectilinear gamma scanner or a gamma camera. The penetration index is the ratio of peripheral to central deposition of the radioaerosol in the lung obtained from an arbitrarily defined central and peripheral lung field. A high penetration index means a high peripheral deposition. The lower the penetration index, the higher the airway resistance. This means the aerosol is deposited more centrally in the bronchial tree. Because the speed of mucociliary transport increases from the peripheral airways to the central bronchi, central deposition leads to comparably higher mc rates than with a more peripheral initial deposition. The penetration index can be measured by outlining the borders of the lungs with ^{81m}Kr gas, with a perfusion scan with another isotope, or by measuring the alveolar deposition. Alveolar deposition is the fraction of the deposited aerosol that remains in the lung after 24 hr of clearance measurements. ^{81m}Kr gas is difficult to obtain (reactor should be near), and the alveolar fraction remaining at 24 hr is inconvenient for the patient. Therefore, the penetration index is mostly estimated by using a perfusion scan or ^{99m}Tc-DTPA as a soluble aerosol for the outline of the lung in patients with obstructive ventilatory defects. To study the influence of different drugs on mc and tc, only an intraindividual crossover design with identical penetration indices should be used.

Breathing Maneuver

Standardization of tidal breathing is difficult to perform with patients and is time consuming. The amount of bronchial deposition is proportional to the tidal volume during inhalation and decreasing breathing frequency, mainly because of higher extrathoracic airway deposition. Increased breathing frequency leads also to a more central deposition within the bronchial tree. For practical and theoretical reasons, repeated, slow, near-inspiratory vital capacity maneuvers are optimal to obtain reproducible deposition patterns. An inspiratory flow limitation of 250 ml/sec is essential to avoid increased upper airway deposition. After an inhalation time of about 2 min, the subject reaches a thoracic activity of 30 to 50 μCi, which is sufficient to begin mc and tc measurements.

In subjects without major bronchial obstruction, there is little visible deposition in the trachea and the main bronchi. This is an additional advantage of the procedure, since it allows the measurement of mucociliary linear velocity toward the larynx by following the progress of the front of activity moving from the lung into the trachea.

AIRWAY GEOMETRY

Ten to sixty percent of the inhaled radioactive particles are deposited in the larynx by impaction because of different sizes and openings of the rima glottidis. Figure 4 shows the intrabronchial deposition of monodisperse erythrocytes (6 ± 1 μm AMMD) in 30 normal subjects. Figure 5 shows the influence of unilateral central and peripheral bronchial carcinoma on both sides of the lung in 64 patients. The penetration index is mainly influenced by the side of the central carcinoma

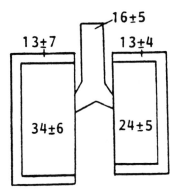

n=30

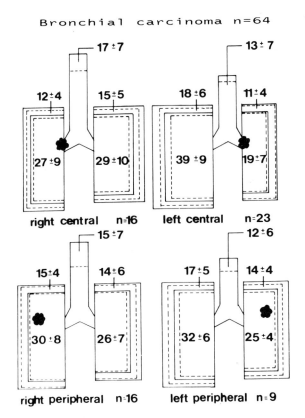

FIG. 4. Deposition of ^{99m}Tc O$_4$-tagged erythrocytes in the trachea, the mainstem bronchi, and the central and peripheral bronchial tree. Mean values and standard deviation in 30 normal subjects. The areas are proportional to the percentage of initial local deposition.

Normal subjects

Bronchial carcinoma n=64

right central n=16   left central n=23

right peripheral n=16   left peripheral n=9

FIG. 5. Deposition of monodisperse particles (erythrocytes) depending on the side of airway obstruction due to carcinoma in the right ($n = 16$) and left ($n = 23$) mainstem bronchi (upper part). The differences are significant ($p < 0.01$). Peripheral right and left bronchial carcinoma (not visible by fiberbronchoscopy) do not influence significantly the initial deposition pattern in relation to normal subjects (see Fig. 4).

TABLE 1. *Influence of inhaled radioactively labeled erythrocytes on lung function measured immediately before and after deposition scan*

	Age (years)	IVC (liters)	FEV$_1$ (liters)	R$_{aw}$ (kPa/liter/sec)
Before inhalation[a]	53.3 ± 11	2.9 ± 0.9	1.5 ± 0.5	0.44 ± 0.12
After inhalation[a]	53.3 ± 11	2.8 ± 0.9	1.3 ± 0.5	0.52 ± 0.21

[a] Differences are not significant in this asthmatic subject, but a trend to increased bronchial obstruction due to unspecific airway hyperreactivity is obvious. $N = 10$.

and by the degree of central airway obstruction. Central carcinoma means visible; peripheral means not visible by bronchoscopy. It is important that the airway obstruction does not change rapidly, especially during the measurement of mc and tc, which can be the case in patients with bronchial asthma.

The inhalation of particles leads to a minor increase of airway obstruction in patients with bronchial hyperreactivity (Table 1). With increasing airway obstruction, the initial deposition pattern becomes more central (Fig. 6), and hence the measured mc increases. The amount of swallowed activity seems to increase with increasing airway obstruction, as shown in Fig. 7. Therefore, in all patients with increased bronchial obstruction, we measure mc rates that are artificially too high and tc rates that are also too high because the downstream segment is cleared better by coughing the nearer the tracer particles are initially deposited to the trachea.

In normal subjects, cough clearance (tc) is zero because there is no mucus that envelops the tracer particle and allows it to be torn from the bronchial wall by the airstream.

Reproducibility

We measured in 14 subjects with different mc rates the elimination of tracer particles twice within 1 week under the same conditions of airway patency (identical

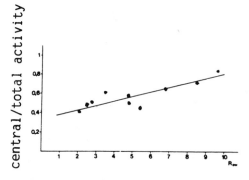

FIG. 6. Amount of central to total tracer deposition on the ordinate as a function of increasing airway resistance (R$_{aw}$) on the abscissa. $y = 0.045x$ & 0.348, $r = 0.80$, $n = 10$ patients.

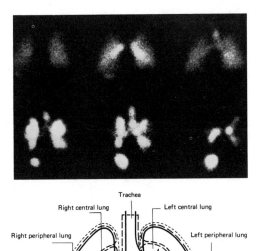

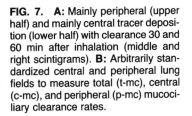

FIG. 7. A: Mainly peripheral (upper half) and mainly central tracer deposition (lower half) with clearance 30 and 60 min after inhalation (middle and right scintigrams). **B:** Arbitrarily standardized central and peripheral lung fields to measure total (t-mc), central (c-mc), and peripheral (p-mc) mucociliary clearance rates.

lung function tests). The range of mc rates in the first hour went from zero to 60% of the initially deposited radioactivity (Fig. 8). The correlation of the first and second measurement was 0.96 and reached practically the line of identity (slope = 1.06).

Normal Reference Values

There is a wide range of different clearance rates in normal subjects. We measured this in 80 subjects (59 men, 21 women) without any respiratory symptoms, normal lung function tests, and X-ray of the thorax during the first hour. We found a clear decrease of mc as a function of age (Fig. 9).* Puchelle et al. (31) found a similar relation. In the same age range, the mc may vary by approximately 10 to 15% (41). Albert et al. (2), Lourenco et al. (18), Camner (4), Sanchis et al. (37), Yeates et al. (45), Wanner (43), and Pavia et al. (28) reported similar interindi-

---

* The normal age-dependent regression lines are as follows:

tmc (1 hr): $y = -0.369x + 53.01 \pm 6.96, r = 0.66, p < 0.001$

cmc (1 hr): $y = -0.45x + 72.75, r = -0.59, p < 0.001$

pmc (1 hr): $y = -0.25x + 37.61, r = -0.59, p < 0.001$

y = elimination in percentage after 60 min (42).

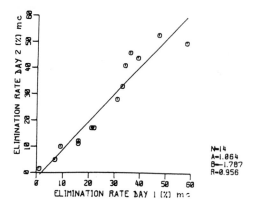

FIG. 8. Elimination rate in percentage of the initially deposited radioactivity of the bronchial tree measured in 14 subjects with different mc rates on two different days within 1 week. The first mc measurement is on the abscissa; the second is on the ordinate.

vidual differences. Exercise increases mc transport (44). The position of measurement (supine, sitting) influences the mc measurement only slightly, but it does influence the tc measurement, which must overcome gravity forces.

Relationship Between mc and tc

We registered during the measurement of mc the number of spontaneous coughs. Figure 10 shows that a decrease in mc transport leads to an increase in cough frequency. This indirectly proves that the tc is a compensatory mechanism for a failing mc transport, at least in patients with chronic bronchitis. This was also the conclusion of Puchelle et al. (31). The number of coughs per hour does not increase the efficiency of cough clearance (Fig. 11). This means that the 22 patients who coughed once in an hour with an mc rate of 11% cleared the same amount of tracer activity from the lung as the 5 patients who had 7 spontaneous cough attacks during the 1 hr of clearance measurements with a similar mean mc rate. This indicates that expectorable mucus is completely eliminated during the first

FIG. 9. Normal values for mucociliary clearance (t-mc). Percentage of eliminated radioactive tracers in the first hour after the initial deposition (mc 1 hr) as a function of age, measured in 21 women and 59 men with an age range from 20 to 80 years. They were all lifelong nonsmokers.

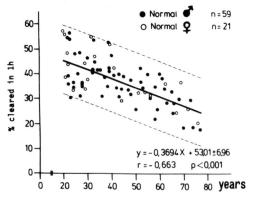

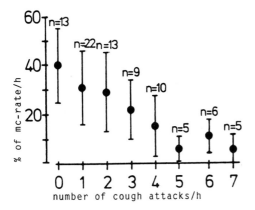

FIG. 10. mc rates in percentage of initially deposited radioactivity are shown on the ordinate; the number of spontaneously occurring cough attacks during the 60 min of clearance measurements is shown on the abscissa in 70 patients with chronic (obstructive) bronchitis with and without bronchial carcinoma. n = Number of patients.

spontanous cough maneuver. Additional coughing is useless, at least in our group of 70 patients with chronic bronchitis with and without bronchial cancer, because spontaneous cough clearance depends on the amount of mucus transported to the central part of the bronchial tree by mc from where it can be expectorated at once by tc. A relatively high mc rate can transport more mucus into the downstream segment ready to be expectorated than a slow mc rate (Fig. 10).

CLINICAL IMPORTANCE OF mc AND tc

mc may be reduced because of acute (extrinsic asthma) or chronic inflammation (chronic bronchitis) or congenital defects of mucus composition [e.g., cystic fibrosis (16,22) and ciliary epithelium (dyskinetic cilia syndrome) (1,9,33)]. The half-life residence time of inhaled particles is a hyperbolic function of the mc rate. If we can, e.g., by medication (22), improve a very low mc rate of 1%/hr to 5%/hr,

FIG. 11. Efficiency of tc. Percentage of spontaneously expectorated activity is shown on the ordinate; the number of spontaneously occurring cough attacks during the 60 min of clearance measurements is shown on the abscissa. Same patients as in Fig. 10. n = Number of patients.

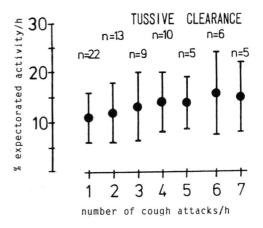

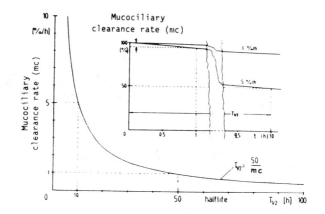

FIG. 12. Hyperbolic relationship between half-life ($T_{1/2}$) (50% elimination of inhaled and deposited particles) and mucociliary clearance rate in %/hr. The example given is for an improvement from 1% to 5% mc rate, which reduces the half-residence time for particles in the bronchial tree from 50 hr to 10 hr.

we reduce the mean half-life for deposited particles from 50 hr to 10 hr (Fig. 12). Like lung function tests, mc rates are not diagnostic in the sense of pathophysiology, but they show that smoking with or without simple or obstructive chronic bronchitis is directly correlated to the number of pack-years smoked as maximal midexpiratory flow (MMEF) (Fig. 13 and Table 2). Furthermore, there is no

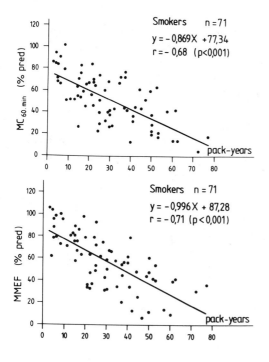

FIG. 13. A: The mc rate as a percentage of that predicated (Fig. 9) for 60 min clearance measured in 71 smokers (ordinate) as a function of pack-years (Table 2). **B:** MMEF of the same patients as a function of pack-years.

TABLE 2. *Correlation of smoking and bronchitis*

	Smokers without chronic bronchitis Group 1 $n = 15$	Smokers with simple chronic bronchitis Group 2 $n = 16$	Smokers with obstructive chronic bronchitis Group 3 $n = 40$	p Groups 1–2	2–3
Age (years)	37.5 ± 16.7[a]	45.4 ± 14.0	60.2 ± 10.7	NS	$p < 0.001$
Smoking interval (years)	14.3 ± 11.1	21.4 ± 9.7	37.5 ± 11.0	NS	$p < 0.001$
Tobacco consumption					
(pack-year: g/day/year)	9.3 ± 6.1	20.5 ± 8.5	40.6 ± 14.4	$p < 0.001$	$p < 0.001$
t mc 60 min[b] (%)	29.5 ± 6.9	19.3 ± 7.7	13.1 ± 6.5	$p < 0.001$	NS
(% pred)	75.5 ± 14.2	52.9 ± 17.7	42.4 ± 20.3		
c mc 60 min (%)	43.0 ± 11.9	29.2 ± 11.9	19.5 ± 9.7	$p < 0.01$	$p < 0.05$
(% pred)	76.3 ± 17.4	55.4 ± 20.7	42.4 ± 19.9		
p mc 60 min (%)	24.8 ± 8.2	16.7 ± 6.8	12.5 ± 7.4	$p < 0.01$	NS
(% pred)	88.5 ± 27.0	62.8 ± 21.9	54.4 ± 31.4		
VC (liter)	4.7 ± 0.7	4.9 ± 1.0	3.6 ± 0.8		
(% pred)	92.0 ± 9.8	92.0 ± 12.0	74.6 ± 15.6	NS	$p < 0.01$
RV (liter)	2.0 ± 0.7	2.2 ± 0.5	3.7 ± 1.0		
(% pred)	115.8 ± 24.6	114.0 ± 24.8	174.6 ± 44.7	NS	$p < 0.001$
FEV_1 (liter)	3.6 ± 0.7	3.6 ± 0.7	2.0 ± 0.8		
(% pred)	98.4 ± 13.2	96.7 ± 11.8	63.5 ± 20.9	NS	$p < 0.001$
MEF (liter sec^{-1})	4.0 ± 1.0	3.4 ± 0.7	1.6 ± 0.7		
(% pred)	86.1 ± 13.8	74.9 ± 10.9	40.4 ± 16.3	$p < 0.05$	$p < 0.001$
R_{aw} (kPa liter^{-1}sec)	0.20 ± 0.05	0.20 ± 0.05	0.40 ± 0.2		
(% pred)	108.1 ± 28.9	110.6 ± 28.4	213.5 ± 108.5	NS	$p < 0.001$

[a] Mean $\pm$ SD.

[b] t mc 60 min, c mc 60 min, and p mc 60 min, total, central, and peripheral mucociliary clearance in the first hour; VC, vital capacity; RV, residual volume; FEV_1, forced expiratory volume in 1 sec; MMEF, maximal midexpiratory flow; R_{aw}, airway resistance.

bronchial cancer without a severe reduction of mc, suggesting that chronic bronchitis is the precursor of bronchial carcinoma due to inhalative toxins (25).

In smokers the central mc is more reduced than the peripheral mc, explaining perhaps why bronchial carcinoma is nearly exclusively located in the central bronchi (first 10 generations of the bronchial tree). In patients with bronchial asthma, mc measurements correlate well with the amount of bronchial inflammation and hyper-reactivity (Fig. 14).

Medications, such as atropine (6,11,29,30,35,46) and β-blockers (24,25) reduce mc. Oxitropium bromide and ipratropium bromide are controversial in different studies but do not reduce mc in a clinically relevant amount (20,23).

β_2-Agonists given subcutaneously, orally, or by inhalation improve in most studies the mc rate (5,10,11,17,19,42,46). Theophylline also increases the mc rate (16,21,38). Mucolytic and secretolytic drugs show no statistical improvement in mc (3,6,8,16,22,26,29,32,40). The optimal rheology of the mucus is difficult to assess. If mucus is too watery or too sticky, the mucus transport rate will decrease (14). In individual patients, secretolytics can interfere with the complicated

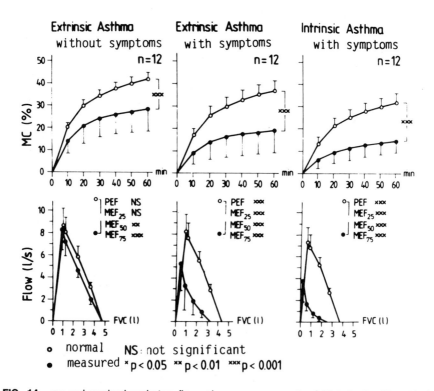

FIG. 14. mc and maximal expiratory flow volume measurements of 12 patients with extrinsic asthma with and without symptoms and intrinsic asthma. The decrease of mc in relation to normal predicted values is proportional to the airway obstruction and a sign of airway inflammation, especially in the symptom-free interval.

interaction between the sol and gel layers of the ciliated mucociliary escalator. The improvement of cough clearance by secretolytic and mucolytic drugs is very controversial; in single patients we often observe a movement in alveolar direction due to such drugs.

Other important issues are to evaluate the efficacy of various types of physiotherapy (forced expiratory treatment, active coughing, high frequency chest wall oscillation and asymmetrical high frequency ventilation) with radioactive markers (12, 13,15,33,34,39) and to follow up patients after single lung or lung/heart transplantation (7).

REFERENCES

1. Afzelius, B. A. (1976): A human syndrome caused by immotile cilia. *Science*, 193:317–319.
2. Albert, R. E., Lippmann, M., Spiegelmann, J., Liuzzi, A., and Nelson, N. (1967): The deposition and clearance of radioactive particles in the lung. *Arch. Environ. Health*, 14:10–15.
3. Aurnhammer, W., Konietzko, N., and Matthys, H. (1977): Problems in evaluating the effect of secretolytic agents on the mucociliary system by means of radioactive particles. *Respiration*, 34:92–99.
4. Camner, P. (1972): The production and use of test aerosols for studies of human tracheobronchial clearance. *Environ. Physiol.*, 1:1–18.
5. Camner, P., Strandberg, K., and Philipson, K. (1976): Increased mucociliary transport by adrenergic stimulation. *Arch. Environ. Health*, 31:79–82.
6. Clarke, S. W., and Pavia, D. (1984): *Aerosols and the Lung*. Butterworths, London.
7. Dolovich, M., Rossman, C., Chambers, C., Grossman, R. F., Newhouse, M., and Maurer, J. R. (1987): Mucociliary function in patients following single lung or lung/heart transplantation. *Am. Rev. Respir. Dis.*, 135(4):A363.
8. Dreisin, R. B., and Mostow, S. R. (1978): Adverse effect of *N*-acetylcysteine on isolated tracheal cilia (Abstr.). *Am. Rev. Respir. Dis.*, 117:109.
9. Elliason, R., Moosberg, B., Camner, P., and Afzelius, B. A. (1977): The immotile-cilia syndrome. A congenital ciliary abnormality as an aetiologic factor in chronic airway infections and male sterility. *N. Engl. J. Med.*, 297:1–6.
10. Fazio, F., and Lafortuna, C. (1981): Effect of inhaled salbutamol on mucociliary clearance in patients with chronic bronchitis. *Chest*, 80(Suppl.):827–830.
11. Foster, W. M., Bergofsky, E. H., Bohning, D. E., Lippmann, M., and Albert, R. E. (1976): Effect of adrenergic agents and their mode of action on mucociliary clearance in man. *J. Appl Physiol.*, 41:146–152.
12. Freitag, L., Long, W. M., Eldridge, M., Kim, C. S., and Wanner, A. (1987): Clearance of excessive mucus in the sheep trachea by asymmetric high frequency ventilation. *Am. Rev. Respir. Dis.*, 135(4):A364.
13. Gross, D., Zidulka, A., O'Brien, C., Wight, R., Rosenthal, L., and King, M. (1985): Enhanced mucociliary clearance from the periphery of the lungs with high-frequency chest wall compression. *J. Appl. Physiol.*, 58:1157–1163.
14. King, M., Gilboa, A., Meyer, F. A., and Silberg, A. (1974): On the transport of mucus and its rheologic simulants in ciliated systems. *Am. Rev. Respir. Dis.*, 110:740–745.
15. King, M., Phillips, D. M., Gross, D., Vartian, V., Chang, H. K., and Zidulka, A. (1983): Enhanced mucus clearance with high frequency chest wall compression. *Am. Rev. Respir. Dis.*, 128:511–515.
16. Köhler, D., App, E., Schmitz-Schumann, M., Würtemberger, G., and Matthys, H. (1986): Inhalation of amiloride improves the mucociliary and the cough clearance in patients with cystic fibrosis. *Eur. J. Respir. Dis.*, 69(Suppl.146):319–326.
17. Lippmann, M., Albert, R. E., Yeates, D. B., Berger, J. M., Foster, W. M., and Bohning, D. E. (1975): Factors affecting tracheobronchial mucociliary transport. *Inhaled Part.*, 1:305–319.
18. Lourenco, R. V., Klimek, M. F., and Borowski, C. J. (1971): Deposition and clearance of 2 μ

particles in the tracheobronchial tree of normal subjects—Smokers and nonsmokers. *J. Clin. Invest.,* 50:1411–1420.

19. Matthys, H., Daikeler, G., Krauss, B., and Vastag, E. (1987): Action of tulobuterol and fenoterol on the mucociliary clearance. *Respiration,* 51:105–112.
20. Matthys, H., Hundenborn, J., Daikeler, G., and Köhler, D. (1985): Influence of 0,2 mg ipratropium bromide on mucociliary clearance in patients with chronic bronchitis. *Respiration,* 48:329–339.
21. Matthys, H., and Köhler, D. (1980): Effect of theophylline on mucociliary clearance in man. *Eur. J. Respir. Dis.,* 61:98–102.
22. Matthys, H., and Köhler, D. (1986): Bronchial clearance in cystic fibrosis. *Eur. J. Respir. Dis.,* 69(Suppl. 146):311–318.
23. Matthys, H., Köhler, D., and Daikeler, G. (1985): Additive actions of bronchodilators on mucus transport. *Prog. Respir. Res.,* 19:369–377.
24. Matthys, H., Vastag, E., Daikeler, G., and Köhler, D. (1983): The influence of aminophylline and pindolol on the mucociliary clearance in patients with chronic bronchitis. *Br. J. Clin. Pract.,* (Suppl.)23:82–86.
25. Matthys, H., Vastag, E., Köhler, D., Daikeler, G., and Fischer, J. (1983): Mucociliary clearance in patients with chronic bronchitis and bronchial carcinoma. *Respiration,* 44:329–337.
26. Melville, G. N., Ismail, S., and Sealy, C. (1980): Tracheobronchial function in health and disease. Effect of mucolytic substances. *Respiration,* 40:329–336.
27. Mercer, T. T. (1975): The deposition model of the task group on lung dynamics: A comparison with recent experimental data. *Health Phys.,* 29:673–680.
28. Pavia, D., Bateman, J. R. M., and Clarke, S. W. (1980): Deposition and clearance of inhaled particles. *Bull. Eur. Physiopathol.,* 16:335–366.
29. Pavia, D., Clarke, S. W., and Thomson, M. L. (1979): Effect of mucolytic and expectorant agents on tracheobronchial clearance in chronic bronchitis (Abstr.). *Am. Rev. Respir. Dis.,* 119:157.
30. Pavia, D., and Thomson, M. L. (1971): Inhibition of mucociliary clearance from the human lung by hyoscine. *Lancet,* 27:449–450.
31. Puchelle, E., Zahm, J. M., and Bertrand, A. (1979): Influence of age on bronchial mucociliary transport. *Scand. J. Respir. Dis.,* 60:307–313.
32. Puchelle, E., Zahm, J. M., Girard, F., et al. (1980): Mucociliary transport *in vivo* and *in vitro.* Relations to sputum properties in chronic bronchitis. *Eur. J. Respir. Dis.,* 61:254–264.
33. Rossman, C. M., Forrest, J. B., Ruffin, R. E., and Newhouse, M. T. (1980): Ciliary motility in bronchiectasis without Kartagener syndrome (Abstr). *Am. Rev. Respir. Dis.,* 122:172.
34. Rossman, C. M., Waldes, R., Sampson, D., and Newhouse, M. T. (1982): Effect of chest physiotherapy on the removal of mucus in patients with cystic fibrosis. *Am. Rev. Respir. Dis.,* 126:131–135.
35. Ruffin, R. E., Wolff, R. K., Dolovich, M. B., Rossman, C. M., Fitzgerald, M. B., and Newhouse, M. T. (1978): Aerosol therapy with Sch 1000. *Chest,* 73:501–506.
36. Rühle, K. H., Köhler, D., Fischer, J., and Matthys, H. (1979): Measurements of mucociliary clearance with ^{99m}Tc-tagged erythrocytes. *Prog. Respir. Res.,* 11:117–126.
37. Sanchis, J., Dolovich, M., Chalmers, R., and Newhouse, M. T. (1972): Quantitation of regional aerosol clearance in the normal human lung. *J. Appl. Physiol.,* 33:757–762.
38. Serafini, S. M., Wanner, H., and Michelson, E. D. (1976): Mucociliary transport in central and intermediate size airways: Effect of aminophylline. *Bull. Physiopathol. Respir.,* 12:415–422.
39. Sutton, P. P., Parker, R. A., Webber, B. A., et al. (1983): Assessment of the forced expiration technique, postural drainage and directed coughing in chest physiotherapy. *Eur. J. Respir. Dis.,* 64:62–68.
40. Thomson, M. L., Pavia, D., Gregg, I., and Stark, J. E. (1974): Bromhexine and mucociliary clearance in chronic bronchitis. *Br. J. Dis. Chest.,* 68:21–27.
41. Vastag, E., Matthys, H., Köhler, D., Gronbeck, L., and Daikeler, G. (1985): Mucociliary clearance and airways obstruction in smokers, ex-smokers and normal subjects who never smoked. *Eur. J. Respir. Dis.,* 66:93–100.
42. Vastag, E., Matthys, H., Zsamboki, G., Köhler, D., and Daikeler, G. (1986): Mucociliary clearance in smokers. *Eur. J. Respir. Dis.,* 68:107–113.
43. Wanner, A. (1977): Clinical aspects of mucociliary transport. *Am. Rev. Respir. Dis.,* 116:73–125.
44. Wolff, R. K., Dolovich, M., Obminski, G., and Newhouse, M. T. (1975): Effect of sulfur dioxide on tracheobronchial clearance at rest and during exercise. *Inhaled Part,* 1:321–332.

45. Yeates, D. B., Aspin, N., Bryan, C., and Levison, H. (1973): Regional clearance of ions from the airways of the lung. *Am. Rev. Respir. Dis.*, 107:602–660.
46. Yeates, D. B., Aspin, N., Levison, H., Jones, M. T., and Bryan, A. C. (1975): Mucociliary tracheal transport rates in man. *J. Appl. Physiol.*, 39:487–495.

ACKNOWLEDGMENT

The author thanks Dr. M. King, Visiting Professor of the University of Edmonton, Canada, for reading the manuscript.

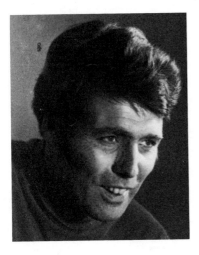

Heinrich Matthys was born in Zurich, Switzerland, in 1935. He received the M.D. degree in 1966 from the University of Basle, Switzerland, and the Ph.D. degree in 1971 from the University of Ulm (FRG). He is currently Professor and Medical Director of the Division of Pneumology of the Department of Internal Medicine, University of Freiburg, West Germany. His interests are in pneumology, nuclear medicine, and occupational medicine.

Subject Index

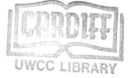